Instant
HEALTH
answers

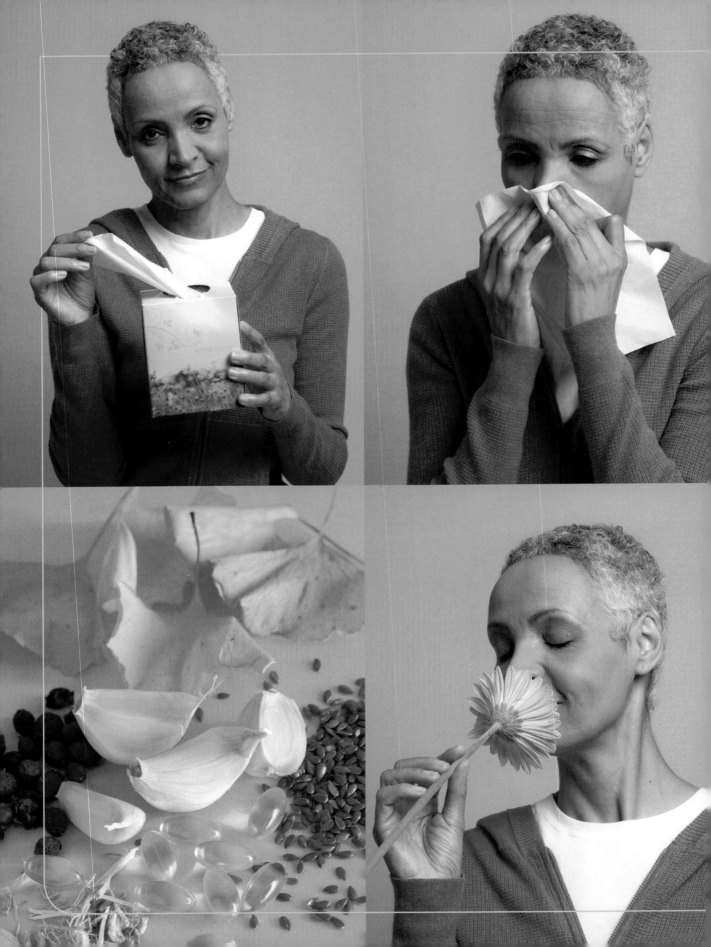

TRUSTWORTHY INFORMATION
THE MOMENT YOU NEED IT

Instant
HEALTH
answers

Feel **Safe, Secure**, and **In Control** of Your Health

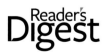
Reader's
Digest

The Reader's Digest Association, Inc.
Pleasantville, NY | Montreal

PROJECT STAFF

Executive Editor
Marianne Wait

Senior Art Director
Rich Kershner

Writers
Debra Gordon,
Timothy Gower,
Sari Harrar,
John Hastings

Copy Editor
Lisa Andruscavage

Indexer
Cohen Carruth Indexes

RDA CONTENT CREATION STUDIO

VP, Editor in Chief
Neil Wertheimer

Creative Director
Michele Laseau

Executive Managing Editor
Donna Ruvituso

Associate Director, North America Prepress
Douglas A. Croll

Manufacturing Manager
John L. Cassidy

Marketing Director
Dawn Nelson

THE READER'S DIGEST ASSOCIATION, INC.

President and Chief Executive Officer
Mary G. Berner

President, Emerging Businesses
Alyce C. Alston

SVP, Chief Marketing Officer President & CEO, Direct Holding
Amy J. Radin

Photography © Jonathan Pozniak

Library of Congress Data has been applied for.

ISBN 978-1-60652-974-4

Address any comments about *Instant Health Answers* to:
The Reader's Digest Association, Inc.
Editor in Chief, Books
Reader's Digest Road
Pleasantville, NY 10570-7000

To order copies of *Instant Health Answers*, call 1-800-846-2100.

Visit our online store at rdstore.com

Photographs © Jonathan Pozniak

Printed in the United States of America

1 3 5 7 9 10 8 6 4 2

US 6070/IC

Note to Readers
The information in this book should not be substituted for, or used to alter, medical therapy without your doctor's advice. For a specific health problem, consult your physician for guidance. The mention of any products, retail businesses, or Web sites in this book does not imply or constitute an endorsement by the authors or by The Reader's Digest Association, Inc.

Medical Consultants

Mary M. Austin, MA, RD, CDE

Barrie R. Cassileth, MS, PhD
Laurance S. Rockefeller Chair
    in Integrative Medicine
Chief, Integrative Medicine Service
Memorial Sloan-Kettering Cancer Center

Tod Cooperman, MD
President, ConsumerLab.com

Steven R. Feldman, MD
Professor, Dermatology, Pathology &
    Public Health Sciences
Wake Forest Health Sciences

Jonathan Fellus, MD
Clinical Assistant Professor,
    Department of Neuroscience
New Jersey Medical School

Leonard G. Gomella, MD, FACS
The Bernard W. Godwin Professor
    of Prostate Cancer
Chairman, Department of Urology
Thomas Jefferson University

Randy C. Hatton, PharmD
Clinical Professor
University of Florida College of Pharmacy

David L. Katz, MD, MPH
Associate Professor, Adjunct
Yale University School of Medicine

Shannon Laughlin, MD, MPH

Daniel Muller, MD, PhD
Associate Professor, Medicine
University of Wisconsin-Madison School
of Medicine and Public Health

Gerard E. Mullin, MD
Division of Gastroenterology and Liver Disease
Johns Hopkins Hospital

Robert Pallay, MD

Anastasia Rowland-Seymour, MD
Assistant Professor of Medicine
Johns Hopkins University School of Medicine

Heather Wakelee, MD
Assistant Professor
Stanford School of Medicine

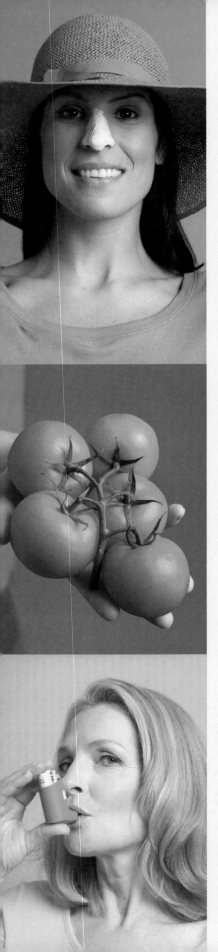

contents

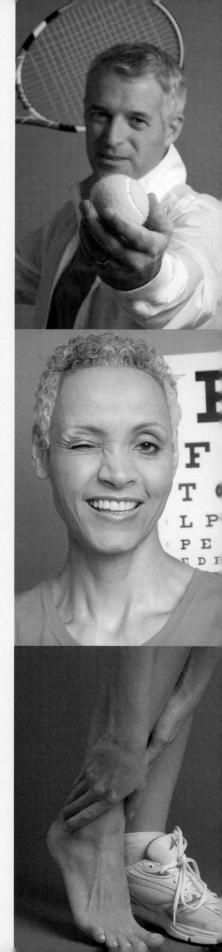

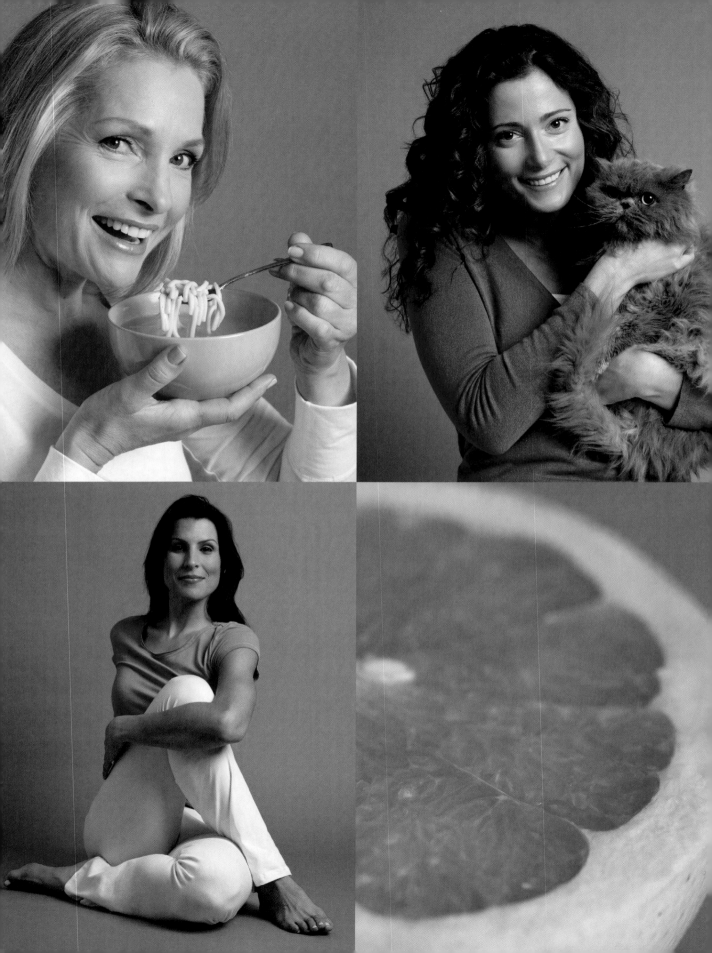

Answers When You Need Them

You just ate a three-egg omelet for breakfast—then remembered your cholesterol test is tomorrow. Should you reschedule? You found a tick on your skin. Does that mean you'll definitely get Lyme disease? Your spouse's snoring could summon wild hogs. Should you stock up on earplugs, or start to worry?

You could call your doctor and ask...but unless it's matter of life and death, getting through is about as likely as erasing wrinkles with wrinkle cream. At Reader's Digest, we think every health question is a matter of life (living a good one) and death (putting it off for as long as possible). That's why we created *Instant Health Answers*. You'll find clear, concise, to-the-point answers to hundreds of health questions— answers that will put your mind at ease (no, that headache doesn't mean you have a brain tumor), help you understand what's going on with your health (yes, a new blood-pressure medicine can make you dizzy temporarily until your body gets used to the drug),

and guide you to action (it's actually okay to keep cold medicines past their expiration date). Every answer is doctor- or pharmacist-approved, so you can be certain the information is 100 percent trustworthy.

Wondering about a weird symptom? Experiencing an unexpected side effect? Confused about a test or treatment? Even if you just want to know how much dark chocolate you can consume and still claim it's good for you, you'll find the answer here. Use the index to make sure you locate all the information you want on a subject, since many topics are covered in more than one chapter. If you have arthritis, for instance, you'll find answers to questions on

symptoms, drugs, supplements, diet strategies, and disease treatment, all in their proper places. We've even devoted a chapter to questions you may be too embarrassed to ask aloud (did someone say gas or itchy private parts?), so don't be shy—no one's looking.

Of course, no book is a substitute for good medical care. Follow up with your doctor whenever you have an ongoing concern, and call 9-1-1 if there's a true emergency. In the meantime, turn to *Instant Health Answers*. There's no paper gown required, and the book will never have to rush off to see the next patient.

Without the facts, you're left to worry, do the wrong thing, or do nothing at all, even when action is warranted. *Instant Health Answers* gives you the right information at the right time. Read it in good health.

—*Marianne Wait*
Executive Editor
Reader's Digest Health Books

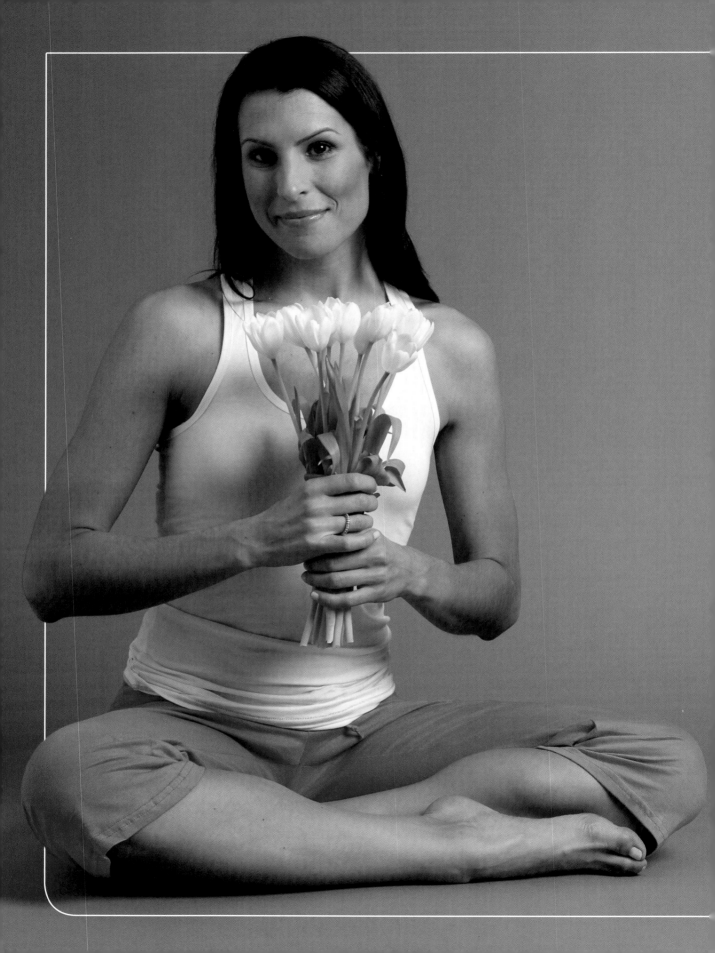

PART ONE

Your General Health

Everyday Health

Should I use antibacterial soap? Can I get chicken pox again? Will walking protect my bones? Will the flu shot give me the flu? Find out here.

Your Most Embarrassing Questions

Stinky feet? Itchy privates? Digestive disturbances? In this chapter, frank answers to the questions you'd rather not ask your doctor.

Common Symptoms and What They Mean

From abdominal pain to appetite loss, hoarseness to headaches, what it means, when it's harmless, and when to see your doctor on the double.

Your Diet

Is coffee good for me? What about carbs? Can I eat meat and still lower my cholesterol? When is it safe to cut mold off cheese? These answers and more.

Everyday Health

☐ **AIR FILTERS**

Do air filters and HEPA vacuum cleaners help with allergies and asthma?

Filters do remove some airborne particles that provoke sneezes and wheezes, but there's scant proof that allergy and asthma sufferers get any real relief as a result. When Canadian doctors reviewed ten air-filter studies, they concluded that filtered air didn't boost lung function and only improved symptoms like coughing, sneezing, watery eyes, and runny noses a tiny bit.

One exception: A filter may help if you have a pet-dander allergy. One study of 30 allergic pet-owners found that two-thirds of those who installed HEPA air filters in their bed-rooms and living rooms needed less allergy medication. Just keep your pets out of your boudoir. Studies suggest that air filters can't keep up with the steady supply of dander in the air when your pooch or kitty is allowed free rein there.

☐ **ANTIBACTERIAL PRODUCTS**

Do I need to use antibacterial soap?

No. Antibacterial soaps are no better than a good scrubbing with regular soap and water for removing disease-causing germs or preventing the illnesses they can cause. Studies show no differences in the number of illnesses suffered by people and families who use these soaps versus regular soaps.

Should I use, or avoid, antibacterial household cleaners?

They probably won't harm you and can reduce the transmission of some germs, which is important when someone in your house has an infection. The drawback? These cleaners fight bacteria but not necessarily viruses, and many common infections such as colds and flu are caused by viruses.

Don't dismiss homemade cleaners, though. Hot water

WHAT YOU DON'T KNOW

Washing Too Quickly May Leave Enough Germs to Get You Sick

To really protect yourself, lather vigorously for at least 20 seconds, the amount of time it takes to sing the "Happy Birthday" song twice. Then rinse and dry with a clean towel. If you're using a public sink, use a paper towel to turn off the tap (and to open the door on the way out). There are an estimated 229,000 germs per square inch on frequently used faucet handles!

and dish detergent has proven effective for killing germs on surfaces in kitchens and bathrooms, for example. And baking soda or vinegar solutions killed 90 percent of bacteria such as *Salmonella, Staphylococcus aureus*, and *E. coli* in another study, though commercial cleaners zapped 99.9 percent. Depending on the germs hanging around, that 9.9 percent difference could mean the difference between staying well and getting sick, and may be especially important if your household includes babies, older people, or anyone with weakened immunity.

Are hand sanitizers as good as soap and water?

Almost. Alcohol-based antibacterial gels and towelettes are a proven, germ-fighting alternative for ridding your hands of bacteria and viruses when soap and water aren't available. In one study of 292 Boston-area families with young children, those who used hand sanitizers for 5 months cut the spread of gastrointestinal infections by 59 percent. In another study, families who washed up with hand gels about five times a day cut the risk for colds by 20 percent, compared to families who scrubbed less often. For best results, squeeze out a half-teaspoonful (about the diameter of a nickel) or grab a towelette, and vigorously rub your hands, front and back. Note that alcohol-based hand gels must contain at least 60 percent alcohol to effectively kill germs.

Tuck an antibacterial cleaner into your child's backpack, too. When 420 kids in elementary school used a hand sanitizer several times a day at school—when coming into the classroom, before eating, and after using the bathroom—for 4 weeks, they got 29 percent fewer gastrointestinal illnesses and 49 percent fewer colds. Kids who used sanitizers also had 31 percent fewer sick days.

☐ BIRTH CONTROL

Are pills that promise "no more periods" safe?

"Continuous" birth control pills deliver a low, steady dose of the hormones estrogen and progestin every day of the month, without a break, so that you never have a period. In contrast, women who take regular birth control pills have periodlike bleeding because every pill pack contains a week's worth of hormone-free pills in addition to three weeks' of hormone-containing tablets.

Having no periods may sound odd, but it's safe. When you take continuous birth control pills, the endometrium, or lining of the uterus, becomes very thin. It's not that menstrual blood becomes trapped in the body, but that it doesn't form in the first place. There are no known health risks associated with putting your monthly menstrual period on hold. And in terms of side effects, these drugs are as safe as standard oral contraceptives. As with regular birth control pills, continuous pills don't seem to have a permanent effect on fertility; once you stop, ovulation returns to normal within 60 days for 95 percent of women. The one difference between the two types of pills: Women taking continuous oral contraceptives have more breakthrough bleeding; 20 percent were still experiencing this unscheduled spotting after a year on the continuous pill.

My periods are just about over. Do I still need to use birth control?

Absolutely. As you approach menopause, conception is still possible because you can continue to ovulate even if your periods are irregular. To avoid unwanted pregnancy, keep using birth control until you've had no periods for at least 1 year. Or, when you think you've stopped your periods, go see your doctor; she can do blood tests to determine if you are, indeed, in menopause.

Perimenopausal women (those approaching menopause) have the second-highest rate of unintended pregnancies, just behind teenagers. And pregnancy at this time carries higher risks: Babies face greater odds for birth defects and death, and women who become pregnant in the years just before menopause have a higher risk for life-threatening complications, including a dangerous type of high blood pressure called preeclampsia.

☐ BLOOD DONATION

Is it harmful to donate more often than the guidelines recommend?

Yes. Organizations like the American Red Cross require a waiting period of 8 weeks between blood donations so that your body has time to replace all of the red blood cells and iron you gave away. While it takes your body just a few days to regenerate plasma, the watery substance that makes blood fluid, you'll need 2 to 4 weeks for your bone marrow to replace billions of red blood cells and up to 8 weeks to absorb enough iron from food and supplements to replace 200 to 250 milligrams of iron. (Most of the body's iron is found in hemoglobin, a component of red blood cells.)

☐ BRUSHING AND FLOSSING

Do I really have to floss every day?

If you want to keep your teeth and body healthy, yes. Cleaning between your teeth and below the gum line with floss not only dislodges the corn that got stuck there at dinner, it also helps protect against gum disease as well as more serious health problems. Flossing helps control bacteria that are linked with chronic, body-wide inflammation, a serious risk factor for heart disease, stroke, lung disease, and preterm births.

Incidentally, don't believe claims that rinsing with mouthwash is just as good as flossing. While one study, sponsored by the manufacturer of a famous antiseptic mouthwash, found that swishing beat flossing, later research found that a dental-care routine that included tooth brushing, flossing, *and* using an antiseptic mouthwash cut dental plaque by 50 percent, better than flossing or mouthwash alone.

Is an electric toothbrush more effective than a regular toothbrush?

Yes, provided that the bristles rotate in one direction, then the other. People who used this type of toothbrush twice daily for 3 months had 17 percent less gum disease than those who brushed with a manual toothbrush, report researchers from the Forsyth Center for Evidence-Based Dentistry in

WHAT YOU DON'T KNOW

What to Eat and Drink Before and After

The Red Cross recommends that you drink extra water and fluids before and after you give blood to replace the volume you will lose, and that you eat iron-rich foods, such as red meat, fish, poultry, beans, iron-fortified cereals, raisins, and prunes, before you donate.

Boston. After reviewing 42 toothbrush studies, they concluded that "rotation oscillation" brushes were the most effective (they are also the most expensive). Ultrasonic brushes and those with brush heads that move side to side or in a circle in just one direction only performed no better than a manual toothbrush.

Of course, a toothbrush works only if you use it. Plan to brush for 2 minutes at least twice a day.

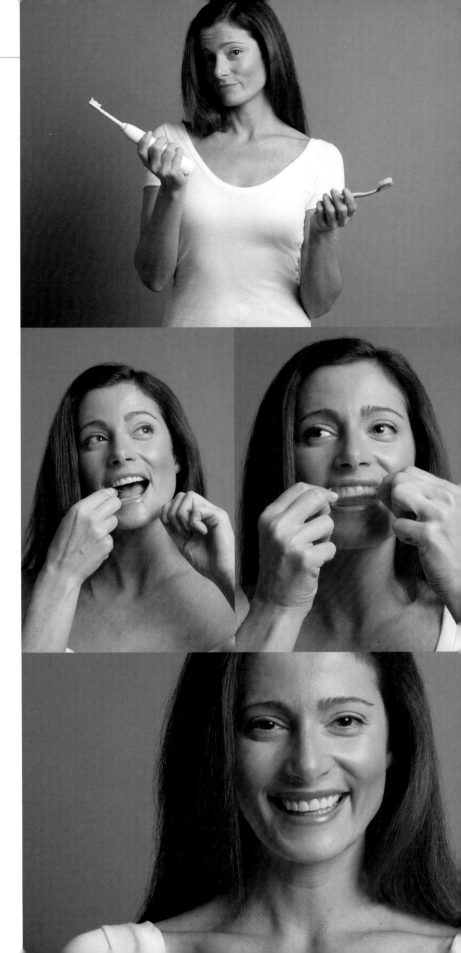

□ CELL PHONES

Do cell phones cause cancer?

A landmark 13-year Danish study of 420,000 cell phone users found no increased cancer risk. But a rare type of salivary gland tumor was 50 percent more likely to occur in people who used a cell phone for several hours a day in one large Israeli study. And odds for a rare, benign tumor called an acoustic neuroma were 2.4 times higher in people who used cell phones regularly for a decade in a study of 4,400 people conducted by the Swedish National Institute for Working Life. Emerging evidence also suggests that children are at greater risk than adults, with European and some U.S. authorities warning against frequent cell phone use in those under 18 years of age.

If you or your kids chat frequently on a mobile phone and

WHAT YOU DON'T KNOW

Not All Cell Phones Are Equal

Swedish cell phone safety researchers say it's smart to choose a phone with a low Specific Absorption Rate (SAR) value, a measure of how much of a phone's radio frequency waves are absorbed into the user's head. But SAR values aren't always easy to find on a phone, or to compare when shopping. Find SAR values for most major phone manufacturers online from the international Mobile Manufacturers Forum at www.mmfai.org/public/sar.cfm.

are worried about the potential effects on your health, consider using an earpiece, or put your caller on speaker and hold the phone away from your head. Text messaging is another alternative as it doesn't involve holding the phone up to your head.

□ **CHICKEN POX**

Can I get chicken pox again if I've already had it?

Yes. Experts once believed that your first feverish, blistery bout of chicken pox was also your last, conferring lifetime immunity against the varicella virus. But recent research suggests that 4 to 13 percent of people may experience a repeat infection. It may be that some people are extremely susceptible, or that their first exposure didn't generate enough antibodies to create complete protection. Infections also hit one in ten people who've been vaccinated against chicken

pox, but these cases are usually extremely mild, involving just a handful of chicken pox "bumps," and last just a few days.

You can find out if your childhood chicken pox shot is still working by getting a blood test, called a titer, that measures levels of antibodies against the varicella virus. If they are still high, then you are probably still immune. If they aren't, you may need a booster vaccine to remain protected.

If I had chicken pox as a child, will I get shingles as an adult?

It's possible. About half of all adults develop shingles by the time they're 85. After a childhood bout of the chicken pox, the varicella virus that causes chicken pox can lie dormant in nerve cells for decades, held in check by your immune system. But weakened immunity, thanks to aging or illness, can allow it to escape later in life,

leading to the tingling, burning blisters of shingles. One in five people with shingles also develops nerve damage that leads to intense, lingering pain. (If you do get shingles, your doctor can prescribe medication to markedly decrease your chances of getting this debilitating side effect, called post-herpetic neuralgia.)

Everyone's risk for shingles is different. Your odds for developing it are 4 times higher than normal if you have one close relative who's had shingles, and 13 times higher if you have two or more. Your best move? Consider the shingles vaccine once you're age 60, the recommended age for receiving the shot (you can get it earlier, but insurance may not cover it). The vaccine can cut your risk for developing shingles by half and lessen the severity of an outbreak if you do have one.

Can I get shingles if I've had the chicken pox vaccine?

Yes. To begin with, the vaccine's protection isn't perfect; about one in ten people who get the chicken pox vaccine can still "catch" a mild case of chicken pox, which means they could potentially get shingles later in life. What's more, since the chicken pox vaccine has only been widely used since the mid-1990s, and because shingles usually strikes after age 60, researchers don't yet know how much protection against shingles a childhood chicken pox vaccine will provide.

You may have heard that shingles is on the rise in people over age 60 *because* of the chicken pox vaccine. Researchers have discovered that adults who in the past would have gotten a subtle "booster shot" against the varicella virus through exposure to kids with chicken pox are no longer getting it because so few kids get chicken pox anymore. As a result, shingles cases could rise by an estimated 30 to 50 percent.

□ **DENTAL FILLINGS**

Are white fillings better than silver fillings?

Cosmetically speaking, they're more appealing because they blend in with your teeth. But they're no safer than old-fashioned silver (amalgam) fillings, and they generally don't last quite as long. While about half of all tooth-colored composite fillings need to be replaced within 10 years, amalgam fillings last about 20 percent longer (their durability depends on the size of the filling, your chewing pattern, and the strength of the tooth surrounding the filling). Composite fillings may also cause more tooth sensitivity in some people, but the effect is usually temporary.

Silver fillings, a mix of elemental liquid mercury with a powder containing several other metals, have been blamed for triggering a wide variety of health problems. While it's true that exposure to mercury vapors on a large scale can lead to health problems, the minute amounts released by metal fillings in your mouth are too small to pose a threat. Studies show that they do not raise the risk for Alzheimer's disease, multiple sclerosis, memory loss, or tremors in adults. And they do not harm intellect, memory, coordination, focus, nerve conduction, or kidney function in children.

My dentist says my fillings have to be replaced. Aren't they permanent?

Alas, no. Amalgam, or silver fillings, may last a little longer than enamel fillings. And if you can afford them, gold fillings may be the most durable of all. But the average lifespan of a tooth filling is about a decade. Thanks to the friction of chewing, temperature changes from eating and drinking hot and cold stuff, and the high-pressure assault of grinding or clenching your pearly whites, fillings wear, chip, crack, and break. Even if you don't feel any pain or notice anything's wrong, tiny cracks and gaps between the filling and your tooth can open up, allowing

food and bacteria to slip down inside, creating the perfect environment for new tooth decay or even infection.

□ **DOCTORS**

Why do I always have to have a follow-up visit with my doctor? Often, it seems like a phone call would do.

Follow-up appointments are important if you have a chronic health condition that needs ongoing attention. This is the time when you and your doctor can discuss test results, review the effectiveness of any medications you're taking, assess whether your condition is improving, and look at your successes and challenges in making healthy lifestyle changes. Follow-ups are also important if the results of a routine screening test reveal that you have a new health problem.

Follow-ups for more minor problems are also useful; your doctor can assess whether or not a treatment has worked and look for complications so that a small issue doesn't become something bigger. But if you have a feeling that a quick phone call might be all that's needed, such as to get the results of a routine test or screening, it never hurts to ask. Don't skip an appointment without calling, though.

Is it rude to ask health-care workers to wash their hands?

A doctor should not be offended by this question if you ask politely. Clean hands save lives: Half of all infections that people pick up in hospitals could be avoided if health-care practitioners washed up as often *and* as well as they should. Yet doctors, nurses, and other professionals scrub up less than 20 percent of the time before meeting a new patient, studies show. That's why hospitals have launched hand-washing awareness campaigns—and sometimes even enlist patients in the effort.

Should I keep my own health records?

Yes. Some day, electronic medical records kept by health-care practitioners and by consumers will make keeping paper records obsolete. Until then, it's smart to keep a file containing important information about your health so that your doctor can make informed decisions about your care, so that any new doctors you see have your complete record, and so that nothing's overlooked if another doctor or health-care practitioner is taking care of you in an emergency. Too often, crucial health data is

scattered among the various doctors and specialists you've seen and hospitals and clinics where you've received treatments. Even when you ask a doctor or medical institution to send your records along to your primary care doctor, most of the time, not everything is copied and forwarded.

Keeping your own records is easier than you may think. Start by jotting down:

- Your name, birth date, blood type, and emergency contact
- The date of your last physical
- A list of your medicines, dosages, and how long you've taken them
- Any chronic diseases and allergies
- Any history of illnesses in your family

- Results of recent routine screenings and of any specially ordered tests. Ask your doctor which results are important for you to keep in your own files and whether the office can provide copies. In the future, ask for copies of results when you have medical tests, scans, x-rays, and screenings.
- Major illnesses and surgeries, with dates. Include the name of the procedure, if you know it, and the medical center where it was performed.

How can I avoid a long wait in the waiting room?

Schedule the first appointment of the day—and arrive early, as some doctors may double-book appointment slots.

 FACT OR FICTION

An Older Doctor Is the Best

Fiction. Younger physicians often deliver better care and have healthier patients simply because their skills are more up to date. In one Harvard Medical School analysis, doctors 20 years out of medical school were 43 percent less likely than recent graduates to follow current patient-care guidelines in important areas such as cancer screenings. Older doctors were less likely to prescribe aspirin for heart patients, more likely to perform unnecessary hysterectomies, and more likely to undertreat conditions, including depression, breast cancer, and high blood pressure. Of course, age isn't what defines a good physician. In the Harvard study, some older doctors outperformed younger colleagues because they kept abreast of new developments in their specialties.

Waiting room times in doctor's offices and clinics are consistently shorter in the morning and get longer as the day progresses simply because many doctors fall behind schedule as the day goes on. Claiming the first appointment after lunch, if your doctor's office closes for lunch, and choosing the day of the week that the staff says is usually the least busy can also help. In addition, it pays to be on friendly terms with the office staff, so that you can call ahead on the day of your appointment to see whether your doctor is on schedule or running behind.

If your doctor repeatedly keeps you waiting a long time, consider finding a new doctor. Today, more and more doctors are being taught to value their patients' time. The result is shorter waiting times in many practices. Note, however, that if you want to see a specialist who's in high demand, long waits can be par for the course.

☐ **EXERCISE**

Is it better to eat before or after exercise?

Before. Exercising on an empty stomach could leave you low on energy just when you need a little more oomph to walk that extra mile or complete that last set of strength moves. Having a small meal 2 to 3 hours before you exercise,

 AVOID THIS MISTAKE

Eating More Because You're Exercising

Don't undo the calorie-burning benefits of exercise by overeating. It would take an hour of walking to burn off the extra 230 calories in a small doughnut, 40 minutes of swimming to burn off the calories in an extra slice of cheese pizza, and 85 minutes of fast dancing to get rid of the 500 calories in a cinnamon roll.

or a light snack such as a piece of fruit 30 minutes to an hour before exercise, can give you the energy you need. A strategic preworkout snack can also keep you from becoming so ravenous that you overeat afterward.

How much exercise do I really need?

Most healthy people should aim for at least 30 minutes, five times a week, of moderately intense activity such as brisk walking, plus 10 to 15 minutes or so of strength-training (digging in your garden counts) 2 or 3 days a week. This is enough exercise to help you lower your risk for health conditions like high blood pressure, stroke, coronary artery disease, type 2 diabetes, colon cancer, and osteoporosis, and to prevent the natural loss of muscle mass that slows metabolism and contributes to weight gain in your thirties, forties, fifties, and beyond.

If you're trying to lose weight, more activity is better. An hour or even 90

minutes of moderate exercise, or 1/2 hour of vigorous activity such as jogging, strenuous aerobics, or fast-paced cycling, is ideal. Of course, anything you do is better than nothing, and consistency counts. Fitting in 30 minutes most days of the week, even in 10-minute bursts, is better than playing the weekend warrior by overdoing it once or twice a week.

If you're the type that just doesn't enjoy going to the gym or using a treadmill, choose an activity you enjoy that you can do for 10 to 30 minutes or longer and that raises your heart rate. This could be dancing, playing tennis, chopping enough wood to heat your house for the winter, or lining up strenuous yard work or housework that feels like a workout.

Do I really need my doctor's okay before I start to exercise?

If you're a starting a low- or moderate-intensity program, you're probably good to go

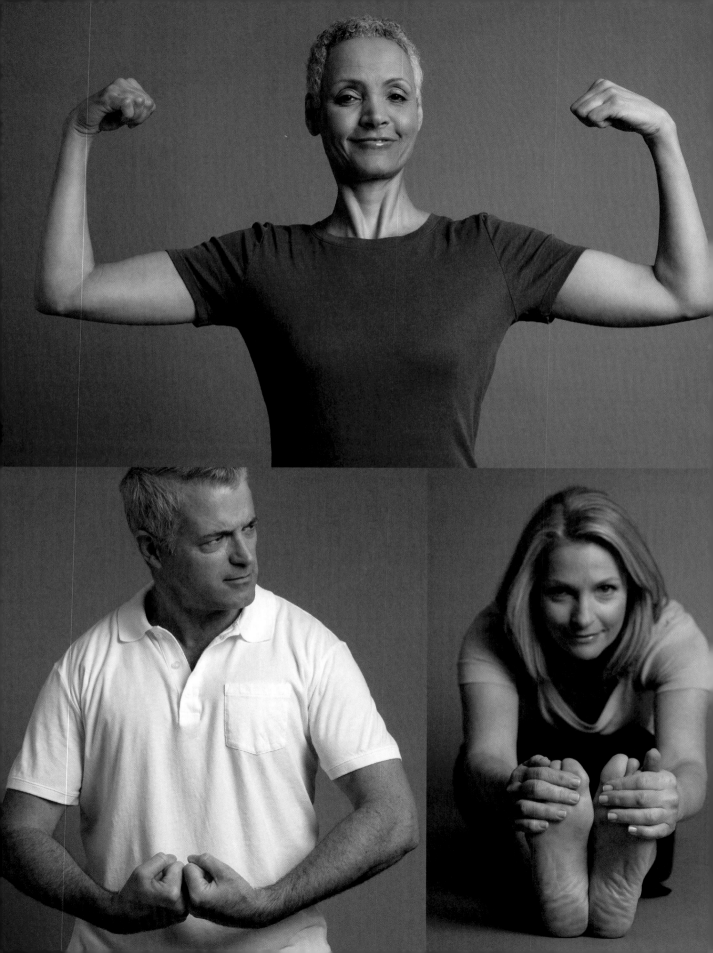

without a doctor's approval. Check with your physician first, though, if you have a heart condition, have had chest pain recently, lose your balance or feel dizzy on a regular basis, have osteoporosis or a joint or back problem, or take medications for high blood pressure or a heart condition. If you're a woman over age 50 or a man over age 40 planning to jump into a vigorous program, such as training for a marathon, get the okay from your doctor first.

Will sit-ups flatten my abs?

They'll tone your abdominal muscles, but no exercise can reduce fat on a single, targeted area of the body. The only way to do that is to lose weight.

Some ab moves are better than others for tightening tummy muscles. Sit-ups and crunches work, but two exercises, known as the vertical leg crunch and the bicycle maneuver, are twice as effective at working the network of muscles in your abdominal area. If you have back pain, talk with your doctor or a trainer before trying either of these.

To perform a vertical leg crunch, lie face-up on the floor. Place your hands behind your head for support. Extend your legs up toward the ceiling, crossing them at the ankles, knees slightly bent. Contract your abdominal muscles to lift your hips slightly off the floor.

For the bicycle move, lie face-up on the floor with your lower back pressed to the ground. Place your hands behind your head. Bend your knees and raise your legs far enough off the floor to do a bicycle pedaling motion, and then bicycle away, touching your left elbow to your right knee, then your right elbow to your left knee, and so on.

Is walking weight-bearing enough to prevent osteoporosis?

Though brisk walking will help, it may not be sufficient. The impact as your feet hit the ground stimulates cells in the bones of your legs, hips, and spine to build new bone, preventing the thinning that can lead to osteoporosis. But higher-impact activities such as dancing, hiking, jogging, jumping rope, climbing stairs, or playing tennis do more to stimulate bone growth and maintain bone density. (Check with your doctor first if your bones are already thinning or if you have joint problems or are prone to falls.)

Strength-training is also important. It stimulates bone growth when muscles and ligaments "tug" on bones as you lift weights, use resistance bands or machines, or do exercises (think push-ups) that rely on your own body weight to build muscle. Your best bet is a combination of high-impact exercise and strength-training; in one study, this strategy pre-

served bone mineral density in women who had just reached menopause, a time when loss of bone density accelerates.

It's also critical to get enough calcium and vitamin D. And even if you do everything right, remember that genetics plays a role in bone strength and fracture risk. Experts believe bone density is about 60 percent controlled by your genes—a reason to get a bone-density test if you have a family history of osteoporosis or bone fractures, and to talk with your doctor about whether you need bone-preserving prescription medications if you're at high risk for fractures.

I'm significantly overweight. Will walking harm my joints?

It could, so take it slowly and pay attention to any pain in your knees, hips, and ankles. With every step, every pound of body weight puts 3 to 6 pounds of pressure on your knee joints. This can damage cartilage, the cushion between bones, and put you at increased risk for arthritis. Overweight people lost cartilage rapidly over 2½ years in one recent Boston University study; for every 11 extra pounds they carried, their odds for cartilage loss rose 11 percent.

If walking hurts, don't give up on exercise. Instead, try something low impact such as swimming or water aerobics, which gives you the benefits of exercising without stressing your joints. Other options include riding a recumbent bike or using an elliptical trainer at the gym or asking a trainer to recommend exercises to strengthen your leg muscles, which will help protect your knees from damage.

I have high blood pressure. Do I have to be careful when exercising?

Exercise is proven to lower high blood pressure, so don't shy away from aerobic activities like walking, jogging, or riding an exercise bike. It's important, of course, to check with your doctor first and, if you have her okay, to start slowly. Overexercising could temporarily raise your blood pressure. It's also important to know when it's time to stop: If you feel short of breath, dizzy, or have chest pain or tightness across your chest, stop and sit down immediately.

Adding strength-training also has benefits; in one study, it lowered blood pressure by 2 to 6 points, a small improvement that can lower odds for a heart attack or stroke. If you'd like to try strength-training, follow two rules. First, don't hold your breath while lifting weights; this could make blood pressure spike. Instead, keep on inhaling and exhaling with each lift. Second, consider lifting lighter weights and doing more repetitions of each exer-

cise, which won't increase your blood pressure as much as using heavier weights.

☐ **EYES**

I want to have laser eye surgery to correct my vision. What type is best?

Wavefront-guided LASIK looks like a winner. This type of laser surgery uses a more detailed map of the imperfections in your cornea (the transparent surface of your eye) than conventional LASIK, so your surgeon can make more customized vision corrections. Research comparing the two suggests that wavefront-guided LASIK can produce sharper, clearer eyesight with less risk for night-vision problems such as glare and halos around lights than conventional LASIK.

You may have also heard about "bladeless" LASIK. Conventional LASIK uses a microkeratome, a surgical instrument with a tiny blade, to create a flap in your cornea; the surgeon then uses a laser to reshape corneal tissue underneath. Newer, bladeless surgery uses a laser to make the flap. In one study comparing bladeless LASIK to conventional LASIK, vision and healing times were similar, but the researchers noted that bladeless surgery could reduce

the already-low risk for vision loss (less than 1 percent) of conventional LASIK.

☐ **FLUS AND PANDEMICS**

How can I protect myself and my family from new strains of flu?

No matter what kind of flu is going around, the advice is the same:

1. Wash your hands thoroughly and frequently with soap and water or with an alcohol-based hand sanitizer when you can't get to a sink. Teach your kids to do this, too; children and young adults, ages 5 to 24, seem most susceptible to swine flu, also called the H1N1 virus.

2. Avoid touching your eyes, nose, and mouth; these are the most common routes of infection.

3. Try to avoid close contact (within 6 feet) with people who have any type of flu. This may include avoiding crowded public areas during the height of flu season. Note that with most flus, people may be contagious from 1 day before they develop symptoms to up to 7 days after they get sick.

If someone in your family does get sick, they should stay home until their fever has been gone for 24 hours, and cover their coughs to avoid spreading the flu to others.

How do I know if it's regular flu or something more serious like swine or avian flu?

Symptoms of seasonal influenza are very similar to those of avian flu and swine flu, also called H1N1 flu. These include fever, cough, sore throat, runny or stuffy nose, body aches, headache, chills, and fatigue. A significant number of people who have been infected with the H1N1 virus also have reported diarrhea and vomiting. If you have flu symptoms, call your doctor and ask if you should be tested to see what type you have.

Call 911 or go to an emergency room if your flu symptoms include trouble breathing, dizziness, confusion, persistent vomiting, or pain or pressure in your chest. Get emergency care for kids whose flu symptoms include a fever with a rash, dehydration, fast breathing, bluish skin, sluggishness or difficulty waking up, severe irritability, or flu symptoms that get better, then return suddenly with more coughing.

Will wearing a mask I buy in the drugstore protect me from the flu?

Probably not. Drugstore face masks don't fit tightly enough around your nose and mouth to

protect against inhaling microscopic, airborne virus particles. But these inexpensive and easy-to-find masks can help prevent someone who has the flu from spreading the virus via coughs and sneezes. If *you* have swine flu, health authorities recommend wearing a mask in the doctor's office or hospital or when you have to be out in your community to help protect other people from becoming infected.

Though it's unlikely that a mask will keep you from getting the flu if you don't already have it, the Centers for Disease Control and Prevention recommends wearing one, rather than doing nothing at all, in certain circumstances if you're at high risk for swine flu infection. You're considered at high risk if you have a medical condition that weakens your immunity. If that's you, consider wearing a mask out in public if swine flu is on the rise in your community or at home if you live with someone who has it.

☐ **HAIR DYE**

Do hair dyes cause cancer?

Probably not. Plenty of research, including a Harvard Medical School study of 99,000 women, has found no cause-

and-effect relationship between hair dyes and bladder cancer, leukemia, multiple myeloma, Hodgkin's disease, non-Hodgkin's lymphoma, lung cancer, breast cancer, oral cancer, or cervical cancer. One review of 79 cancer/hair dye studies concluded that no strong link existed, though it noted that women who used hair dyes before 1980 seem to have higher rates of two types of non-Hodgkin's lymphoma. Another study found that long-term use of hair dye might raise bladder cancer risk.

If you want to color your hair and at the same time limit your exposure to hair dye ingredients, leave the dye solution on your hair for the shortest time possible, rinse thoroughly, and wear gloves during the process. Permanent dyes have the greatest levels of potentially harmful chemicals so stick with semi-permanent dyes or go with highlights or streaks instead of a full-head treatment. Or opt for a plant-based dye containing henna.

Is it safe to dye my hair while I'm pregnant or trying to get pregnant?

There's no evidence that the chemicals in hair dye can harm

an unborn baby, but no one knows for certain because very few studies have been done in humans. One study of 174 pregnant hairdressers, who handled hair dyes at work almost daily, found no increased risk for miscarriage or birth defects. Another small study—it included only 18 women, but it's the only study of its kind—looked at women who colored their hair during the first trimester of their pregnancies and found no problems. But some animal studies that exposed mice to large doses of hair-dye ingredients have detected an increased incidence of birth defects.

To be on the safe side, it may be smart to stick with your natural hair color while you're pregnant or even until you're done breast-feeding, to switch to a vegetable- or henna-based dye, or to opt for highlights instead of a full dye job.

☐ **HOSPITALS**

How can I avoid picking up an infection while in the hospital?

The most important thing you can do is to ask doctors, nurses, and other health-care practitioners to wash their hands with soap and water or to use an alcohol-based hand sanitizer before they take care of you. This one step can help reduce risk for the most common infec-

tions picked up in hospitals, including staph infections, urinary tract infections if you have a catheter, diarrhea from *Clostridium difficile* if you're taking antibiotics, and even bloodstream infections if you have a central line placed in a vein to deliver medications or fluids. Keeping your own hands clean is also important, so be sure to wash up or use a hand sanitizer after using the bathroom, before eating, and even after touching the TV remote.

But there's more you can do. Ask family and friends to wash their hands right away when they visit you in the hospital. If you have a catheter, central line, or surgical dressings, ask visitors not to touch them. If you're wearing a catheter, be sure it stays below the level of your bladder; don't pull, twist, or kink the tubing. Ask your doctor or nurse every day whether you still need it—the sooner a catheter is removed, the lower your chances for infection. If you have a central line, let a nurse know right away if the bandage around it comes off or becomes wet or dirty or if the skin around it becomes red or sore.

Is "medical tourism"—going abroad for surgery—really a smart move?

Big savings and exotic locales send hundreds of thousands of people on globe-trotting trips

for medical procedures each year. The cost savings can be dramatic; everything from a nose job or a knee replacement to a heart bypass, cancer therapy, and brain surgery may cost one-half to one-tenth as much in places like Thailand, Brazil, the United Arab Emirates, or Costa Rica. Some health insurance companies are even beginning to cover some of the costs and have developed contracts with some overseas medical centers. If you're contemplating medical tourism, your insurer may be able to help you set it up.

But healthcare isn't just about saving money. Safety and a doctor's expertise can be difficult to assess from a distance, especially if there's a language barrier. Recovery far from home and far from your own doctor can be risky, as can long airplane journeys home after a procedure, when risk for dangerous blood clots rises. If you want to become a medical tourist, these strategies can help you ensure the best possible care:

● *Choose a medical center accredited by the Joint Commission International,* a branch of the Joint Commission on Accreditation of Healthcare Organizations at www.joint-commissioninternational.org.

● *Work with your doctor at home, before you go, to be sure you're a good candidate.* Are you healthy enough not only to travel great distances but also to recover in a hotel room far from home and to travel back home after your procedure? Is the treatment something that should be ongoing, such as cancer care, and better provided at home? If you are a good candidate, ask your doctor to help you arrange for follow-up care via appointments with them or with a specialist at home. Get copies of medical records you'll need, and ask if your doctor at home can arrange a conference call with your doctor abroad.

- *Look for a reputable medical tourism agency.* There are plenty of medical tourism "middlemen" out there who will plan your trip for you. A good one will match you with an accredited hospital that's best for your needs and help arrange follow-up care.

- *Interview the prospective doctor.* Call and find out how experienced the doctor is and what his or her success and complication rates are.

I'm about to be released from the hospital and am worried that my health (or my spouse's) will decline without all the care and attention. What's my best plan?

Ask your doctor for a written discharge plan. This should include a review of the medications you'll be taking, any special home care you'll need, symptoms to watch out for, and a 24-hour phone number you can call if you encounter any problems. A nurse or your doctor should review the plan with you; it's smart to have a relative or close friend there, too. Also have a loved one schedule a follow-up visit with your own doctor. Good plans cut your odds for winding up back in the hospital by 30 percent, research shows.

Before you leave the hospital, make sure you figure out how you'll get by in the days after your release. Don't be shy about asking relatives and friends for assistance with meals, laundry, grocery shopping, transportation to medical appointments, and simply for friendly checks to see that everything's okay. Ask hospital staff involved with your discharge to help find out whether your health insurance will cover the cost of a visiting nurse or home health aid if you or your doctors think you'll need one. There also may be free or low-cost community organizations that can help.

In most hospitals these days, a care coordinator will help set up ways to meet your post-hospital stay needs before you leave. But it never hurts to ask about these plans as soon as your doctor or nurses begin discussing your eventual hospital discharge. If there's just not enough help available, it's smart to ask if you or your spouse can spend time recovering in a short-term-care nursing center before moving back home.

☐ HOT TUBS

How can I tell if a hot tub is clean enough to use?

You can't tell by looking, only by asking questions. Bacteria that can cause skin rashes (especially red, itchy bumps around hair follicles) and lung infections thrive on pipes, filters, tiles, and other surfaces of hot tubs, especially if they aren't cleaned regularly. The bacteria rise to the surface on bubbles and are dispersed into the air, and into your lungs, when the bubbles burst.

If you want to know if the hot tub in a spa, gym, or campground is safe, you'll have to ask to see the inspection records. The chlorine and pH levels should be tested twice daily and at times when the tub is heavily used. (The more bodies in the tub, the faster the disinfectant is depleted.) When in doubt, stay out. When inspectors from the Centers for Disease Control and Prevention checked 5,000 public hot tubs in the United States, they concluded that more than half were not maintained safely. Some problems are out of sight, such as dirty drains and pipes.

If you own a hot tub, follow the manufacturer's directions for water changes, cleaning, and disinfection.

☐ **ILLNESS**

How do I know if I or someone else is still contagious from a cold or other illness?

In general, adults are contagious for about 5 days after developing symptoms of a cold or stomach bug; kids and people with weakened immune systems may be contagious for longer than a week. A cold is most contagious 2 to 3 days after sniffles begin; some people stay contagious longer, perhaps a reflection of lower immunity or the virulence of a particular cold. In any case, you can safely assume you are absolutely no longer able to give it to other people 7 to 10 days later. If you have a strep infection, you're contagious until you've been on antibiotics for 24 hours. Seasonal flu is contagious from the day *before* symptoms appear until 5 to 7 days after you first notice symptoms. To be safe with stomach flu, consider yourself contagious from the moment you feel ill until at least 3 days after you recover.

How can I avoid catching a bug on a plane?

Start your trip in good health. Be sure you're well-rested, well-fed, and well-hydrated and you'll be less susceptible to any bugs you're exposed to in the air. While on board, wash your hands with soap and warm water or with an alcohol-based hand sanitizer before you eat or drink, after using the restroom, and, if it's a long flight, several times in between (especially after you touch surfaces such as a your seat belt buckle). Avoid touching your nose, mouth, or eyes. If you're sitting beside a passenger who's coughing and sneezing, ask the flight attendant if you can change seats. If your plane is delayed on the ground for more than 30 minutes, ask the crew to turn on the ventilation system; in one famous 1979 incident, 72 percent of passengers caught the flu when their plane was grounded for 3 hours with no extra ventilation.

Stay alert to signs of flu once you reach your destination. If you develop a headache, cough, fever, chills, or body aches, get to a doctor fast and ask for an antiviral medication such as oseltamivir (Tamiflu) or zanamivir (Relenza). These

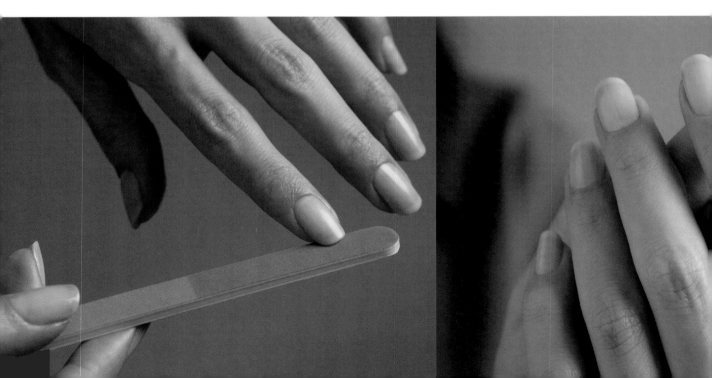

drugs can shorten a bout of flu if taken within 2 days of the start of symptoms.

What is the best way to boost my immunity?

The most effective measures don't involve buying anything in the supplement aisle, but rather, tweaking a few habits in your everyday life:

- *Find ways to alleviate stress.* In more than 300 studies, researchers have found that while short-term stress, such as rushing to meet a deadline, can boost levels of natural killer cells, which battle bacteria, viruses, and other invaders, chronic stress reduces immunity.

- *Devote 8 hours a night to sleep.* Plenty of research suggests that shortchanging yourself on slumber diminishes your body's ability to fight off bacteria and viruses. In one study, for example, getting less than 7 hours of shut-eye per night tripled the risk for catching a cold.

- *Exercise on most days.* Getting about 45 minutes of moderate-intensity aerobic exercise 5 days a week cut risk for a cold by two-thirds in a recent study from the Fred Hutchinson Cancer Research Center in Seattle. Other studies show that regular exercise helps battle gastrointestinal infections, too.

- *Eat a healthy diet.* That includes plenty of fruits, vegetables, beans, fish, yogurt with active cultures, and whole grains.

☐ **MANICURES/PEDICURES**

Do I have to worry about getting an infection from a manicure or pedicure?

Yes, if the salon you go to doesn't practice proper sterilization techniques. Spa footbaths can harbor bacteria that trigger boils, ulcers, and skin infections. And you can catch a nail fungus from clippers, files, and cuticle pushers that haven't been properly disinfected. For a safe pedicure, ask your nail salon if they disinfect the foot bath or foot spa after each customer and again at the end of business. Skip it if you have any broken skin on your feet or legs, and don't shave, wax, or use hair-removal creams for a day before your pedicure. To protect against nail fungus, bring your

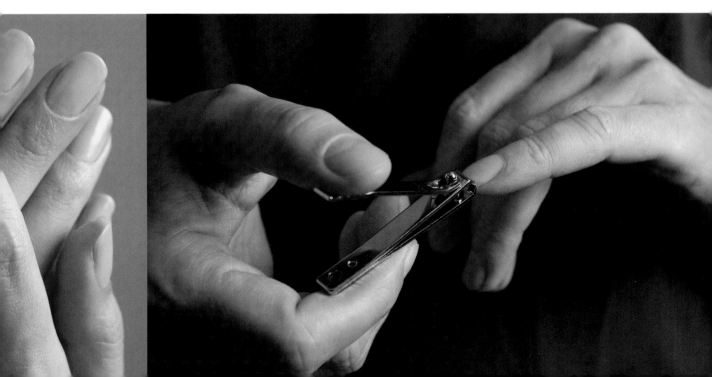

own nail-care tools. Or ask your manicurist if the salon's tools are sterilized in an autoclave or disinfectant between uses, not simply wiped down with alcohol.

□ **NONSTICK PANS**

Are nonstick pans safe?

When heated to 500°F and higher, the coating inside nonstick cookware begins to break down, emitting fumes that cause "polymer fume fever," flulike symptoms that subside quickly if you get some fresh air. Heated to 680°F, some nonstick pans release toxic gases that may include carcinogens, according to the Environmental Working Group, a nonprofit watchdog organization. Pet birds are very sensitive to nonstick pan fumes so, if you overheat your pan, make sure you remove your bird from the kitchen.

One nonstick substance, perfluorooctanoic acid (PFOA), will be phased out of nonstick cookware made and sold in the United States by 2015. In animal studies, PFOA has been linked with cancer, liver damage, growth defects, and immune-system damage. (Meanwhile, we're exposed to PFOAs more often from micro-wave-popcorn bags, fast-food packaging, shampoo, carpeting, and clothing.)

Manufacturers of nonstick cookware recommend never preheating it on the stove or in the oven. In one independent test, even pans containing butter, oil, and some foods topped 500°F in a matter of minutes on the stove. Heavier, more expensive pans are slower to overheat and may be a better choice. Opening a window and turning on the exhaust fan during cooking can also dissipate any fumes. Avoid scratching the pan's surface; if your favorite pan is scratched, it's time for a new one.

□ **PLASTICS**

Which plastics can I safely reheat and store food in?

We recommend using a glass or ceramic bowl to heat foods and drinks in the microwave, rather than plastic, just to be on the safe side, since some plastics, even those labeled microwave-safe, may leach compounds into foods when heated. To figure out what's safe for storage, use the recy-cling number found inside a small triangle on the bottom of most plasticware to help guide your choices.

Safest for storage: #2, #4, or #5. Most name-brand food-storage containers are made of these stable plastics, including high-density polyethylene (#2), low-density polyethylene (#4), or polypropylene (#5).

Don't reuse: #1, #3, or #6. Water, soda, and juice bottles are usually made from #1, or polyethylene terephthalate eth-ylene. Their shape can make them tough to clean thoroughly, which could allow bacteria to thrive inside. There's some evi-dence that styrene, a toxic chemical, may leach from Styro-foam containers, made with #6 polystyrene containers. Environ-mentalists also warn that reusing #3 polyvinyl chloride containers, such as peanut butter jars, may be risky, too.

Replace polycarbonate water bottles, pitchers, and other hard, clear, shatterproof food containers. These may have a "PC" or a #7 on the bottom. Polycarbonates contain bisphe-nol-A (BPA), linked in animal studies with cancer, miscar-riage, and obesity. Many countries now ban the sale of baby bottles containing BPA, and plenty of BPA-free prod-ucts, such as shatterproof water bottles, are now on the market. Newer types of polycarbonate are BPA-free but have not been fully tested for other leaching properties. The best option for drinking-water bottles may be stainless steel types.

□ **SLEEP**

I'm getting older. Do I need fewer hours of sleep?

Not necessarily. In fact, many older adults get less sleep than they need. They have more diffi-culty falling asleep, wake more often during the night, and have more trouble getting back to sleep. They may also wake ear-lier in the morning. One reason for these sleep changes seems to be that our bodies produce less melatonin, the sleep hor-mone, as we get older. But that doesn't mean we require less sleep. Sleep-deprived older people have more memory prob-lems, depression, and falls than their well-rested counterparts.

□ SMOKING CESSATION

How do I know what dose nicotine replacement patch to use?

The milligrams of nicotine in your patch should be the same or slightly more than the number of cigarettes you smoked per day. If you smoked 30 a day, for example, you'd need a 21-milli-gram patch plus a 14-milligram patch. If you're still craving ciga-rettes or feel irritable, anxious, or unable to concentrate, you may need a slightly higher dose. Don't be afraid to also use nico-tine products like gums and sprays for extra ammunition when the urge to smoke strikes. If you're using too much nico-tine, you'll know it: You'll feel nauseated and very shaky. After a month, your doctor may rec-ommend beginning to reduce your dose by 7 to 14 milligrams every 2 weeks.

Nicotine-replacement products, combined with a stop-smoking program, coun-seling, the smoking cessation drug bupropion (Zyban), or a mix of these strategies, can double your chances for suc-cess compared to relying on nicotine replacement alone.

How can I avoid gaining weight when I quit?

Take advantage of quitting strategies such as nicotine-replacement patches, cognitive behavioral therapy, and the anti-depressant bupropion (Zyban). Studies show that quitters who used one, two, or all three of these gained less weight than those who tried going cold turkey, presumably because their cravings were less intense and they didn't have to compen-sate by eating more snacks or bigger meals. Exercise helps, too. Women who worked out for 30 to 40 minutes three times a week gained 5 pounds less than nonexercisers in one study a year after quitting. They were also twice as likely to be smoke-free after a year.

Among people who quit smoking, about one-third lose weight, one-third stay at the same weight, and one-third initially gain weight. Keep in mind that the health benefits of quitting far outweigh the dangers of putting on a few pounds.

Why am I cough-ing more since I quit smoking?

Because your body's cough reflex is returning to normal. A constant stream of cigarette smoke turns off sensory nerve cells known as cough receptors in your throat and airways. The receptors begin to function again about 2 weeks after you quit and become increasingly sensitive over the next few months. At the same time, microscopic hairs lining your airways, which are paralyzed by tobacco smoke, begin to function again. Once the cilia have been restored, coughing subsides. In the meantime, sip-ping water or using cough drops may help.

Can I take bupropion (Zyban) to help me quit smoking if I'm already taking another anti-depressant?

Talk with your doctor first. It's often okay to do this, with your doctor's permission, but you should know that taking this stop-smoking drug along with another antidepressant could increase the risk of side effects from bupropion, such as dry mouth, insomnia, dizziness, upset stomach, and anxiety.

☐ **SUN PROTECTION**

Is an SPF-80 sunscreen better than an SPF-50?

Yes, but only by a tiny bit. Protection doesn't increase in proportion to the SPF number; the higher you go, the less the added benefit. An SPF-15 protects against about 93 percent of UVB rays; an SPF-30, 97 percent; an SPF-50, about 98 percent; and SPF 100, about 99 percent. More important than what SPF you use (assuming you use at least 30) is how much sunscreen you use, how often you reapply it, and whether the sunscreen is broad-spectrum—that is, in addition to protecting against UVB rays, the kind that cause sunburn, it protects against UVA rays, the kind that cause skin cancer.

To ensure the best UVA protection, look for the ingredients zinc oxide, titanium dioxide, sulisobenzone, meradimate (methyl anthranilate), ecamsule (Mexoryl SX), dioxybenzone, or avobenzone. And slather yourself well. It takes about an ounce of sunscreen, an amount that will fill your entire palm, to adequately cover an average-size adult. Apply the first coat 20 to 30 minutes before going outdoors so your skin can absorb sun-blocking chemicals. Reapply every 2 hours even on cloudy days, sooner if you've been swimming or are sweaty. Even water-resistant and waterproof types can stop working after about 40 to 80 minutes.

Can I get sunburned through a window?

No. Window glass in cars, homes, and buildings blocks the sun's UVB rays, the ultraviolet light responsible for sunburn—but it doesn't stop UVA rays. These penetrate deep into the skin, damaging the collagen fibers that keep skin looking firm and increasing risk for skin cancer. If you spend a lot of time close to a sunny window or driving in the car, wear a broad-spectrum sunscreen.

☐ **SURGERY**

Is it okay to take my usual supplements and medications before surgery?

Don't decide on your own to continue taking any supplements, over-the-counter remedies, or prescription drugs before surgery. Talk with your doctor when you decide to have surgery about the medications and supplements you take so he can decide if you need to continue on them or when to stop taking them before the procedure. Everything from herbal remedies to prescription meds could interact with your anesthesia or interfere with healing in the hours and days after your procedure. For example, ginkgo biloba, garlic, ginseng, fish-oil capsules, and others may increase risk for excess bleeding; St. John's wort and valerian may interact with anesthesia.

I'm not supposed to eat or drink before surgery. Does coffee count?

If you are told not to eat or drink before surgery, it's best to skip coffee, too. But if you've had some, tell the medical staff. You may still be able to have your surgery, especially if the coffee was black (no cream, milk, nondairy creamer, or sweetener). In recent years, anesthesiologists have had a lively debate about whether coffee counts as a clear liquid that you may safely sip up to 2 to 3 hours before surgery, or if it belongs on the list of foods and drinks to avoid for 6 to 8 hours before a procedure. Many now conclude that black coffee is okay if you drink it at least 2 hours beforehand.

If you've had some java closer to the time of your surgery, that may pose a problem. Doctors want your stomach empty to avoid problems in the rare event that you vomit while the anesthesia is taking effect or wearing off. Your cough reflex may be immobilized and you could inhale particles into your lungs, which could lead to pneumonia.

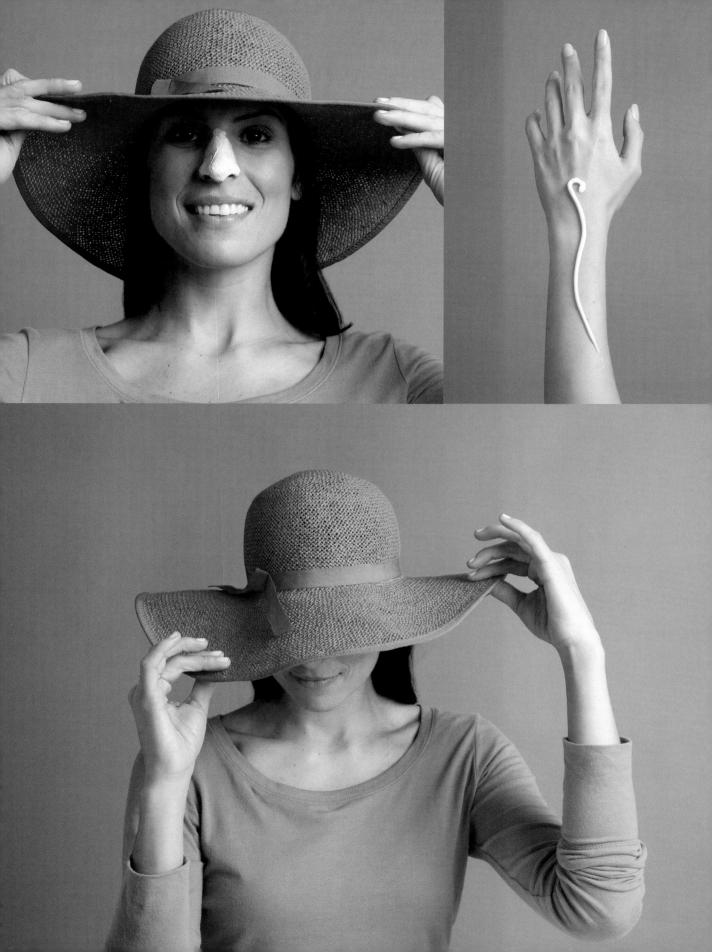

☐ TICKS AND BUG BITES

What's the best way to remove a tick from my skin?

Skip the hot matches, nail polish, and petroleum jelly. Instead, use fine-tipped tweezers to grab the tick as close to your skin as possible and pull it out slowly and steadily. Don't twist; this can leave the mouth-parts of the tick, which are barbed, stuck in your skin. If the tick doesn't come out right away, hold the tension until the tick releases. When it comes out, wash the tick down the drain or flush it down the toilet. You can also keep it in a jar or zip-close bag or stick it to a piece of tape to show to your doctor if you later suspect you have a tick-borne illness. Wash the bitten spot and your hands right away with soap and water. If you can't remove the tick, call your doctor.

What's riskier: A tick or mosquito bite or using an insect repellent?

The bite. Ticks can carry Lyme disease as well as Rocky Mountain spotted fever, babesiosis, ehrlichiosis, and human anaplasmosis, all of which can cause serious symptoms, including nerve damage, paralysis, and in some cases, death. Mosquitoes may harbor West Nile virus and viruses that cause encephalitis (brain inflammation).

WHAT YOU DON'T KNOW

Ticks Take Time to Transmit Lyme

A tick must be attached to you for about 24 hours or more before it begins to transmit Lyme disease.

The repellent DEET sets up a mosquito- and tick-repelling vapor barrier that was more effective and long-lasting than 15 other insect-stopping products in one study. DEET is safe even for kids when used as directed, which means using the lowest dose that will keep bugs away (kids should use a 10 percent or lower concentration), not reapplying more often than directed, and washing it all off at night, researchers report. If you don't like the smell, try products containing picaridin, which is odorless. Used around the world since 1998, it's considered safe by the World Health Organization.

For more tick protection, spray your shoes, socks, pants, and shirt—but never your skin—with permethrin, an insecticide that kills bugs within seconds after they land on you.

☐ TOOTH WHITENING

Is tooth whitening safe?

Generally, yes. The active ingredient in home and dentist's office tooth-whitening bleaches is carbamide perox-

ide, which breaks down into hydrogen peroxide in your mouth. Studies show that this chemical does not raise your risk for oral cancer, which had been an early concern. However, it can temporarily make teeth more sensitive for up to 78 percent of people who have their pearly whites lightened.

Your teeth become sensitive because the hydrogen peroxide in whiteners soaks through the protective outer coating of enamel and into the softer layer of dentin underneath, irritating the nerve-rich dental pulp at the core. Microscopic cracks and leaks along dental fillings increase your odds for tooth sensitivity. Up to 40 percent of people who use whitening trays also experience temporary gum irritation as well. It goes away in a few days or at most in a week or so.

Don't use tooth-whitening bleaches more often than recommended. Research shows that these products do wear away microscopic amounts of tooth enamel, which could increase tooth sensitivity and in rare cases, even tooth decay.

□ VACCINES

What vaccines and vaccine booster shots do adults need?

There are some shots and boosters that virtually all adults need, and others that only certain people need.

VACCINES AND BOOSTERS FOR ALL ADULTS:

- *Tetanus, diphtheria, pertussis (Td/Tdap):* Every 10 years.
- *Varicella (chicken pox):* Two doses if you have no immunity to the chicken pox virus (you were never vaccinated before and you never had the virus).
- *Zoster (shingles):* One dose if you're age 60 or older. Lasts at least 7 years. Ask your doctor if you need a booster after that.
- *Measles, mumps, rubella (MMR):* One or more doses if you have no immunity to these illnesses. You may need it if you were born after 1957 or have had only one shot in the past.

- *Influenza (flu):* Once a year for most adults, best in fall or early winter.
- *Pneumococcal:* Get a dose at age 65, younger if you smoke or are at risk for lung infections. Get a one-time booster shot 5 years later.

EXTRA VACCINES AND BOOSTERS YOU MAY NEED:

- *Hepatitis A:* A two-shot series. Ask about it if you have a history of illegal drug use, if you're a health-care worker, or if you have signs of chronic liver disease. You may also need a hepatitis A vaccine before traveling to certain countries.
- *Hepatitis B:* Three-shot series. You may need it if you're a health-care worker, have a history of injected drug use, or are sexually active and not monogamous.
- *Meningococcal:* One or more doses. Recommended for college freshman who will be living in dormitories, military recruits, people whose spleens have been removed,

and those with a weakened immune system.

- *Human papilloma virus:* Three-shot series. Recommended for girls as young as 9 and young women through age 26 to protect against four strains of HPV that can cause cervical cancer.

I had my last tetanus shot 5 years ago, but I just stepped on a nail and the emergency room doctor wants to give me a booster shot. Do I really need it?

Yes. Tetanus, also known as lockjaw, can be deadly. While adults need routine boosters of the tetanus vaccine every 10 years, if your last shot was roughly 5 or more years ago, it's worth the extra insurance that an early booster can provide if you've stepped on a rusty nail or had any other type of puncture wound or deep, dirty cut that could let this bacterium enter your body. To avoid unnecessary shots, be sure to keep up-to-date vaccination records in a handy place for all family members.

Can you get the flu from a flu shot?

No. The virus particles in injected vaccines for seasonal flu are dead and can't give

WHAT YOU DON'T KNOW

There Are Many Ways to Get a Tetanus Infection

Stepping on a rusty nail or getting a puncture wound raises the risk for a tetanus infection, but this bacterium can also enter the body through a tiny pinprick, a scratch from an animal, a splinter, a bug bite, and even a burn that breaks the skin. Head to the emergency room right away if you experience warning signs of tetanus such as neck stiffness, difficulty swallowing, rigidity of abdominal muscles, spasms, sweating, and fever.

you the flu, though you may feel a little achy and even run a low-grade fever for a day or two afterward. Viruses in the nasal-spray flu vaccine FluMist are live but are weakened and may cause minor symptoms but not full-blown flu.

☐ **WATER**

Is it true that I'm supposed to drink 8 glasses of water a day?

No. "Eight a day" is a myth. What you really need is enough fluid to replace what you lose each day in your sweat, urine, breath, and other bodily excretions. That's about 8 to 10 cups of water. Since we get about 4 cups' worth from fruits, vegeta-bles, and other foods, that leaves 4 to 6 cups for you to make up with beverages. Tea, coffee, juice, even soda count (though it's also smart to avoid empty calories) toward your total. Of course, you may need more in hot weather or if you're exercising or being more physically active than usual. So if you're still thirsty, sip more.

Why can't I cook with hot tap water? Why must it be cold, even if I'm going to heat it anyway?

Hot water can dissolve tiny amounts of lead from your plumbing system. Older homes may have lead pipes, but even new plumbing that's lead-free can still contain lead in brass fittings or faucets or in copper pipes with soldered joints. In one study, tap water accounted for up to 20 percent of human exposure to lead. Boiling doesn't help; in fact, it can further concentrate lead, which can damage your brain and nervous system. If you're using a faucet that hasn't been in use for the past 6 hours or more, first flush the pipes by letting the cold water run until it's as cold as it will get.

Should I use a water filter at home?

Yes, if water tests show that your drinking water contains pollutants or if it has an unpleasant taste or color. The right filter can remove impurities and toxins, including bacteria, copper, lead, mercury, parasites such as Giardia and Cryptosporidium, pesticides, radon, and volatile organic chemicals such as methyl-tert-butyl ether (MTBE) and dichlorobenzene and trichloroethylene (TCE).

There are many types of filters on the market, from activated carbon filters that fit on your faucet to whole-house "anion exchange" systems, so your first step is to learn what you need to filter out of your water. Ask your local water-treatment authority for a report on your water quality. If you're on a private well or want more in-depth information, consider hiring a private water-testing company.

 FACT OR FICTION

Drinking Too Much Water Is Dangerous

Fact. "Water intoxication" is common among marathon runners, but it can also happen to anyone who's exerting themselves for an extended period and guzzling lots of H_2O. Physical stress like exercise reduces the kidneys' ability to send urine to the bladder for excretion. Drink too much, and fluid levels could build in your body and brain, making brain cells swell and leading to headaches, nausea, vomiting, disorientation, and in some cases, death. To avoid it, drink enough to quench your thirst, not gallons. And if you need to drink large amounts of fluid, use Gatorade, Propel, Powerade, or other similar drinks that have vitamins and electrolytes besides just water.

If you simply don't like the way your water smells or tastes, an activated carbon filter may be all you need in order to enjoy your drinking water again.

How can I tell if I have a slow metabolism?

You can decide if your metabolism is generally fast, slow, or in between based on a combination of experience and honesty. If you can eat more than anyone else and never gain an ounce, your metabolism is fast. If you gain weight by just smelling food, your metabolism is slow. Most of us are in between. Honesty is key to making the call: Most people overestimate the calories they burn and underestimate the calories they take in.

Everyone's basal metabolic rate (BMR), or the number of calories they burn at rest, is different. Your BMR, responsible for about 65 percent of the calories you burn each day, is largely determined by your genes, but it changes with your body composition. The more muscle mass you have, the faster your metabolism. Whatever your metabolism, you can manage your weight by strength-training two or three times a week to build muscle and consuming fewer calories than you expend.

If you've noticed that you're not eating any more than usual yet you've been steadily gaining weight over the past few years, you may be in the midst of a metabolic slowdown brought on by the natural, age-related loss of muscle mass. Starting in your mid-thirties, your metabolism slows by about 5 percent each decade as muscle mass declines. After menopause, a woman's body burns about 30 percent less fat than it did before menopause, further slowing metabolism.

If you're gaining weight and you also have other symptoms, such as dry skin, constipation, and increased sensitivity to cold, ask your doctor to check your thyroid level. Hypothyroidism can cause you to burn fewer calories than normal.

What is the best weight-loss diet?

The one you can stick to, as long as it's healthy and cuts calories. When 811 overweight women and men tried one of four healthy, calorie-restricted eating plans for a landmark 2-year study, all lost an average of 13 pounds in 6 months and kept most of the weight off for 2 years. Dieters tried low-fat, low-carb, high-carb, and high-protein plans that shared two things: Moderate calorie-cutting (nobody ate fewer than 1,200 calories per day) and a mix of healthy foods including plenty of fruits, vegetables, whole grains, fiber, and low levels of artery-clogging saturated fat.

Your Most Embarrassing Questions

☐ ANAL ITCHING

My bottom is extremely itchy; what will relieve it?

Gentle cleaning after a bowel movement. Itchiness means the sensitive skin of your anus is irritated, most often by sweat, bits of feces left behind after an incomplete wiping, hemorrhoids, a dry-skin condition such as psoriasis, or even by too-enthusiastic hygiene, harsh soaps, or ingredients in scented toilet paper. Often we wipe too hard and try too hard to clean with the toilet paper and that leads to worsening irritation. Using soft, unscented toilet paper or baby wipes treated with a soothing, nonirritating moisturizer, such as lanolin, instead of toilet paper can help,

as can applying a dab of over-the-counter hydrocortisone.

Opt for loose cotton under-wear instead of tight synthetics, which trap sweat. If itching persists, skip coffee, tea, colas, beer, chocolate, tomatoes, spicy foods, and excessive amounts of vitamin C for a week or two; these

culprits can irritate delicate rectal tissues. See your doc if nothing helps, or if you also have a fever, rash, or discharge. Itching can also be a symptom of a bacterial or yeast infection, warts, or even pinworms. Finally, if you start to notice any bleeding accompanying the itch, you certainly should see a doc as that can be a sign of other problems like an anal fissure or worsening hemorrhoids.

DRUG-FREE FIX

Witch Hazel

A dab of witch hazel, applied with a cotton ball, helps to shrink swollen blood vessels. For extra relief, chill the bottle of witch hazel in the fridge; the cold helps reduce swelling and stops itching and discomfort fast.

☐ BAD BREATH

Nothing I do— brushing, flossing, mouthwash—gets rid of my bad breath. What *will* work?

Brush your tongue or clean it with a tongue scraper. Bad breath usually means bacteria are munching on food residue in your mouth, then emitting nasty-smelling sulfur compounds. Cleaning the tongue removes the film of microscopic food particles and also evicts some of those ill-mannered microbes before they can gas again. In one New York University study, people who brushed their teeth *and* tongues twice daily for 60 seconds had a 53 percent reduction in breath-souring sulfur compounds after 2 weeks.

Rinsing with a mouthwash containing a germ-fighting ingredient, such as chlorhexidine, cetylpyridinium chloride, zinc lactate, or chlorine dioxide, is also effective. If these strategies don't work, check your dinner plate: Garlic and onions contain odoriferous oils which, when digested, wind up in your bloodstream; they're released in your lungs and can sour your breath for up to 3 days.

Talk with your doctor or dentist if nothing seems to help. Stubborn bad breath can be a symptom of advanced gum disease, dry mouth, a sinus infection, tonsillitis, cryptic tonsillitis (when white debris collects in pockets in the tonsils), acid reflux, or a gastrointestinal or respiratory infection.

☐ BELCHING

My husband claims he can't control his loud, frequent belches. Should he see a doctor?

Rafter-rattling burps can be a sign of acid reflux or even an infection with the ulcer-causing bacterium *Helicobacter pylori*. But it's more likely that your spouse is simply swallowing more air than he realizes. We suck in about a teaspoonful with every swallow; body heat makes the extra air expand in our stomachs, creating the perfect set-up for an explosive belch.

Gum chewing, sucking on hard candy, smoking, drinking carbonated beverages, gulping down food and beverages, and even things like excess saliva generated by poorly fitted dentures and sinus drainage (due to an infection or allergy) can lead to an excessive intake of air. Try to correct those problems first. If belching continues, your husband may need relief for reflux or an *H. pylori* infection, especially if he also has abdominal discomfort, indigestion, a bloated feeling, or frequent, mild nausea.

☐ BODY ODOR

Nothing helps my BO. Am I doomed to stink?

Stubborn body odor can be caused by bacteria that live on your sweat, by the foods you eat, even by your emotions. Start by washing your armpits—and a wide area around them—with antibacterial soap twice a day. If BO returns during the day, clean up again with alcohol wipes—portable, individually wrapped alcohol-drenched pads.

After you wash up, apply a clinical strength antiperspirant/deodorant; these contain higher concentrations of sweat-inhibiting aluminum compounds, plus ingredients that make your skin more acidic, discouraging bacteria. Also apply it after bathing at night to keep the pores of your sweat glands closed. Keeping underarms shaved also helps discourage bacteria.

Wear loose, natural-fiber shirts that allow sweat to dry; a moist environment encourages bacteria to grow. Check your diet, too. Garlic, onions, chili peppers, black pepper, vinegar, blue cheese, cabbage, radishes, and marinated fish can all make BO stronger. In one study from Czechoslovakia, so did red meat.

If BO persists, talk to your doctor. She can rule out medical causes such as hyperhidrosis (excessive sweating) as well as an abscess under your arm. While you're there, ask about a prescription antibiotic cream containing clindamycin (such as Cleocin) or erythromycin (such as E-Mycin, Erythrocin, or Ilosone) to fight underarm bacteria.

If your problem is excess sweating, another option is a drug containing oxybutynin (Ditropan) or glycopyrrolate (Robinul). These drugs are normally used for other purposes but have the side effect of drying up sweat. Unfortunately, they dry up all sorts of other secretions, too, and can have side effects including dry mouth and vaginal dryness. Another solution is botox. Injections of this toxin stop nerve impulses that trigger overproduction of sweat. In one study, botox reduced sweat production by up to 70 percent. You may need repeat injections to keep your shirts dry, however.

☐ BOILS

I had a painful, embarrassing boil. How can I prevent another one?

A boil is a hair follicle that's become infected with the highly contagious *Staphylococcus aureus* bacteria. These "staph" bugs live on the surface of human skin and even in our respiratory systems. Normally, the immune system keeps them in check. You can't wipe them out, but there's plenty you can do to prevent their spread.

● *Wash your hands regularly* and thoroughly with soap and water, and use an alcohol-based hand sanitizer gel when you can't get to a sink.

● *Bathe or shower daily* and after using a hot tub, a swimming pool, a sauna, or a steam room. Use a mild antibacterial soap and clean towels and washcloths.

● *Don't use oils, oily moisturizers, or greasy sunscreen—they can trap bacteria.* Opt for oil-free lotions and sunscreens instead.

● *If boils return in an area that you shave, use a clean razor blade every time you shave.* That means replacing the blade or soaking it in alcohol before reuse. Or opt for a hair-removal cream instead.

● *Rinse scrapes and cuts,* apply an antibiotic ointment, and keep them covered with clean bandages until healed.

● *Don't share razors, towels, clothes, or athletic equipment* (at the gym, use germ-killing cleaner on equipment seats and handles).

● *Avoid using powder in those areas that seem to build up sweat.* The powder holds onto moisture, which breeds bacteria.

☐ BOWEL MOVEMENTS

What's a normal frequency for bowel movements?

Whatever feels comfortable for you. Anywhere from three bowel movements a day to one every 3 days is generally considered normal, but the real test isn't frequency, it's how easily you pass that stool. A normal bowel movement is soft—not hard and lumpy or watery—and most of the time can be passed without straining, and without laxatives.

Of course, some variation is also normal. Stress, travel, hormone shifts during a woman's menstrual cycle or pregnancy, aging, a bout of heavy exercise, certain medications, and diet changes can all throw things off temporarily. But if the frequency of your bowel movements starts to change for no obvious reason or any constipation you might have doesn't respond to easy fixes such as consuming more fiber and drinking more water, see your doctor.

I can't hold a bowel movement long enough to get to the bathroom anymore. What can I do?

Don't panic. Fecal incontinence is usually caused by constipation or diarrhea. If you have constipation, big, hard stools may be blocking the exit, allowing watery stuff to seep out around the sides. Constipation also stretches and weakens the ring of muscles (the anal sphincter) that normally holds a bowel movement in.

The fix includes eating more high-fiber foods (such as beans, whole grains, and vegetables) and drinking more water. Fiber can also help watery stools hold together, so they're easier to control. And drinking plenty of water keeps all the fiber moving through your system. Skip coffee, tea, and chocolate, all of which can relax the anal sphincter, and eat smaller meals.

Setting up a regular bathroom schedule can also help. Make it a habit to spend a little time on the toilet about a half-hour after meals, when the gastrocolic reflex—the wave of muscle activity along the intestines that leads to a bowel movement—usually occurs. If nothing happens, try again after your next meal.

Steer clear of diarrhea-provoking trigger foods like sugar-free treats containing the sugar alcohols sorbitol, xylitol, mannitol, and fructose; sausages and other cured meats; fatty and greasy foods; alcoholic beverages; dairy products; and even peaches, pears, and apples.

If these changes don't help, talk with your doctor. He may suggest biofeedback to help you strengthen the rectal muscles, as well as antidiarrheal medication. If you have diabetes, high blood sugar can

damage nerves that govern your digestive system; getting blood sugar under control is critical. Finally, sometimes this problem can stem from anxiety and stress. If that is the case, biofeedback, psychotherapy, and even short-term antianxiety drugs from your doctor can help.

☐ **DANDRUFF**

When I wear a dark shirt, there's a snowstorm on my shoulders. What will get rid of serious dandruff?

Start with a new shampoo, something mild; overenthusiastic washing simply may have dried out your scalp. If dandruff persists, use trial and error to find the right flake-fighter. Dandruff may be the result of anything from a desert-dry scalp to a skin condition called seborrheic dermatitis to eczema, psoriasis, or, very commonly, an overgrowth of a yeastlike fungus called malassezia. Different dandruff shampoo ingredients do different things. Zinc pyrithione targets fungus and bacteria; ketoconazole also fights fungus; coal tar and selenium sulfide slow the growth and die-off of skin cells on your scalp; salicylic acid loosens flakes so they can be washed away. If one doesn't work, buy

two or three different types and alternate between them.

Still flaky? If nothing's helped after a few weeks of shampooing with various formulas or if your scalp is irritated, see your doctor. She may prescribe a prescription-strength dandruff shampoo or another treatment if a skin condition like seborrheic dermatitis, eczema, or psoriasis is the real cause.

☐ **ERECTION PROBLEMS**

I have difficulty becoming erect and staying that way. Is it time for Viagra?

Not just yet. Actually, the most common causes of erectile dysfunction (ED) are psychological issues, such as too much stress in your life, performance anxiety, guilt, or depression. A few sessions with a therapist may help. Another common culprit is that good old spare tire: Four out of five men with ED are overweight, and high blood pressure and high cholesterol associated with extra pounds can interfere with erections. Losing weight and becoming more physically active cured ED for one in three men in an Italian study. Get a med check, too; certain drugs used to treat high blood pressure, depression, allergies, ulcers, and anxiety can all interfere with your sex life. Your doctor may be able to prescribe an alternative.

☐ FOOT ODOR

My feet stink so much that I'm afraid to take my shoes off in public. What will stop the odor?

Beating "toxic sock syndrome" involves keeping your feet as well as your shoes and socks clean, dry, and bacteria-free. Controlling moisture is crucial; your feet have more sweat glands than any other body part, with the exception of the palms of your hands. Trapped in footwear for hours on end, sweat builds; bacteria feed on a protein in sweat and emit stinky isovaleric acid.

For drier feet, change your socks at least once a day, wear shoes made from natural, breathable materials such as leather or canvas, and let shoes air out for at least a day before you wear them again. Knock out bacteria by washing your feet every day (some foot doctors recommend using an antibacterial soap). If foot odor persists, try soaking your feet in a solution of 1 part vinegar to 2 parts water once a day for a week; the acidity helps kill bacteria. Foot odor can also be caused by a bacterial infection

set off by an advanced case of athlete's foot. If you've noticed peeling skin between your toes or on the soles of your feet, see your doctor if an athlete's foot cream or spray doesn't solve the problem.

☐ GAS

I'm frequently gassy. What can I do?

Nobody's gas-free. From prim-and-proper Aunt Martha to your gassy teenage nephew, everybody releases intestinal gas 13 to 21 times a day. Reduce your personal emissions by cutting back on beans, broccoli, Brussels sprouts, cabbage, and

asparagus, all of which contain an indigestible sugar called raffinose that's broken down by bacteria in your digestive tract. The by-product: stinky hydrogen sulfide. Taking a remedy like Beano before you eat may help; it contains an enzyme that breaks down raffinose. You can also reduce the raffinose in beans by thoroughly rinsing dried beans after soaking and by rinsing canned beans just before eating.

Have heartburn? Stay away from sodium bicarbonate (the stuff in baking soda), found in some products such as Alka-Seltzer. It produces carbon dioxide, a gas that's gotta go somewhere!

If gas won't quit, talk with your doctor. Medical conditions such as lactose intolerance (the inability to digest sugars in milk), gluten intolerance (the inability to digest the gluten protein in wheat and other grains), and irritable bowel syndrome may be behind it.

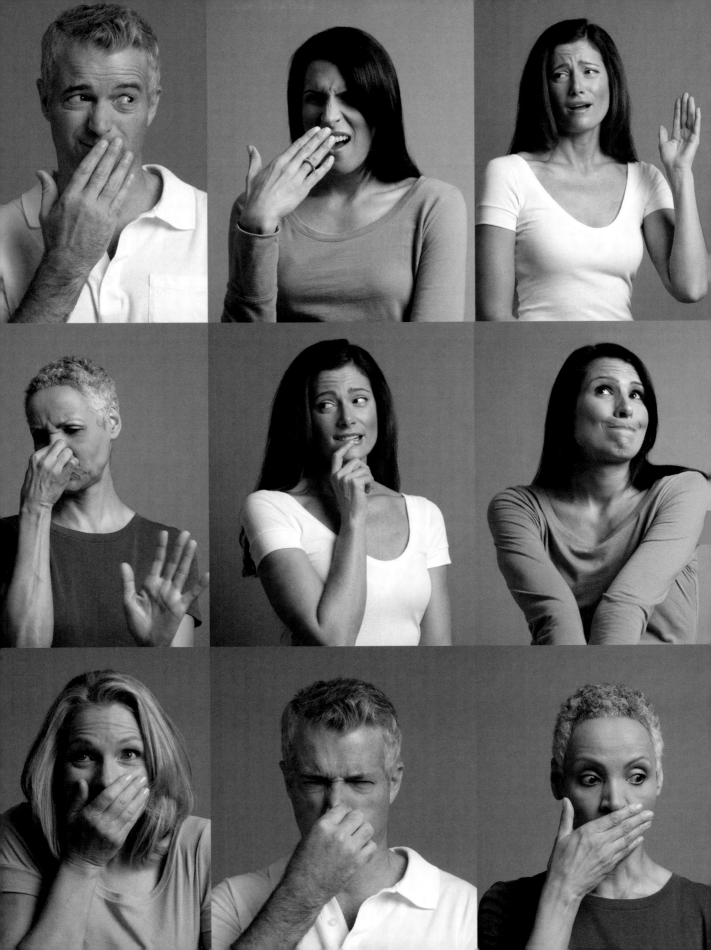

☐ GENITAL DISCHARGE

Does a weird genital discharge mean I have an STD?

Any unusual discharge merits a trip to the doctor's office, pronto! For women, a milky, mild-smelling discharge is normal. A thick, whitish discharge could be a sign of a yeast infection; a thin, dark discharge accompanied by a fishy odor could be a sign of a bacterial infection; and a yellow, gray, or green discharge could be a sign of infection with the parasite *Trichomonas vaginalis* or of gonorrhea, a sexually transmitted disease. For men, a discharge from the penis, other than ejaculate and urine, isn't normal. A greenish or yellowish discharge could mean you have a bacterial infection of the urethra, the fragile tube through which urine exits the bladder.

☐ GENITAL ITCHING

My private parts won't stop itching. What's going on?

If you're a woman, it's most likely a yeast infection. If you're a man, it's most likely jock itch. In either case, you can find relief with an over-the-counter antifungal product—if you're sure that's what you have. Other possibilities include genital herpes (which many men and women have but don't know it), pubic lice, a skin

disorder requiring a doctor's care such as Lichen sclerosus (affecting the vulva), or an irritation caused by harsh soaps, vaginal douches, or sweat. It's best to see your doctor for a diagnosis. Meanwhile, here are some clues.

● *If it's a vaginal yeast infection:* You may also have a burning sensation, a red, swollen vulva, and whitish, lumpy discharge. Over-the-counter antifungal creams and suppositories that contain yeast-fighters such as miconazole (Monistat), clotrimazole (Gyne-Lotrimin), and tioconazole (Vagistat) work. So do prescription antifungal pills such as fluconazole (Diflucan). If these infections come back over and over again despite treatment, be sure to tell your doctor. Sometimes they're a sign of type 2 diabetes.

● *If it's jock itch:* You may also have a patchy red rash. Changing out of sweaty underwear immediately after a workout and wearing boxers instead of sweat-trapping briefs are your best defense. Using an antifungal powder such as Cruex, Desenex, or Zeasorb in skin

folds at your groin can help discourage itchy fungal growths and keep you dry. If you're already itchy, apply an over-the-counter antifungal treatment such as terbinafine (Lamisil), naftifine (Naftin), miconazole (Micatin, Monistat-Derm), and clotrimazole (Lotrimin AF). If it doesn't help, you may need a prescription-strength product. Once you've had jock itch, you may want to continue using an over-the-counter product every day to prevent a recurrence.

If it's lice: You'll also be able to see crablike critters and tiny white or yellow eggs in your public hair. Get rid of them with an over-the-counter louse-killing shampoo or mousse containing permethrin and piperonyl butoxide.

☐ INCONTINENCE

How do I avoid "leaks" when I laugh, sneeze, or pick up a grocery bag?

Lose weight, quit smoking, and exercise your pelvic floor

AVOID THIS MISTAKE

Dusting Yourself with Cornstarch to Stay Dry

Guys, some docs do recommend this, but skin experts warn that some yeast strains thrive on the stuff and can cause infections similar to jock itch. Stay dry with an antifungal powder instead.

muscles every day. Carrying extra pounds and smoking both increase the risk for embarrassing stress incontinence. Age, hormonal changes, and pregnancy also contribute by weakening pelvic muscles and reducing the ability of the urethra (the fragile tube that lets urine exit from your bladder) to close tightly.

Strengthening your pelvic floor muscles helps support the urethra and can reduce leaks by up to 60 percent. The trick? Working the right muscles. For women, it's those that stop a stream of urine. For men, it's the muscles you use to stop the passage of urine. The exercise: Contract your pelvic floor muscles for 3 seconds, then relax them for 3 seconds. Do ten repetitions, three times a day. Build up to 10 seconds for each contraction and each relaxation. Men should feel their penises pull in slightly toward their bodies.

It's also smart to go to the bathroom more often. If you empty your bladder regularly, it will less often fill up to a point of overflowing.

If leaks continue, women can wear a disposable "incontinence tampon" available by prescription. Inserted in the vagina to press against the urethra, they can be helpful during physical activities such as tennis. A pessary is another possibility. This is a stiff ring placed in the vagina that presses on the urethra,

repositioning it to reduce leaks. Wearing a pessary can increase your risk for vaginal and urinary tract infections, so be sure to talk with your doctor about symptoms to watch out for.

If low-tech strategies don't keep you dry, surgery may. For women, several procedures are available using surgical threads, transvaginal positioning tape, or even sections of your own tissue to hold the bladder and urethra in position. A simpler procedure injects bulking agents into the urethra and neck of the bladder, to make them close more tightly. Medications called anticholinergics may also help by preventing bladder spasms.

For men, an enlarged prostate may cause "urge incontinence," leakage after a sudden, strong need to urinate. Your doctor can diagnose this condition and discuss options with you such as medications for prostate enlargement and surgery.

☐ MEMORY PROBLEMS

I keep forgetting names, words, appointments, and even where I've left the car. How do I know if it's Alzheimer's?

Everybody forgets things once in awhile, and aging, stress, multitasking, and even some common medications can make

memory lapses a little worse. It's normal to occasionally forget names, appointments, or where you put those pesky car keys, and then remember the information later on. But one potential early warning sign for Alzheimer's disease is forgetting important dates and names as well as new facts you've just learned (such as how to work the new TV), and then asking for the information over and over again. While it's normal to lose your car keys, it's not normal to forget how to use them. Forgetting why you've opened the refrigerator on a busy morning is normal, but forgetting how to find the kitchen in your home isn't. Forgetting a name on the tip of your tongue is not a problem, but failing to recognize a close friend is. Other red flags include trouble doing familiar things like balancing a checkbook or following a recipe, losing track of what day it is, difficulty following a conversation, mood changes, and poor judgment. All are signs that its time to see a doctor for an evaluation.

☐ NOSE AND EAR HAIR

My ears and nose are sprouting hair like weeds. Do I get out the garden tools?

Leave the lawn trimmer in the garage. And forget about plucking; it hurts like heck and can lead to infection. The best way to trim an unfortunate outcropping is with a nose and ear hair trimmer. These devices protect your skin from the cutting blades and are cleanable (a must!); some even have tiny headlights or can suck shorn locks out of your nose, so you don't inhale them.

☐ RECTAL GROWTH

There's a growth on my rectum; is it a hemorrhoid or anal cancer?

The odds are overwhelmingly in favor of the hemorrhoid. But since symptoms of the two are so similar, it's worth asking your doctor to take a look if the "growth" persists. Itchy, painful, hemorrhoids usually clear up in a week or two; anal cancer is rare (your lifetime risk is 1 in 624, according to the National Cancer Institute). Caught early, survival rates are high; they plummet to 20 percent if the cancer is advanced. Smoking, multiple sex partners, and anal sex all raise your risk. Doctors check for signs of anal cancer during a woman's annual pelvic exam or a man's digital rectal exam. But if you experience bleeding, itching, a lump that doesn't go away, anal discharge, or an unexplained change in bowel habits (such as narrowed stools), ask for a check-up.

☐ SEX

I'm never "in the mood" anymore. How can I increase my desire?

Skip the libido-boosting supplements and aphrodisiac foods (though feeding strawberries and chocolate to your sweetheart *is* sexy). If you're a woman approaching menopause, know that hormone shifts during this period can torpedo desire and also dry up the vagina. While you can't do much about the hormone shifts but ride them out, you can make sex more comfortable—and therefore desirable—by using an over-the-counter vaginal lubricant. Otherwise, look for other common culprits.

● *Medications:* Talk to your doctor about a drug switch if you take a selective serotonin reuptake inhibitor (SSRI) for depression, a blood pressure–lowering drug, an oral contraceptive, estrogen, an opioid pain reliever such as codeine, or an antianxiety medication such as Valium.

● *Stress:* Find ways to de-stress. Half of the people in one British survey said work, financial worries, and fatigue had flatlined their sex lives. Iron out issues with your partner outside the bedroom, too. In one study, women who said their relationships with their spouses or partners was good were 50 times more likely to be happy with their sex lives.

● *Boredom:* It may take some effort to keep your excitement about sex new in an old relationship. Dare to have more fun during foreplay. Slow it down by sharing an erotic fantasy with your partner, playing with a sex toy or vibrator, or grabbing some massage oil and rubbing each other down. In addition, take breaks from your normal routine. Even a change of venue can help.

My spouse wants to have sex every day. Is that abnormal?

Daily sex is perfectly normal; in one recent survey of married couples, 7 percent rang each other's chimes four or more times a week. Another study showed that the average couple has sex once a week.

Of course, quality counts. A couple is having the "right" amount of sex if both partners are happy with how often they make love and how much both of you enjoy it. If your partner wants sex more often than you do, open the lines of communication. Finding the right balance may require some give and take from both of you, and getting the issue on the table is the best first step.

I find sex painful. Can this problem be solved?

Painful sex can be the result of anything from not enough foreplay to infection, injury, muscle spasms, and fibroid tumors. The most common cause is a lack of vaginal lubrication. Sometimes, the fix is as simple as taking things slowly until you're sufficiently aroused. Personal lubricants such as Astroglide and K-Y Jelly provide instant relief. Personal moisturizers (Replens, Lubrin) can keep your vagina moist for up to 3 days.

If you've reached or are nearing menopause, hormone replacement therapy (HRT) can help, too. But your best bet for better lubrication is vaginal estrogen, not hormone pills. A vaginal estrogen cream (such as Estrace or Premarin), vaginal estrogen ring (Estring), or tablet you insert into your vagina (Vagifem) can prompt vaginal tissues to secrete more lubrication. These topical estrogen treatments won't reduce testosterone levels the way oral hormone therapy can; that's important because libido depends on testosterone. HRT comes with health risks such as an increased risk of heart attack and breast cancer, and using vaginal estrogen instead reduces these risks because less of it enters the bloodstream.

Changing positions can also ease discomfort. If you're on top, you'll have more control of the pace and depth of penetration. If sex irritates your vagina or vulva, you may just need a different type of condom or spermicide. But sharp pain in your vulva or muscle spasms

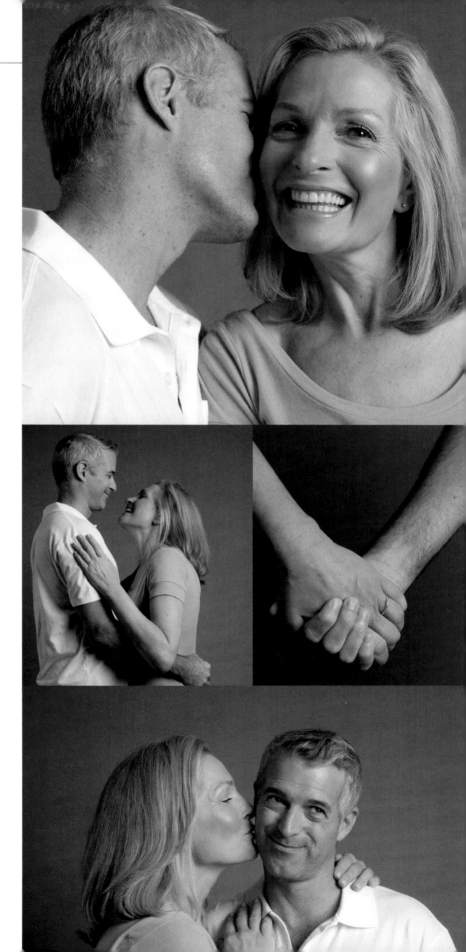

WHAT YOU DON'T KNOW

Postpartum Vaginal Dryness Is Common

New mothers sometimes experience vaginal dryness due to a drop in estrogen after they give birth. Lubrication usually returns as hormonal levels normalize.

of the vagina that make penetration nearly impossible can be caused by infections, scars from surgery, or childbirth. And fibroid tumors, endometriosis, and pelvic inflammatory disease can also make sex painful. Talk with your gynecologist.

Will a "sexual enhancement" cream help me have orgasms more easily?

With come-hither names like Dream Cream, O'My pleasure gel, and Excite, these drugstore creams for women promise more arousal, more pleasure, and, oh yes, easier orgasms. Applied to the clitoris before sex, many contain the amino acid l-arginine. In the body, it's converted to nitric oxide, which dilates blood vessels—and according to manufacturers, boosts sensitivity and lubrication. Some creams also contain menthol or peppermint, which warms the skin but could also lead to irritation.

Do they work? In one manufacturer-funded study of 20 women ages 33 to 62, half reported that a cream containing l-arginine improved lubrication, orgasm, and overall sexual experience.

A larger study is underway. But without solid and unbiased research, the most anyone can promise is that if you believe these creams help, they're okay to use.

Should I worry about sexually transmitted diseases? I'm not promiscuous.

Newly single, more and more people over age 50 are dating, making new connections—and contracting sexually transmitted diseases (STDs). The most common of these are herpes and the human papilloma virus (HPV), which can cause cervical and anal cancer and genital warts. But people over age 50 also account for one in ten new cases of HIV/AIDS. The STD danger is especially high if you're entering new sexual relationships but never had to worry about practicing safe sex before. You may not know what to do; one survey of single women ages 58 to 93 found that 60 percent hadn't used a condom during their most recent sexual encounter.

Make sure you know the safe-sex rules. Find out your partner's sexual health history before having oral, anal, or vaginal sex. Get tested for AIDS and other STDs, and ask your partner to do the same before you're intimate. And use a condom every time you have sex, even if you're in a monogamous relationship.

Is there any need for condoms with anal sex between a man and a woman?

Anal sex probably won't lead to pregnancy (though sperm released anywhere near the vagina could find its way to a waiting egg). But there are still good reasons for wearing a condom. They're effective at preventing the spread of STDs, including HIV (the virus that causes AIDS), HPV (human papilloma virus), and other viral and bacterial infections. HPV, the most common and "silent" of all STDs, is spread by genital and anal sex; 50 percent of sexually active people will have an infection at some point in their lives. This is the same virus responsible for genital warts and cervical cancer. Infections are usually short-lived and symptom-free, but some types seem to raise the risk for anal cancer.

Can you break your penis?

There are no bones in the penis. Nevertheless, you can indeed fracture this organ.

Acrobatic sex, or even a mis-timed thrust that meets firm tissue instead of a moist vagina, can rupture a membrane inside the penis called the tunica albuginea. You may hear a loud pop and feel a sharp pain as this tissue breaks, allowing blood contained in the penis' spongy core to leak out into surrounding tissue. Hurry to your doctor's office or emergency room; often, a penile fracture requires surgery to heal properly. You can usually resume sexual activity in about a month, depending on the severity of the injury.

☐ THINNING HAIR

I'm a woman with thinning hair. Are there any medical ways to regrow it?

Try minoxidil (Rogaine). This over-the-counter hair restorer works by slowing down hair loss and encouraging the growth of new hair. In studies, 50 percent of the women who tried it for hair loss saw at least a little hair regrowth and 13 percent reported moderate regrowth. Developed originally for men, a 2 percent minoxidil solution is FDA approved for women, too. The 5 percent strength is not; it's more likely to cause side effects like itching, irritation, and hair growth in unexpected places such as the face. Some dermatologists

AVOID THIS MISTAKE

Using an Over-the-Counter Nail Fungus Product

These don't penetrate the nail and therefore won't work, even if they list nail fungus among their uses.

use the stronger formula but suggest doing so only under a doctor's care.

Women should steer clear of another male hair restorer, finasteride (Proscar). It is not FDA approved for women and can cause birth defects if used during pregnancy.

Sometimes thinning hair is a sign of an underlying medical condition, like thyroid problems. It's a worth a mention to your doctor.

☐ TOENAIL FUNGUS

What's the best way to clean up crusty, yellowed toenails?

Prescription antifungal pills. They clear up 50 to 75 percent of nail infections, which are usually caused by dermatophytes, the same fungus responsible for athlete's foot. The best of the bunch contain the fungus-zapping active ingredient terbinafine (Lamisil), which studies show is more effective than two other types, itraconazole (Sporanox) and fluconazole (Diflucan). But these oral medicines can cause liver damage, raise risk for heart problems, and may interact with other drugs. If you'd

rather not risk complications and interactions, ask your doctor about a prescription antifungal toenail "polish" containing ciclopirox (Penlac). This clear lacquer cleaned up crusty, fungus-ridden nails for 36 percent of the people who tried it in one 48-week study.

Your treatment may work better if you also see your doctor several times during the 12-week treatment to have infected areas of your nails debrided, or cut away.

☐ WARTS

I have a wart on my finger. Is it contagious?

Yes, but not very. All warts are infections caused by 1 of over 100 varieties of the human papilloma virus (HPV). In contrast to the highly contagious HPV types that cause genital warts, the types behind common warts of the hands and fingers are much less so. Still, direct contact could spread the virus to another person or to another part of your body. To treat one, try an over-the-counter remedy containing 17 percent salicylic acid. In one review of 13 wart-removal studies, salicylic acid cured 75 percent of warts.

Common Symptoms and What They Mean

☐ ABDOMINAL PAIN

I have bad indigestion and a pain along my arm. Should I take Tylenol or Tums?

You should call 911 and then chew an aspirin. You could be having a heart attack.

Why do I have a burning pain in my stomach even when I haven't eaten in hours?

You could have a peptic ulcer. Symptoms include burning or gnawing pain, cramps, nausea, and vomiting. The pain may get worse or better with eating depending on where the ulcer is located. If you have an ulcer, your doctor can prescribe medicines to treat it. You'll also want to stop smoking, avoid alcohol and any foods that trigger symptoms, and steer clear of nonsteroidal anti-inflammatory drugs such as ibuprofen (Advil, Motrin), which can irritate the stomach lining.

Another possibility is gastritis, or inflammation of the stomach lining. This can be brought on by regular use of anti-inflammatory drugs such as aspirin, ibuprofen, or naproxen (Naprosyn); by infection with the bacteria *Helicobacter pylori*, which causes ulcers; by overuse of alcohol; and sometimes, by surgery. Your doctor will diagnose it by ruling out more serious conditions like an ulcer. The solution may include eating smaller, more frequent meals and, if necessary, using a proton pump inhibitor such as esomeprazole (Nexium), lansoprazole (Prevacid), or omeprazole (Prilosec) to reduce acid production in your stomach.

I have a sharp pain in my abdomen. Could it be appendicitis?

Where exactly does it hurt? Appendicitis typically involves a dull pain that begins around the belly button but becomes sharper as it moves to the lower right. It is often accompanied by fever, nausea, and vomiting. If these are your

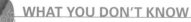

WHAT YOU DON'T KNOW

Bariatric Surgery Can Cause Gallstones

Very rapid weight loss, like the kind that occurs after bariatric surgery to shrink the stomach, leads to gallstones in up to 60 percent of people. If you are contemplating such surgery, ask your doctor about possibly starting you on ursodiol (Actigall), a medication used to help dissolve gallstones.

symptoms, call your doctor immediately as appendicitis is a life-threatening condition. If the pain is severe, get to the ER. Fever and stomach pain can also be signs of other gastrointestinal conditions, including diverticulitis, in which pouches in the intestine become inflamed. This pain is usually felt in the lower *left* side of the abdomen. Diverticulitis requires prompt treatment but is not usually a medical emergency. Call your doctor.

I love fried food. But a half-hour after eating, I sometimes get intense stomach pain. Do I have to give up fried food forever?

Actually, you may need surgery for gallstones. These are hardened deposits of bile, a liquid your body makes to help you digest fat. Many people have gallstones and never know it; they don't need treatment. But if a stone gets stuck in the passageway to the liver, gallbladder, or bile duct, it can cause a gallstone attack. Symptoms include pain in the right upper abdomen that intensifies quickly, pain between the shoulder blades, and pain under the right shoulder (which some people mistake for a heart attack symptom). Depending on your age and medical condition, your doctor may recommend surgery to remove the gallbladder or medication to dissolve the stones.

Help! I can't eat ice cream anymore without developing terrible gas and belching. Is there any cure?

Sounds like you may be lactose intolerant. That means your body lacks the enzyme required to digest lactose, a sugar found in most dairy. Ice cream could still be a part of your life, however. Try an over-the-counter supplement like Lactaid when you eat dairy. Such supplements provide the missing enzyme (lactase) required to digest lactose. You can also find lactose-free dairy products (including ice cream) in many supermarkets.

☐ APPETITE LOSS

I've noticed that I'm much less hungry than I used to be. Should I worry?

While many of us may wish we suddenly lost our urge to eat, appetite loss could be a symptom of numerous conditions, including cancer, infection, liver or kidney disease, low thyroid, and even some medications. Another common cause is depression, especially in older people. Make an appointment with your doctor, and be ready to accurately describe how much you eat in a day; you may want to keep a food diary for several days in advance.

DRUG-FREE FIX

Yogurt

Eating yogurt with live, active cultures may improve your ability to digest lactose and reduce symptoms of lactose intolerance.

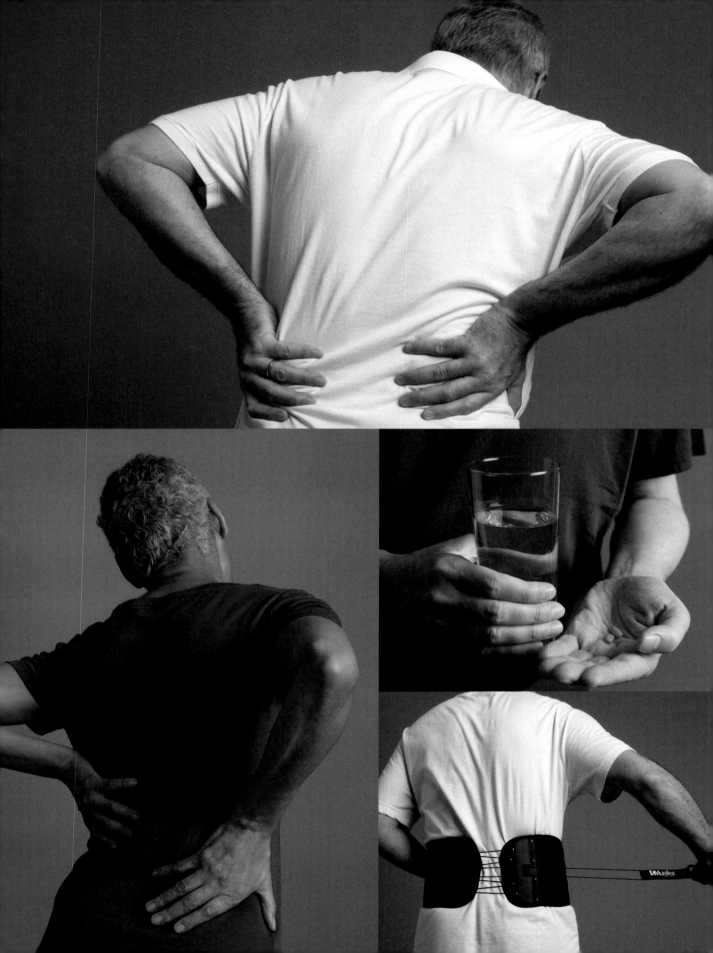

☐ **BACK PAIN**

How do I know if I have a herniated disk?

A physical exam from your doctor followed by an MRI, if needed, will tell you whether you've herniated a disk, the spongy cushion that sits between the vertebrae of your spine. When a disk herniates, it ruptures, allowing part of the disk to slip out and potentially press on nerves in the spinal cord. Symptoms vary depending on where the herniation occurs, but may include back pain, often radiating down to your pelvis, buttocks, and upper thigh. You may also have some numbness or weakness in those areas. Even if your disk is herniated, rest, physical therapy, and exercises to strengthen the back and abdominal muscles can help you avoid more intensive approaches like surgery. Your doctor may prescribe an anti-inflammatory drug, an oral steroid to reduce swelling, or a muscle relaxant to calm spasms of the back muscles.

☐ **BOWEL MOVEMENTS**

When I went to the bathroom this morning, my stool was bright red! Do I have cancer?

If you ate a lot of beets last night, relax. A compound in beets can stain some people's stool bright red. If you didn't, the bleeding is probably a sign of hemorrhoids, or swollen veins around the anus, often caused by straining during bowel movements (and by pregnancy), or tiny tears along the lining of the anus, known as anal fissures. If hemorrhoids get irritated during a bowel movement, they can bleed. It's a good idea to mention the problem to your doctor, though; other causes of visible blood in the stool include diverticulosis (pouches along the wall of the intestine) and infection. By the way, colon cancer more often causes blood in the stool that you can't see.

Why does it hurt when I have a bowel movement?

Most likely you have hemorrhoids. Try a stool softener such as docusate (Colace, Fleet) to reduce straining and sitz baths for the pain. To take a sitz bath, sit in warm water that covers your buttocks. You can buy a plastic tub made for this purpose—it fits over your toilet—at the drugstore. If the pain continues, an over-the-counter hemorrhoid ointment may help reduce the itching and swelling. If your hemorrhoids are caused by frequent constipation, up the amount of fruit and vegetables you eat and drink more water. If the pain continues after trying these approaches for a few days, see your doctor. More serious causes of anal pain during bowel movements include an anal fissure, inflammation of the rectal lining, an abscess (pus-filled cavity), or fecal impaction, in which dry, hard stool is "stuck" in the rectum.

Lately I am terribly constipated. Could it be from one of my medications?

Yes. Many medications can cause constipation, including opioids like morphine and oxycodone (OxyContin), antihistamines, antipsychotics, iron, and calcium channel blockers such as amlodipine (Norvasc) and diltiazem (Cardizem). That's why it is important that you take both a stool softener and a laxative such as senna while taking opioids. Studies find that typical lifestyle approaches to constipation—drinking water, exercising, increasing the amount of fiber, fruits, and vegetables in your diet—are not very effective with opioid-induced constipation.

The senna may make your urine red—nothing to worry about. But you shouldn't take senna for a long time; it can cause serious changes to the lining of the colon, diarrhea, and bone weakness, and can leave your bowels unable to work normally. Make sure your doctor tracks your use.

☐ **BREAST LUMPS**

I felt something. Is there any reason *not* to panic?

Yes. You could have fibrocystic breasts, literally "lumpy" breasts that usually are also painful and tender. Doctors don't know what causes them, although they are likely related to hormones since they tend to wax and wane with a woman's menstrual cycle. The lump could also be a fluid-filled cyst. If you press on a cyst, it feels kind of like a water balloon. It might also move around or change size throughout your menstrual cycle. Both fibrocystic breasts and fluid-filled cysts are benign. However, you should see your doctor as soon as possible for a clinical breast exam and mammogram.

☐ **BREATHING DIFFICULTY**

The other day when I went to lunch with my girlfriends, I suddenly felt like I couldn't breathe. They had to take me to the restroom and lay me on the floor. Was I having a heart attack?

It sounds like you may have had a panic attack, which can be mistaken for a heart attack.

A panic attack is a case of extreme anxiety in which the body is flooded with stress hormones that increase your heart and breathing rates. They may occur for no known reason or if you suddenly feel anxious or claustrophobic. Panic attacks are treatable with medication and therapy. You should make an appointment to see your doctor to rule out any heart conditions and get a firm diagnosis.

Why would I have trouble breathing after a bout of laughter or crying?

You may have asthma. Contrary to what many people think, asthma can develop in middle age. And while you may rarely experience any wheezing or shortness of breath, hearty laughter or crying, as well as exercise, can trigger an attack. If this breathlessness is a common occurrence, see your doctor for an evaluation.

☐ **BRUISING**

I bruise very easily; sometimes the bruises are so bad my friends think someone is beating me. What causes easy bruising?

Many people think they bruise easily or have a bleeding disorder when they actually don't.

So what you think is easy bruising may, in fact, be quite normal, particularly as you age and your skin thins, making the bruises more obvious. Easy bruising could, however, be caused by certain medicines including blood thinners such as warfarin (Coumadin). Even taking a daily aspirin or two, which interferes with the ability of blood to clot, can lead to easy bruising.

If you tend to bruise easily, it is important that you get enough vitamin K in your diet. This vitamin, found in cabbage, cauliflower, spinach, and other green leafy vegetables, fortified cereals, and soybeans, is critical for normal blood clotting. Make sure you get at least one food that's high in vitamin K a day.

Other causes of easy bruising include clotting disorders such as hemophilia and von Willebrand syndrome, hormonal changes, and vitamin C deficiency.

☐ **CHEST PAIN**

My chest hurts but it's not bad enough to be a heart attack—or is it?

Any chest pain is cause for concern. If it's a crushing pain that extends to your jaw or arm, call 911 immediately. You may be having a heart attack. Even moderate pain could be a sign of a heart attack, particularly in women or in people with diabetes, who

WHAT YOU DON'T KNOW

Antibiotics Can Trigger Easy Bruising

Antibiotics interfere with your body's absorption of vitamin K, important to blood clotting.

often don't have significant pain during a heart attack. Other symptoms of a heart attack include shortness of breath, fatigue, weakness, nausea and vomiting, extreme sweating, and dizziness. Pain that comes on with exertion, like shoveling snow, but improves when you rest may be angina. Angina results from narrowed coronary arteries and reduced blood flow. While it's not a heart attack, it is a warning sign of heart disease. See your doctor as soon as possible.

☐ COLDS

How do I know if it's a cold or the flu?

Take your temperature and assess how you feel. If you have influenza, you will likely have a temperature (101°F or higher) and terrible headache, feel achy all over, and be incredibly tired. It's rare to have a significant fever with a cold. The primary symptoms of a cold are a stuffy and/or runny nose, cough, and sore throat, which rarely occur with the flu. While you may feel tired if you have a cold, with the flu, you probably won't be able to get out of bed.

☐ COUGH

I can't seem to shake this cough. It's particularly bad after eating and at night. Do I need a chest x-ray?

A common cause of chronic cough is gastroesophageal reflux disease (GERD), which occurs when acidic stomach contents back up into the throat and esophagus. This type of cough is particularly bad in the early morning and at night. One way to find out if GERD is causing your cough is to decrease the acid in your stomach by taking a histamine-2 receptor antagonist such as cimetidine (Tagamet), ranitidine (Zantac), or famotidine (Pepcid), or a proton pump inhibitor such as esomeprazole (Nexium), lansoprazole (Prevacid), or omeprazole

(Prilosec), for 2 weeks. If your cough clears up, then GERD was probably the problem. Other causes of chronic cough include allergy-induced post-nasal drip, asthma, and chronic obstructive pulmonary disease, a lung condition common in smokers. If you feel like you can't breathe when you cough, are coughing up blood, or have lost weight without trying, see your doctor. Taken together, these symptoms could be a sign of something more serious like tuberculosis or cancer.

I just started taking a new blood pressure medication and now I can't stop coughing. Is there any relation?

There could be if your doctor put you on an ACE inhibitor such as enalapril (Vasotec) or lisinopril (Prinivil, Zestril). A common side effect of ACE inhibitors is cough. It is also the main reason people stop taking them. If the cough is related to the ACE inhibitor, ask your doctor about switching to

AVOID THIS MISTAKE

Calling Family and Friends First

If you have chest pain, don't call friends or family until *after* you've called for an ambulance and then chewed an aspirin (aspirin reduces the risk of blood clots and significantly improves the likelihood of surviving a heart attack).

an angiotensin II receptor blocker, or ARB, which studies find are just as effective at reducing blood pressure but carry little risk of cough.

I'm coughing up green stuff. Do I need an antibiotic?

Maybe, but not necessarily. Green mucus often signifies a bacterial infection, most likely bronchitis. An antibiotic may help, although, in most cases, the infection will clear on its own in a week anyway. However, even if you're coughing up green or brown mucus, your infection could be caused by a virus, not bacteria, in which case an antibiotic will be useless.

☐ **CRAMPS**

I get terrible cramps about 10 days before my period. Why?

You may be experiencing a condition called *mittelschmerz*, a German word meaning "middle pain." The pain tends to occur on one side of the pelvic area and is caused by the release of an egg from your ovary. About one in five women experiences this pain, which can be excruciating. Over-the-counter anti-inflammatory drugs like ibuprofen (Advil, Motrin) can help. To get rid of the pain altogether, talk to your doctor about oral contraceptives. Because they prevent ovulation, they eliminate the root cause of the pain.

12 Symptoms You Should Never Ignore

If you experience any of the following symptoms, call 911 or have someone drive you to the nearest emergency room.

IF YOU EXPERIENCE ...	IT COULD BE ....
1 Coughing up or vomiting up blood	Tuberculosis, lung cancer, internal bleeding
2 Pain, swelling, redness, or warmth in your leg, possibly with night cramps and/or bluish or white coloration of skin	A blood clot
3 Sudden, severe headache unlike any you've had before	Stroke, aneurysm
4 Loss of consciousness	Dehydration, stroke, seizure, irregular heartbeat or other heart problem, anemia, low blood sugar, drug overdose
5 A wound that gets hot and red, particularly if you also have a fever	Systemic infection
6 Difficulty breathing or shortness of breath that makes you feel as if you're suffocating	Asthma attack, anaphylactic shock, collapsed lung, pneumonia

Last night I had leg cramps so bad they woke me up. What causes this?

These sudden muscle contractions may seem like a bad dream, but they're quite real. Leg cramps typically occur for no reason. Sometimes, however, they are related to underlying problems such as an electrolyte imbalance (electrolytes include minerals such as sodium and potassium) caused by dehydration, clogged arteries in your legs, or diabetes. Other possible causes include an underactive thyroid or chronic kidney failure.

Try stretching your leg muscles, especially by flexing your foot toward the ceiling, before bed or taking a hot shower or warm bath to relax muscles. Also make sure that you're drinking plenty of water throughout the day. If the leg cramps continue, affecting your ability to function the next day, see your doctor.

☐ DEPRESSION

Lately, I just haven't been feeling myself. I'm always tired and I don't feel like doing much. What's going on?

You could be depressed. Common symptoms of depression include fatigue, lack of interest in normal activities, irritability, anxiety, difficulty concentrating, changes in sleep

7	Sudden increase in the number or size of "floaters" in your vision and/or flashes of light in your peripheral vision	Retinal tear or detachment
8	Chest pain or pressure with or without nausea or clamminess; the pain may radiate to your jaw, upper back, shoulders and/or arms	A heart attack
9	Weakness, numbness, tingling or a feeling of heaviness on one side of your body, or a sudden inability to move one side of your body; may be accompanied by problems seeing, speaking, or understanding words, dizziness, fainting, or confusion, and all symptoms may disappear in a minute or two	A stroke or transient ischemic attack (TIA)
10	Loss of appetite, nausea/vomiting with abdominal pain, abdominal swelling, fever, inability to pass gas	Appendicitis, bowel obstruction
11	Sudden change in mental status, such as not knowing where you are or not recognizing people you should know	Stroke or other neurological problem, head injury, infection, seizure, low blood sugar
12	Sudden, severe dizziness	Stroke, heart attack, reaction to medication

and eating habits, and feeling worthless. Depression can be caused by a traumatic event, such as the death of a loved one, but also by some medications, medical conditions such as hypothyroidism, or simply by an increasing unhappiness with one's life.

If your sadness isn't enough to make you get help, know that depression is linked with numerous medical conditions, including diabetes and heart disease. Whether the depression "causes" the disease or vice versa isn't clear, but experts know that depression can make the physical disease worse. For instance, people with heart disease are more likely to die from it if they are also depressed. The good news is that depression is treatable with medication and/or therapy. Call your doctor and be honest about what's bothering you so you can be treated.

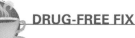

DRUG-FREE FIX

Exercise

In one study that pitted brisk walking or jogging against the antidepressant sertraline (Zoloft) or a combination of the drug plus the exercise, after 4 months, all three groups had about the same improvement in their depression, but at 6 months, the people who kept up the exercise, had the lowest rates of remission.

□ **DIARRHEA**

I constantly seem to have diarrhea and sometimes cramps. What could be causing it?

Numerous conditions can cause chronic diarrhea, including inflammatory bowel diseases like Crohn's disease and ulcerative colitis, irritable bowel syndrome, hyperthyroidism, and certain cancers. Other causes include an inability to digest certain foods, such as wheat or dairy. Your doctor should evaluate you for these and other conditions to get at the root of your problem.

□ **DIZZINESS**

I feel dizzy when I stand up suddenly. Is my blood pressure too low?

Getting dizzy upon standing is common. The phenomenon even has a name: postural hypotension. When you stand up, gravity pulls blood to your legs, and your body may not have enough time to compensate by pumping blood faster or constricting blood vessels to get more blood to your head. It doesn't necessarily mean that you have low blood pressure. In fact, there's actually no such thing as blood pressure that's too low, unless it's causing uncomfortable symptoms, in which case you could probably benefit from drinking more liquids and consuming more salt. Dehydration and certain medications, especially heart drugs known as beta-blockers, can make you more prone to this type of dizziness, as can heart failure, diabetes, and other conditions that affect the nerves. If the problem bothers you, it's worth mentioning to your doctor.

Lately I'm dizzy a lot. What's going on?

Have you recently begun taking a new medication? Numerous prescription and over-the-counter drugs can cause dizziness, including certain antibiotics and antivirals, nonsteroidal anti-inflammatory drugs (even aspirin), narcotic pain relievers, chemotherapy, high blood pressure drugs (diuretics, beta-blockers, ACE inhibitors, angiotensin II receptor antagonists), antidepressants, anxiety-relieving medications such as diazepam (Valium), muscle relaxants, corticosteroids, bisphosphonates (taken to treat osteoporosis), and anti-ulcer drugs like cimetidine (Tagamet). Dizziness related to medication usually goes away after a few days once your body gets used to the medicine. If it doesn't, give your doctor a call.

☐ **DRY MOUTH**

Why is my mouth dry all the time?

The most common cause of dry mouth is medication. Drugs prescribed for asthma and other lung conditions, such as ipratropium (Atrovent) and tiotropium (Spiriva), those used to relieve gastrointestinal symptoms, such as dicyclomine (Bentyl) and hyoscyamine (Levsin), anti-Parkinsonian medications, certain antidepressants, and chemotherapy drugs can all result in dry mouth. Dry mouth is more than annoying; the lack of saliva to clear out bits of food and bacteria can lead to tooth decay and gum disease. Talk to your doctor about possible changes in your medication if the dry mouth persists. Also see your doctor if you also have dry eyes and skin and a rash or joint pain. These could be signs of the autoimmune condition called Sjörgen's syndrome.

☐ **EAR PROBLEMS**

I went swimming and now I have water stuck in my ear. How do I get it out?

The water may be stuck behind a plug of earwax. Try putting several drops of hydrogen peroxide or an over-the-counter earwax softener in your ear,

then tilt your head for several minutes to keep it in while it goes to work. Use an ear bulb syringe (available at the pharmacy) to flush the ear with warm water until the wax comes out, at which point the trapped water should drain. (You may have to repeat this process several times.) For stubborn earwax, see your regular doctor or even an ENT (ear, nose, and throat doctor). Your regular doctor can use suction or use a cotton cloth like a wick to draw the water out of the ear. An ENT has special equipment that can grab stubborn wax blocks and pull them out.

It's also possible that the water just got stuck in the curves of your ear canal. Try using a hair dryer on the cool setting to dry out the water. (Hold it a foot away from your ear to avoid burning yourself.)

I swam a lot this weekend, and now my ears itch and hurt a little. Why?

Sounds like you may have swimmer's ear, also known as external otitis—basically, an infection of the outer ear. Don't try to clear the water yourself by poking your ear with a cotton swab. Instead, make an appointment to see your doctor (and take ibuprofen if the pain is bad). The doctor will remove any trapped water and may prescribe medicated eardrops.

To prevent swimmer's ear next time you hit the pool, mix equal parts rubbing alcohol and vinegar and put several drops in each ear before and after swimming. The solution alters the normal acidity of the ear to prevent the growth of bacteria from pool water.

I hear this weird humming noise in my ear all the time. Why?

It could be tinnitus, in which you hear a ringing, buzzing, swishing, or other noise when there are no external sounds. It's fairly common and may be caused by noise-induced hearing loss or by abnormal nerve firings in the part of the brain responsible for hearing, a phenomenon somewhat similar to the phantom pain that some amputees feel where their limbs used to be. Other causes include ear infection, certain medications, tumors, or Ménière's disease, an inner ear condition that also leads to vertigo and hearing loss. If it doesn't improve in a week or so, see your doctor for an evaluation. There's no cure for tinnitus, but there are various approaches that can help make the noise less bothersome. In some people, stress worsens tinnitus, so find a relaxation technique that works for you.

☐ EYE PROBLEMS

I have a gritty feeling in my eyes. Did I scratch something?

Quite possibly. Do you wear contact lenses? You may have contact lens keratitis, an infection that results from wearing your contacts too long. A corneal abrasion, on the other hand, typically occurs when a foreign body—even a fingernail—scratches the cornea. Of course, a fairly simple cause of gritty eyes is dry eyes, in which your eyes don't make enough oily fluid to keep the cornea lubricated.

One not-so-common cause is a temporary condition called superficial punctate keratitis, in which groups of cells on the surface of the cornea die. Other symptoms of this condition include red, watery eyes that are sensitive to light. Numerous factors can cause it, including infections, dry eyes, wearing your contacts too long, or getting too much sun exposure.

Prescription eye drops, ointments, and over-the-counter artificial tears can all help with these conditions, but see your doctor first for the correct diagnosis.

My eyes are red and itchy. Is it allergies?

It could be, but if your eyes are red and itchy and it's not pollen season, or they remain red and itchy even when you're not around allergens, it could also be conjunctivitis, an inflammation of the white part of the eye. Conjunctivitis—also known as pinkeye—can be caused by allergies, a virus, or bacteria and may cause sensitivity to light. If you have it, you'll likely wake up with crusty eyelids. See you doctor; you may need prescription antibacterial eye drops or ointment. Meanwhile, stop wearing your contacts and apply warm compresses to your closed eyes. Be very careful to wash your hands before touching the other eye and other people.

☐ FAINTING

I've fainted a few times lately. How serious is it?

Fainting is always serious because you could fall and hurt yourself. If you've fainted even once, you should be checked by a doctor. Numerous conditions cause fainting, including low blood sugar, low blood pressure, erratic heartbeat (arrhythmia), or a condition that obstructs blood flow to the brain, such as in a stroke. Medications that lower blood pressure may also make fainting more likely.

☐ FATIGUE

I am tired all the time, even when I think I've gotten a good night's sleep. What's going on?

While a host of medical conditions can lead to fatigue, including anemia, low thyroid production, depression, and even heart disease, sleep problems are the most likely cause. Just because you *think* you got a good night's sleep doesn't mean you did. If you snore, for example, and you find yourself exhausted during the day, you could suffer from chronic obstructive sleep apnea, which repeatedly interrupts your breathing and causes you to momentarily awaken many times throughout the night, though you may not realize it. Your exhaustion could also be related to your

WHAT YOU DON'T KNOW

You Could Have a "Silent" Stroke and Not Even Know It

Called transient ischemic attacks (TIA), symptoms of these mini-strokes can include brief loss of consciousness or fainting, slight numbness in an arm or leg, loss of strength in the legs, and loss of balance. A TIA is a major risk factor for a more serious stroke in the next week or two, so make sure you see a doctor right away.

heart medicine if you take beta-blockers, which are notorious for causing fatigue. Definitely mention your fatigue to your doctor.

☐ FEVER

I have a fever of 103°F. Should I go to the emergency room?

No. A fever of 103°F is not typically something to worry about in an adult; although any fever over 100.4°F in a child younger than 3 months old or over 102.2°F in an older child should trigger a call to the doctor. You should take some ibuprofen (Advil, Motrin) or acetaminophen (Tylenol) if you feel uncomfortable. They will bring your fever down. (Never give aspirin to a child with a fever.) If you also have a headache, stiff neck, rash, low blood pressure, rapid heartbeat, or your temperature is higher than 104°F, call your doctor or, if you can't be seen immediately, go to the emergency room. These suggest a serious condition such as meningitis.

☐ FLUSHING

Why does my face get really red after a glass of wine?

You could have a skin condition called rosacea. Symptoms include flushing like you describe, the appearance of small, broken blood vessels on

your face and, over time, clusters of pimples on your cheeks and nose. Alcohol, spicy foods, and emotional excitement can trigger an attack. Rosacea can be treated with prescription creams you apply to your face.

☐ FOOT PAIN

My heel hurts. Should I see a podiatrist?

Yes. Pain on the bottom of the heel that tends to be worst first thing in the morning is usually plantar fasciitis, the most common cause of heel pain. It results when the thick band of tissue that connects the heel bone to the bottom of the toes (the plantar fascia) becomes inflamed. Runners and people who are overweight are more likely to suffer from this condition. You may need anti-inflammatory drugs and heel-stretching exercises. It could take several months or even longer for the pain to go away. To help prevent plantar fasciitis, wear shoes with good arch support when you're going to be spending a lot of time on your feet.

Another possible cause is a heel spur, a hook of bone protruding from the bottom or back of the heel. These can

occur alone or in conjunction with plantar fasciitis. You may need shoe inserts, ice, and anti-inflammatory drugs. Surgery isn't usually necessary.

☐ HAIR LOSS

My hair is falling out like crazy. I'm not taking any medications. Is this related to age or to some disease?

Ask your doctor to test your thyroid hormone levels. An underactive thyroid (hypothyroidism) or pituitary gland can lead to hair loss. A serious illness, particularly if you had a high fever, can also cause hair loss, so make sure you get a thorough checkup.

☐ HEADACHES

Why do I often get headaches in the late afternoon?

Sounds like you're experiencing tension headaches, which tend to occur near the end of the day. They can result from numerous causes, including stress, your posture (strained neck muscles can cause headaches), and eyestrain. If you haven't had your eyes examined in a year, make an appointment. If you work at a computer, make sure your workstation is set up ergonomically. It should include a keyboard tray that allows you to set the keyboard on an angle and adjust the height so that when you type, your forearms are parallel to the floor with your shoulders relaxed, not hunched. Make sure you can sit with both feet flat on the floor and look straight—not up or down—at your monitor. And take frequent breaks; every 15 minutes is a good idea. These will help you avoid eyestrain, too.

Also ask yourself how often you've been taking aspirin or other pain relievers. Your headaches could be "rebound" headaches that occur after the drugs wear off. Try laying off the drugs for 3 to 4 days to see if that helps. And cut out the caffeine, too: A serious coffee habit can cause headaches.

I have had a headache for 2 days on one side of my face. I'm scared I have a brain tumor.

More likely you're having a very bad migraine. Migraines are headaches that typically occur on one side of the head or face and they can last for up to 3 days. The pain gets worse if you continue your normal activities and with bright light and loud noises. The pain may be throbbing or not, and you may or may not feel nauseated. Over-the-counter pain relievers often don't help, but prescription medications called triptans can be very effective. If it is the worst headache of your life, it could be a brain hemorrhage; get to the emergency room immediately. Otherwise, make an appointment with your doctor to be evaluated for migraine.

☐ **HEARING PROBLEMS**

I have to keep turning the television up loud. Am I losing my hearing?

It's likely, yes. Do you find yourself asking people to repeat themselves a lot? Have trouble differentiating consonants? Feel that words often "run together"? Do you keep trying to increase the volume on your cell phone? If so, then

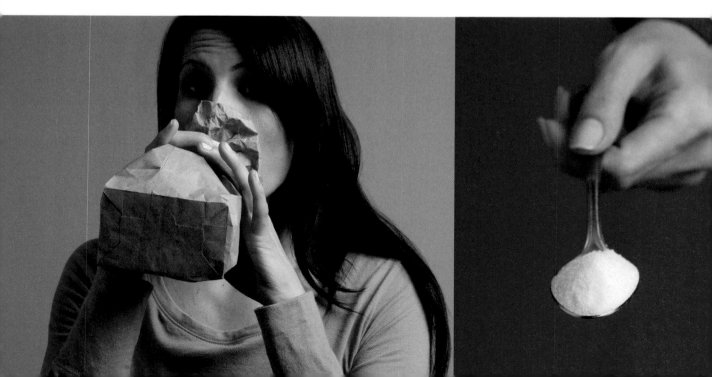

you've probably experienced some hearing loss, either due to plain old age or to years' worth of listening to high-volume music on your stereo or iPod. High blood pressure and diabetes, not to mention smoking, can also dim your hearing. Other, more serious causes of hearing loss include tumors, infections, and autoimmune disorders. Start by asking your doctor to send you for a hearing test.

☐ HICCUPS

I get hiccups a lot, sometimes for hours. Should I see a doctor?

If you can get rid of them on your own, then no. Most likely, you ate too much or too fast or you simply gulped too much air while talking, eating, or drinking. Those beers you slurped down last night could also be to blame. Another culprit is acid reflux, when stomach acid pushes up into your esophagus and throat. Stress and excitement can also bring on hiccups.

The traditional home remedies—pulling on the tongue, swallowing a teaspoon of sugar, gargling with water, sipping ice water, drinking from the "wrong" side of a glass—can all help. So can biting on a lemon or sniffing ammonia. If those approaches don't work, try holding your breath, breathing very fast until you hyperventilate, or breathing into a paper bag to increase the amount of carbon dioxide in your blood. If your hiccups last more than 2 days, however, see your doctor. Persistent hiccups can be caused by a number of underlying health conditions, some of which are serious.

☐ HOARSENESS

Why is my voice so hoarse?

Assuming that you didn't strain it yelling or singing loudly, you may have a virus that's inflamed your larynx (vocal cords). Even a chronic postnasal drip from allergies or a runny nose can lead to a hoarse voice. But if you've been sounding as if you live in a smoke-filled room for more than 2 weeks, something else is going on. Gastrointestinal reflux disorder (GERD), in which the acidic contents of your stomach reflux into your throat, is one possibility. The acidity of the stomach contents can irritate the vocal cords,

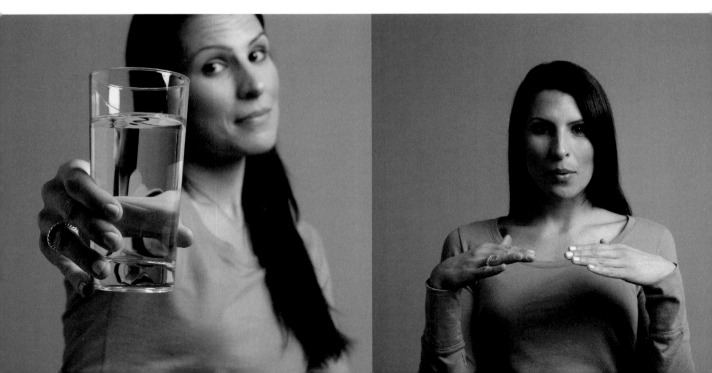

If You Have Laryngitis, You Should Speak in a Whisper

Fiction. Whispering is one of the worst things you can do; it strains your vocal cords more than talking does.

leading to polyps, nodules, or even tiny ulcers. Other clues that GERD may be to blame include a chronic cough plus lots of throat clearing and mucus production. You may also feel like you have a lump in your throat. See your doctor if the hoarseness lasts more than 2 weeks.

☐ ITCHY SKIN

If I scratch a mosquito bite until it bleeds, will it get infected?

Probably not. The major risk of mosquito bites is infection with diseases like West Nile virus, St. Louis encephalitis, and other viruses the blood-sucking insects carry. To reduce your risk of becoming a mosquito feeding ground, stay inside at dusk and dawn when the buzzers are most active, cover your arms and legs, and spray an insect repellent containing DEET on any exposed skin. One application should protect you for up to 5 hours. Oil of citronella or lemon eucalyptus may also provide some minor protection, but not nearly as much as DEET repellants.

I was hiking last weekend and now there is a red spot on my leg with a circle around it. Could it be Lyme disease?

It could, indeed, be a bite from the tick that carries Lyme disease. That rash is characteristic of the first stage of the disease. Sometimes these rashes appear as a solid red circle; sometimes they look like a bull's-eye after the middle begins to fade. Other early symptoms include a low fever, fatigue, neck pain, joint and muscle stiffness and soreness, and swollen lymph nodes. Antibiotics can eradicate the infection, but only if taken early in the disease. Call your doctor right away.

☐ JOINT PAIN

One of my joints sometimes hurts. How do I know if it's arthritis?

Only a doctor can tell you. There are two main types of arthritis: rheumatoid arthritis, the result of an autoimmune disease, and osteoarthritis, the

more common type in which the joint's cartilage wears down over time. If it's the former, you'll notice swelling, redness, and warmth around the joint, particularly around the toe and finger knuckles, as the result of inflammation. It also hurts no matter what you're doing, even while resting. Osteoarthritis typically affects the larger weight-bearing joints, such as hips and knees, as well as the hands. If your joints hurt on both sides (i.e., the right *and* left knees), then you may have rheumatoid arthritis. If it affects the joints randomly, it's more likely osteoarthritis. Also, while you may feel some stiffness with osteoarthritis, it usually improves once you begin moving.

Another possible explanation is gout, a disease in which uric acid crystals accumulate around the joint. Gout usually affects the big toe, ankle, knee, wrist, and elbow, but usually involves only one or two joints at a time, and rarely occurs in the hip, shoulder, or spine. Symptoms develop suddenly and are often excruciating.

☐ LEG PAIN

Why do my legs ache so much when I walk?

Your pain warrants a visit to your doctor. If your legs stop hurting when you stop walking you may have a condition called peripheral arterial disease (PAD). It's a form of atherosclerosis, in which plaque builds up in your arteries (the same process that occurs in heart disease, except in your legs). The achiness you feel is called intermittent claudication and occurs when you walk because your narrowed leg arteries aren't allowing enough blood to reach your legs. You may also experience numbness in your legs or feet when you're resting, and the skin of the affected leg may be cooler and paler. See your doctor, who may prescribe blood thinners to reduce the risk of a potentially fatal blood clot and a cholesterol-lowering drug. Medical attention is a must: PAD increases your risk of heart attack and stroke, and extreme cases can even cause the loss of a limb.

Why do the front of my legs ache after I take a long walk?

What you describe sounds like shin splints, common in runners. They occur when you overstress the muscles on either side of your shin, the long bone in the front of your lower leg. Once shin splints occur, rest, ice, and anti-inflammatory medications such as ibuprofen are the best way to relieve the pain. To prevent shin splints, strengthen your shin muscles by rising up on your

toes, holding for a count of 10, then slowly rolling down. Complete three sets of 10 with 1 minute of rest between each set at least twice a day. And check your walking shoes; they may not be providing enough support, allowing your foot to roll inward. Replace your shoes often, and ask the salesperson at a specialty shop to help you choose a pair that prevents your foot from pronating. Also consider using shock-absorbing insoles.

I have this feeling like someone is sticking pins into my lower left side. Sometimes I get a shooting pain down my leg. Should I have an MRI?

Try this first: Lie flat on your back with both legs extended. Have someone place their hand under your left ankle and lift your left leg. Do you feel any pain? Now try it with the right leg. This test, called the straight-leg raise, helps diagnose a problem involving the sciatic nerve, which runs from the spinal column to the pelvis and down each leg. If you have pain when your leg is lifted, you may have sciatica. It is often caused by a herniated disk pressing on the sciatic nerve. Other symptoms include weakness in the leg or foot. Make an appointment with

your doctor, who will decide whether you need an MRI. Normally, the pain goes away on its own within a month or two, especially with exercise or physical therapy.

☐ MOLES

How can I tell if a mole is cancerous?

You can't tell for sure without a biopsy, so see your doctor if you notice new moles or a mole that's changed in shape, size, or appearance. However, the ABCD test can provide some basic clues.

- *Asymmetry:* Is one side of the mole bigger or different than the other?
- *Borders:* Are the mole's borders uneven or irregular?
- *Color:* Does the color vary?
- *Diameter:* Is the diameter larger than a pencil eraser?

These, along with changes in the mole such as color, itching, or bleeding, are all signs of melanoma, a very serious skin cancer. Start with a full skin examination by your doctor or dermatologist, which should include hidden parts of your body, such as between your fingers, on your scalp, and between your buttocks.

☐ **MOUTH AND GUMS**

I just brushed my teeth and my gums were bleeding. Do I have gum disease?

Possibly. Of course, you could be just brushing too hard. Gums can also bleed if you're taking medications or supplements that thin the blood, such as warfarin (Coumadin), aspirin, or coenzyme Q10. Still, bleeding gums usually means you're not getting rid of all the plaque at the gum line, where the tooth meets the gum. The best way to do this is with regular flossing in addition to brushing.

I often have cracks at the corners of my mouth. What causes them?

If the skin there is often wet from saliva (maybe you have poorly fitting dentures, for instance, or you simply lick your lips too much), it can become cracked, which can open you up to a yeast infection. (Having diabetes increases a person's susceptibility to yeast infections.) Ask your doctor what to do. She may suggest applying an over-the-counter antifungal cream and perhaps some hydrocortisone or may give you a prescription for topical medicine. To keep the cracks away once they're healed, dry the skin and apply petroleum jelly or lip balm to protect the area. Less commonly, the cracks are caused by a nutritional deficiency, such as a lack of certain B vitamins or iron.

☐ **NOSEBLEEDS**

My nose bleeds in the winter. Is this something to worry about?

No. Both indoor and outdoor air is dryer in winter. That dries the mucous membranes in the nose, which can lead to bleeding. Running a humidifier indoors can help, as can smearing petroleum jelly just inside your nostrils. You might also try using a saline nasal spray several times a day to keep your nasal passages moist. And don't forget to open your mouth when you sneeze! If you are taking a blood thinner like warfarin (Coumadin) and you experience nose bleeding that doesn't stop, call your doctor.

☐ **NUMBNESS**

This morning, my feet felt slightly numb. They've also been tingling. Why?

Tingling and numbness in your feet are signs of nerve damage. While numerous conditions can cause this symptom, the most common one is type 2 diabetes. Undiagnosed or poorly controlled diabetes exposes you to unhealthy levels of insulin and blood sugar, which can damage nerves throughout your body, particularly in your feet and hands. Other symptoms of diabetes include excessive thirst and urination, increased hunger, blurred vision, a slow-healing wound, and frequent urinary tract infections. Another possible cause is sciatica, in which the sciatic nerve that goes from your spine to your legs and feet becomes compressed, often by a herniated disk. It's time to call your doctor.

 WHAT YOU DON'T KNOW

There Are Two Types of Nosebleeds

The common type, called an anterior nosebleed, occurs below the septum. A rare type called a posterior nosebleed occurs high up in the nose and causes blood to flow down the back of the mouth and throat. It's more common in older people with high blood pressure, and it requires immediate medical attention. The broken blood vessel may need to be cauterized.

I just had this sudden numbness in my left leg and I couldn't move it. Then it went away. What happened?

Call your doctor immediately or get to an emergency room. You may have had a transient ischemic attack (TIA), also called a ministroke. These can cause sudden numbness or weakness in the face, arm, or leg as a blood clot temporarily clogs an artery in the brain. A TIA is no small problem; there's a 10 percent chance that in the next week it will happen again, only this time the clot *won't* clear and you'll have a major stroke. You need tests to determine if you did have a TIA. If you did, you may need medication to break up and prevent blood clots. Depending on your age, blood pressure, and whether you have diabetes and other medical symptoms, you may need to be hospitalized.

□ PALPITATIONS

I swear I felt my heart skip a beat the other day. Should I see a cardiologist?

Palpitations—the feeling that your heart "skipped" a beat, fluttered, or raced—are quite common. (What you felt as a skipped beat may actually have been an extra beat.) Often a palpitation is nothing more than your own sudden awareness of your heartbeat. In other cases, they are caused by a benign form of arrhythmia, or irregular heartbeat. However, arrhythmias can also be a sign of heart disease or other medical conditions. If you have lightheadedness or fainting, chest pain, a family history of sudden death, or underlying heart disease in addition to the palpitations, go to the emergency room. Otherwise, make an appointment with your doctor.

□ PERIODS

I stopped menstruating 5 years ago, I'm bleeding again. Is that normal?

Absolutely not. Vaginal bleeding after menopause is a sign of a problem in the reproductive system, such as inflammation, infection, injury, or uterine cancer. See your gynecologist for a pelvic exam as soon as possible.

□ RASH

I have an itchy rash on my hands. What is it?

It could be any number of things, including eczema, one of the most common skin rashes. People who have it may experience flare-ups on and off. Eczema can occur elsewhere as well, typically on the face, knees, or feet. It's thought of as an allergic condition, but it's usually not clear what sets it off. An over-the-counter hydrocortisone cream may help, though you may need a prescription-strength product to get rid of the rash and the accompanying itching. Moisturizing frequently with a thick cream can help keep future episodes at bay.

Another possibility: You may be allergic to something you touched, such as poison ivy or nickel. Call your doctor, and apply cold compresses in the meantime to stem the itching. You might also take an oral antihistamine.

□ SKIN PROBLEMS

Why is the skin on the bottom of my feet peeling off?

You might have a fungal infection, also known as athlete's foot. Other symptoms include itching, redness, burning, and blisters or sores. Try an over-the-counter antifungal cream and keep the foot dry and clean. If it doesn't clear within 2 weeks, see your doctor.

I'm 42 years old. What's with the acne?

We tend to think of acne as a teenage problem, but, in reality, it can occur at any age. Middle-age, when hormone levels begin fluctuating, is prime time. Manufacturers have caught on, and today you can find products designed to fight acne in older women that aren't as drying to your skin as those for teens. If over-the-counter options don't do it for you, see a dermatologist. Prescription drugs such as antibiotics can do wonders, while creams or lotions containing retinol, a form of vitamin A, can not only clear up the zits but smooth out the wrinkles, as well.

□ SORE THROAT

My throat is sore. How do I know if it's strep throat?

The only way to know for sure is with a test for the streptococcus bacteria that causes strep. Most sore throats, however, are caused by a viral infection. That's probably the case with your throat, especially if you also have cold symptoms, which don't usually accompany strep. Strep usually entails a fever of at least 101°F. Your doctor can give you a rapid strep test, which should provide an answer on the spot, though you may also need a throat culture. Even though the infection will usually go away on its own, your doctor may prescribe antibiotics so that you are no longer contagious after 24 hours. Meanwhile, ibuprofen (Advil, Motrin) or acetaminophen (Tylenol) can help relieve the pain.

DRUG-FREE FIX

Saltwater

Gargling with warm saltwater really does soothe a sore throat.

□ SWEATING

I keep waking up drenched in sweat. What could cause this?

How old are you? Night sweats are particularly common in women just before and after menopause; they are the evening form of hot flashes. Other causes include low blood sugar (a concern if you have diabetes and use insulin), tuberculosis (usually accompanied by fever and weight loss), hormonal disorders such as hyperthyroidism, and certain cancers, particularly lymphoma (usually accompanied by fever and weight loss). Night sweats are also a side effect of certain medications such as antidepressants, niacin, and the anticancer drug tamoxifen.

My sweat has been smelling, well, *different*. Is something wrong with me?

Changes in body odor are one of those subtle symptoms, like changes in your fingernails, that are your body's way of telling you something isn't right. Possible problems include diabetes or kidney failure. Of course eating a lot of onion- or garlic-rich foods, will make you smell of them. In addition, body odor changes slightly with age as you produce more fat-related by-products, resulting in a "greasier" smell.

□ SWELLING

Why are my fingers and ankles so swollen?

You may be eating too much salt. High-salt diets lead to fluid retention, resulting in swelling. The easiest way to cut back on sodium is to stop eating processed (boxed, packaged, and canned) foods and fast food. Of greater concern is that the swelling might be a sign of congestive heart failure, in which a weakened heart muscle is not able to effectively pump blood. The extra fluid collects in your fingers and ankles. Kidney and liver problems can also lead to swelling.

□ THIRST

I can't seem to quench my thirst, no matter how much I drink. What's wrong?

One possibility is a relatively rare form of diabetes called diabetes insipidus. There are four different types of this disease, but the most common one, central diabetes insipidus, occurs when the body doesn't make enough of a hormone that's needed to let your kidneys conserve water as they're meant to. It's triggered by damage to the hypothalamus or pituitary gland, both in the brain. The other most common type, nephrogenic diabetes insipidus, is caused by a defect in the parts of the kidneys that reabsorb water back into the bloodstream. It can also be caused by certain drugs, such as lithium, and by high levels of calcium in the body.

Other causes of unusual thirst include some cancers, infections, congestive heart failure, and type 1 and type 2 diabetes. It's time to see your doctor.

□ **TREMORS**

Why are my hands trembling?

That depends. Do they tremble all the time, even when you rest them on your knees? Or do they only shake when you do something like thread a needle? Does any other part of your body shake, like your head or leg? Does the trembling occur only when you're anxious or excited? Your answers will help your doctor hone in on a diagnosis. Most likely, the trembling is nothing to worry about; everyone's hands shake at times, particularly if you're tired or you drank too much the night before.

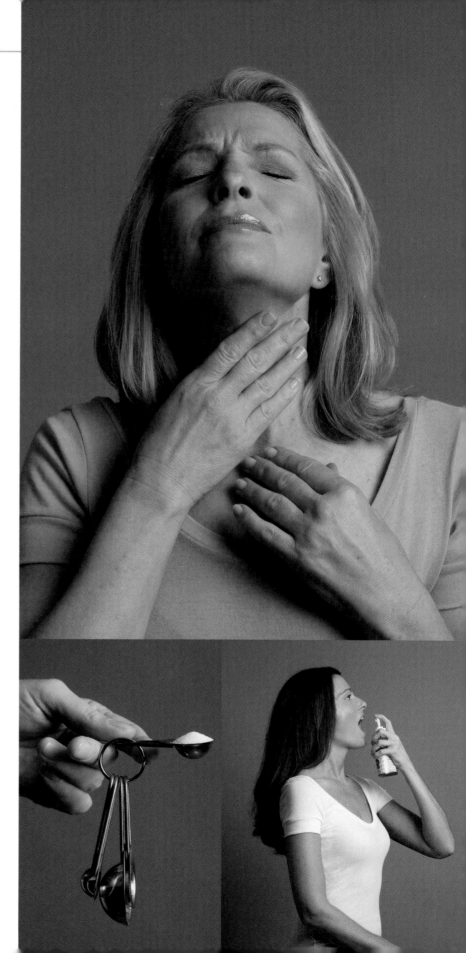

However, the tremble could be a sign of a neurological condition such as essential tremor or Parkinson's disease.

☐ URINATION

It hurts when I pee, and even though I feel like I have to urinate a lot, just a trickle comes out.

This sounds like a urinary tract infection or bladder infection. You likely need antibiotics, so call your doctor.

My urine is a funny color, so dark it's almost brown. Should I worry?

Before you start worrying, start drinking—you're probably dehydrated. Dark yellow or orange urine can also result from taking laxatives, B-complex vitamins, beta-carotene supplements, the drug phenazopyridine (Pyridium) for urinary tract infections, the medication rifampin (Rifadin), or the blood thinner warfarin (Coumadin). Even certain foods like beets or blackberries can leave your urine dark-colored. If, after avoiding those foods and drinking more for 2 days, your urine remains dark, see your doctor immediately. The dark color could be caused by blood or it could be a sign of a liver problem, a urinary tract infection, an enlarged prostate, or a kidney infection.

In the past few weeks, I find I have to pee every hour or so. I'm afraid to leave the house!

You could have urge incontinence, which is when you leak some urine after feeling that you have to go *right now*. However, the fact that this came on suddenly suggests something else, such as a bladder infection, especially if it hurts when you pee. The sudden urge to pee could also be a sign of diabetes, particularly if you are also drinking a lot of water. Has your doctor started you on any new medications? Diuretics, typically prescribed for high blood pressure, increase urination. Finally, you may have an overactive bladder. This is definitely one for your doctor.

Why does my husband get up two or three times a night to go to the bathroom?

The most likely cause is an enlarged prostate. Normally, this is nothing to worry about and can be managed with medication. However, he should be evaluated to rule out prostate cancer or other serious conditions such as congestive heart failure, kidney problems, or hormonal abnormalities that can also cause nighttime urination.

☐ VISION

When I wake up in the morning, it takes nearly an hour before I can see clearly enough to read the paper. What's wrong?

Your eyes are drying out. Chalk this one up to age. As you age, your eyes produce less fluid to keep the cornea and surrounding areas lubricated. The dryness is particularly bad first thing in the morning. You can try over-the-counter artificial tears or even prescription eye drops, but if you're only bothered in the morning, try this: Roll up a washcloth and soak it in hot water, then wring it out. Close your eyes and place the cloth over your eyelids until the cloth cools. Repeat one or two times. This should get the tears flowing.

I can see things on the side of my vision, but not straight ahead. Am I going blind?

What you describe could be age-related macular degeneration (AMD). It is the leading cause of blindness in most industrialized countries. It occurs when cells in the central part of the retina become damaged. Smoking, a family history of AMD, and heart disease all increase your risk. You'll need a complete eye exam to determine if you have AMD and, if you do, whether you have the wet or dry type. Dry AMD is more common and gets worse more slowly than the wet type. While there are several medications that doctors are using to treat wet AMD, the only treatment so far for dry AMD is supplementing with antioxidant vitamins A, C, and beta-carotene, as well as zinc. But don't supplement on your own; see your doctor.

My vision is getting blurrier, and I sometimes see halos around lights. Am I just getting older?

We're all getting older! Seriously, though, the first thing you should do is have an eye exam. Blurry vision and halos around lights sound like nearsightedness. Even if you already wear glasses or contact lenses, you may need your prescription changed. Cataracts could also cause the blurriness. About half of all people have cataracts by age 80. Another symptom of cataracts is a brownish tinge to the view and being unable to see the colors blue or purple. Blurriness could also be related to an underlying medical condition, such as diabetes or uncontrolled high blood pressure.

I see "floaters" in my eyes. Should I worry?

Floaters are those little specks that drift to and fro in your field of vision. They are more common with age, occurring as the vitreous, a jellylike substance that makes up most of the eye, shrinks. While surgery to remove the vitreous can get rid of floaters, it can also severely damage your vision. So just learn to ignore them. If they suddenly increase in number, however, and you see flashes of light in your peripheral vision, that could signify a retinal tear or detachment. Have someone drive you to the emergency room.

☐ WEIGHT

I've suddenly gained a lot of weight (about 10 pounds in the past month). I haven't changed how I'm eating or exercising. What is going on?

Did you just quit smoking? The nicotine in cigarettes not only suppresses appetite, but speeds metabolism, which is why many people gain weight when they quit. If smoking isn't the problem, you may have a hormonal condition. For instance, hypothyroidism, in which your thyroid gland doesn't produce enough hormone, can slow your metabolism significantly, leading to sudden weight gain. Other causes include diabetes and other insulin abnormalities, Cushing's syndrome (caused by an overabundance of the hormone cortisol), and low testosterone levels (in men). Certain medications can lead to weight gain, including corticosteroids and some antidepressants and antipsychotics. Make an appointment to see your doctor.

I've suddenly lost a lot of weight without trying. Could it be cancer?

It could be a lot of things. Maybe your appetite is off due to intense stress or anxiety, or you've been getting more exercise than you think. Certainly, however, there are medical conditions that can lead to sudden weight loss, including gastrointestinal cancer, diabetes (often accompanied by excessive thirst), depression, inflammatory bowel disease (Crohn's disease or ulcerative colitis), or malabsorption diseases such as celiac disease, in which the body is unable to metabolize wheat products. Make an appointment to see your doctor and keep a detailed food diary in the meantime.

Your Diet

□ ALCOHOL
Is alcohol good or bad for me?

Alcohol can be a disease-fighter in moderation, but drinking too much poses a long list of health threats. If you're a woman and you enjoy alcoholic beverages, one per day is the max, while men should have no more than two (one drink is 12 ounces of beer, 5 ounces of wine, or 1.5 ounces of liquor). Drinking within these limits may lower your risk for several diseases, including the following:

● *Heart disease.* Moderate drinking cuts the risk for heart attacks by 30 to 50 percent. Alcohol raises HDL cholesterol—the good kind—by about 12 percent, makes blood less likely to clot, and has other heart-friendly qualities. Any type of alcohol helps, but some research suggests that wine protects the heart better than beer and liquor. That may be because wine, particularly red varieties, contains a potent anti-oxidant called resveratrol.

● *Strokes.* Researchers have also found that up to two drinks per day may slash in half the risk for ischemic strokes, the most common type, which occur when arteries that feed blood to the brain become blocked.

● *Diabetes.* People who drink small amounts of alcohol are more likely to maintain healthy blood sugar levels, research suggests. A Harvard study found that men who had one or two drinks per day cut their risk for type 2 diabetes by 36 percent.

● *Dementia.* Compared with abstainers, people who drink alcohol are 34 percent less likely to develop Alzheimer's disease and nearly 50 percent less likely to be diagnosed with other forms of dementia, such as those caused by diseased blood vessels. It's not clear why drinking guards against dementia, though it may be alcohol's capacity to maintain healthy blood flow to the brain.

Drinking too much alcohol increases the risk for these conditions, not to mention abuse accidents:

● *Liver disease.* Between 10 and 20 percent of heavy

drinkers develop cirrhosis, a serious condition caused as healthy liver tissue is replaced by scar tissue.

- *Cancer.* Drinking alcohol has been linked to many forms of this disease, including cancers of the mouth, throat, liver, colon, rectum, and, in women, breast. As for the latter, a 2009 study determined that alcohol abuse may be responsible for up to 11 percent of all breast cancer cases.

- *Obesity.* Wonder where beer bellies come from? Each can of ale or lager contains about 150 calories. A glass of Cabernet will set you back 127 calories.

- *High blood pressure.* If you have high blood pressure, cutting back on booze could produce a small but significant drop of 2 to 4 mm Hg systolic (the top number) and 1 to 2 mm Hg diastolic (the bottom number).

How much alcohol can I drink if I have diabetes?

If your blood sugar is well-controlled—that is, your A1C is in an acceptable range—you can drink in moderation, defined as two drinks a day if you're a man and one if you're a woman. Just keep in mind that drinking heavily or on an empty stomach can cause people with diabetes to become shaky, dizzy, or confused, or to experience other symptoms of low blood sugar. Normally, when blood sugar begins to drop between meals, the liver releases stored glucose (sugar) to bring levels back to normal. Alcohol temporarily shuts down that process. Lower blood sugar is a concern particularly for those who inject insulin or take certain oral diabetes medications (especially sulfonylureas and meglitinides), which are already working to lower blood sugar. If you choose to drink alcohol, make sure your blood sugar isn't low, sip slowly and in moderation, and only with food.

Many diabetes experts today discourage the practice of swapping booze for food since it increases the risk for hypoglycemia. If you're counting calories or carbs, consider a cocktail or glass of wine as an addition to your daily total.

How much alcohol is safe for pregnant women?

Officially, none. Major medical organizations strongly recommend total abstinence, though some doctors privately tell pregnant women that it's okay to have half a glass of wine with dinner now and then. Most of the worries about alcohol increasing the risk for learning disabilities and other problems in children come from studies of women who drank heavily while pregnant. Studies of women who drank modest amounts of alcohol are less consistent in their results.

How can I sober up a drunk person?

You can't. Popular remedies such as coffee and cold showers do little if anything. Time is your only ally. It takes about 1 hour for the average person to metabolize a single drink, so the number of cocktails your tipsy pal tossed back will dictate how long it takes him to sober up. In the meantime, you can take steps to make sure the person remains unharmed. For instance, you can lay him on his side in case he vomits so he won't choke on it. And, of course, don't let him drive.

☐ ARTIFICIAL SWEETENERS

Are certain artificial sweeteners safer than others?

Not as far as anyone knows. One of the most common concerns people have about saccharin (Sweet'N Low and other brands), aspartame (NutraSweet, Equal, and others), and other artificial sweeteners is that they may cause cancer. But those claims have never been confirmed, according to the National Cancer Institute, so choosing one sugar substitute over another won't make much difference. One exception: Sorbitol and other sugar alcohols, which are often used to sweeten sugar-free gum and some diet foods, can cause diarrhea, bloating, and other digestive distress.

Does Stevia lower blood sugar?

Some diabetes patients use this natural sweetener (sold as Truvia, PureVia, and SweetLeaf) in the belief that it lowers blood sugar. But a 2008 study by Italian researchers found that the sweet-tasting herb had no benefit for patients with type 1 or type 2 diabetes.

□ CARBOHYDRATES

Are low-carb diets best for people with diabetes?

Not necessarily. Since carbo-hydrates raise blood sugar, a low-carb diet might seem the logical way to go. But the research is inconsistent: Some studies show that cutting carbs produces a healthy drop in blood sugar, but others don't. In fact, one study that compared four popular diet plans (two low-carb, two low-fat) found no difference in their effect on blood sugar or insulin levels, another impor-tant measurement for people with diabetes. If you have dia-betes and need to drop some weight, any low-calorie diet you can stick with will work. The American Diabetes Association says that either a low-carb or low-fat diet is acceptable.

I get shaky and light-headed after eating too many carbs or sugary foods. What's up?

You may be experiencing a condition called reactive hypo-glycemia, which occurs if your blood sugar drops too low a few hours after a meal, usually one that includes sugar or other easily digested carbohydrates such as potatoes or rice. In most cases, experts can't say what causes reactive hypogly-cemia, though it may be due to a glitch in the hormonal system that controls blood sugar. In any event, reactive hypoglycemia is usually not serious, and you can probably clear up the problem with a few simple strategies.

- Eat smaller, more frequent meals.
- Include a variety of foods in your diet, including plenty of fiber.
- Cut back on sugary foods and never eat them on an empty stomach.
- Don't drink alcohol on an empty stomach.
- Get plenty of exercise.

If the woozy episodes persist, talk to your doctor. Hypoglyce-mia could be a sign of certain disorders, including diabetes.

What is the glyce-mic index and how do I use it?

The carbohydrates in food break down into sugar during diges-tion, but there is great variety in how rapidly this happens. The glycemic index (GI) is a system that ranks how high and how fast various foods raise your blood sugar. Sugary and starchy foods—such as white bread, white rice, and mashed pota-toes—tend to rank high on the GI, since they produce a quick spike in blood sugar. Studies show that eating too many high-glycemic carbs may make you gain weight and increase your risk for type 2 diabetes, heart disease, and several other seri-ous conditions.

Some experts suggest using the GI to plan meals, but others

FACT OR FICTION

You Can't Eat Potatoes on a Low GI Diet

Fiction. Most potatoes have a high GI ranking, but eating modest portions of spuds is acceptable. Just have a low-GI dish along with them, such as peas or beans, which helps to blunt potatoes' effect on blood sugar. Also, cooling potatoes lowers their GI; try potato salad made with a mix of low-fat mayonnaise and yogurt.

feel that it's too complicated and could lead to some poor food choices. For instance, fat slows your body's ability to absorb sugar, so chocolate ice cream actually has a low GI ranking, as does steak and fried chicken, but you certainly wouldn't be doing yourself any favors by eating a diet that relied heavily on these foods. Still, you'd be smart to cut down on foods that boost blood sugar the most, including hot cooked potatoes, white bread, muffins, white rice, some breakfast cereals (especially rice- and corn-based cereals), and soft drinks. Find a comprehensive list of GI rankings at www.glycemicindex.com.

In general, filling up your weekly menu with plentiful servings of low-glycemic carbohydrates—including most whole grains (especially barley and bran), beans (except black-eyed peas), and most fruits and vegetables—should help keep your blood sugar down without doing any math.

□ CHOCOLATE
How much dark chocolate is good for you?
To reap the health benefits of dark chocolate—which may help lower blood pressure, cool inflammation in the arteries, and improve circulation, all thanks to powerful antioxidants called flavonoids—research shows that you only need a little more than 1.5 ounces per week. That's roughly equivalent to ten Hershey Kisses (dark chocolate, of course). Go overboard and the calories quickly outweigh the benefits. You'll get the most health benefits from chocolate with the highest cocoa content. Look for brands that contain at least 60 percent cocoa.

□ CHOLESTEROL
Will eating shrimp raise my cholesterol?
Shrimp may be high in cholesterol, but eating these delicacies from the sea won't send your levels soaring. In fact, shrimp probably does your heart some good. One study found that eating about 10 ounces of shrimp every day for 3 weeks did not worsen the ratio of LDL ("bad") cholesterol to HDL ("good"), an important measure of heart disease risk. What's more, the study found that eating shrimp actually lowered blood levels of artery-clogging fats called triglycerides.

Shrimp are relatively high in cholesterol, but they contain almost no saturated fat, the real villain when it comes to your cholesterol. And they offer some heart-smart omega-3 fatty acids.

What about eggs?
Eggs are another food that many people fear, but most can enjoy, at least in moderation. Although eggs are high in cholesterol, they contain relatively little cholesterol-raising saturated fat. And of course, they're an excellent source of protein. Studies at Harvard have shown that eating up to one egg per day does not raise your risk for heart attacks and strokes. However, the same research found that eating eggs every day may lead to heart trouble for people with diabetes. Scientists need to learn more about this connection, but in the meantime, people with diabetes should eat no more than three egg yolks per week. (The cholesterol is all in the yolk.)

Can I eat meat and still lower my cholesterol?
Yes. You don't need to swear off beef and burgers if your cholesterol is creeping upward. Lean cuts of meat can fit into a diet designed to lower cholesterol, according to a study by scientists at the Chicago Center for Clinical Research. They asked one group of men and women to adopt a diet heavy on lean beef, pork, veal, and lamb for 6 months. At the end of the study, the meat-eaters' cholesterol levels had dropped a few percentage points, the same reduction as a similar group of subjects who ate mostly chicken and fish.

The leanest cuts of beef include round steaks and

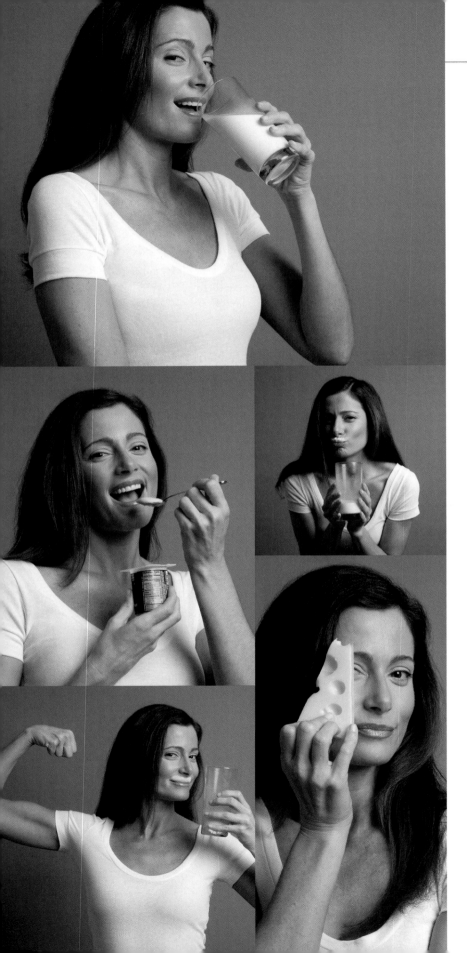

roasts, top loin, top sirloin, and chuck shoulder and arm roasts. Trim any visible fat before cooking.

Are there any foods that will raise my HDL cholesterol?

The only consumable that has been shown to raise heart-healthy HDL cholesterol is alcohol. Research has established that having one drink (for women) or two (for men) daily can raise HDL by about 5 mg/dL. (Heavy drinking, on the other hand, can damage your heart.) A few other foods and beverages, from fish to cranberry juice, have boosted HDL in some studies, but not in others.

If you don't drink alcohol, there's no need to start; regular exercise does the job, too. In one study, men who started jogging three times a week raised their HDL by 8 mg/dL.

☐ **COFFEE**

Is it bad or good for you?

We used to worry that drinking too much coffee might cause heart disease, cancer, and other diseases. However, solid research shows that the dark brew is loaded with antioxidants and may have major health benefits, though drinking too much can have some drawbacks.

Pros: Coffee may lower the risk for type 2 diabetes, gallstones, Parkinson's disease (in men only), liver disease, Alzheimer's disease, and other conditions. A cup or two may also sharpen memory and improve other cognitive skills.

Cons: Caffeinated coffee may keep you up at night or make you feel anxious. Some women find that it increases fibrocystic breast pain, though many experts question whether the link is real. Drinking more than three cups per day may weaken bones, according to some research. French press and boiled coffee may raise cholesterol. And most experts agree that pregnant women should limit their caffeine intake to the amount in one 12-ounce mug of coffee per day.

I switched to decaf, so why am I still having trouble sleeping?

It could be that you're still consuming small amounts of caffeine with each cup. Most coffee sold as decaffeinated still contains at least a little bit of the stimulant. University of Florida scientists found that decaf sold at a variety of coffee shops and fast-food restaurants had as much as 14 milligrams per 16-ounce cup. That's a far smaller jolt than you'll get from caffeinated coffee; a similar serving of brewed joe at Starbucks has at least 20 times more caffeine. However, if you drink several cups of decaf per day you may be downing enough caffeine to make you wide-eyed at night. You might try limiting yourself to one cup a day or switching brands.

☐ DAIRY

Is dairy the best source of calcium for my bones?

Milk and other dairy foods are an excellent source of calcium. Depending on your age, an 8-ounce glass of low-fat milk provides about one-third to one-quarter of the calcium you need each day for good bone health. (The National Osteoporosis Foundation recommends 1,000 milligrams of calcium a day for men and women under 50 and 1,200 milligrams for all other adults.) But dairy isn't your only source of calcium—and it's not even clear that guzzling milk is even necessary for stronger bones. (Asian women are half as likely as American women to develop osteoporosis, yet they consume little dairy.) In fact, there are enough suspicious clues that drinking too much milk might raise the risk for certain cancers (particularly ovarian and prostate) and that getting some of your daily dose from other sources makes sense. Ask your doctor if calcium supplements are an option and eat more:

- **Leafy greens.** Kale and collard greens are the best choices. (Spinach, beet greens, and rhubarb have modest amounts of calcium, too, but they also contain a chemical called oxalate, which keeps your body from absorbing the mineral efficiently.)

- **Beans, peas, and other legumes.** Caution: After soaking dried beans, always discard the water and start with fresh water before cooking to lower levels of phytate, a chemical that makes it harder for the body to absorb calcium.

- **Fortified foods.** Manufacturers now offer calcium-fortified versions of everything from orange juice to soy milk, breakfast cereal, bread, and even bottled water.

 WHAT YOU DON'T KNOW

Coffee Contains Fiber

And not just any fiber—coffee contains the soluble form, which is the artery de-clogger found in oatmeal. According to a study by Spanish researchers, it makes no difference what type of coffee you prefer: Six ounces of drip, instant, or espresso all contain 1 to 1.5 grams of soluble fiber.

I have a cold. Will drinking milk make my congestion worse?

Believe it or not, a group of scientists actually studied this by giving people colds, tracking their milk intake, and measuring the weight of their nasal secretions. Bottom line: Milk didn't increase congestion, though people who believed in the milk-congestion link were more likely to think that it did.

You also can stop worrying about drinking milk if you have asthma. Studies show that people with asthma—who are often advised to avoid dairy—can consume milk without worry.

How do I know if I'm lactose intolerant?

If you have been experiencing gastrointestinal problems, stop consuming dairy products and see if your symptoms improve. Bloating, cramps, diarrhea, flatulence, and other forms of GI distress are classic symptoms of lactose intolerance, which occur in people who lack enzymes necessary to digest the sugar in milk and other dairy foods. You may also feel an urgent need to have a bowel movement shortly after a meal that includes dairy foods. However, other conditions, such as irritable bowel syndrome, may also cause these symptoms.

Doctors can test for lactose intolerance by having a patient blow into a breath analyzer that measures hydrogen given off by undigested lactose (or, with infants and small children, by testing stool samples for the presence of lactic acid). But the simplest step is to cut out all dairy products and other foods containing lactose for 3 to 4 weeks. If you feel better, lactose intolerance is most likely the culprit. Some people find that adding lactase supplements to milk and other foods makes them tolerable; lactose-free dairy foods are available, too. Note that if you're lactose intolerant and you avoid dairy foods, you may need to take calcium supplements.

Does buttermilk contain butter? Is it bad for me?

There is no butter in the buttermilk you'll find at your local supermarket. Buttermilk got its name because it was the liquid left over after milk or cream was churned to make butter. However, modern dairies make buttermilk by fermenting low-fat or nonfat milk, giving it a distinctive sour flavor and thick consistency. Far from being bad for you, buttermilk can replace higher-fat milk or cream in biscuits, mashed potatoes, and other dishes. Some research suggests that fermented dairy products such as buttermilk and yogurt can improve digestion.

Will yogurt really help my digestion?

Yes. Yogurts that contain live and active bacteria cultures may help prevent and relieve digestive problems such as diarrhea, constipation, abdominal pain, and bloating. These bacteria cultures, known as probiotics, behave like the naturally occurring "good" bacteria in your gut that help maintain digestive order. Although scientists are still studying probiotics, different strains appear to offer unique benefits. Certain strains of *Lactobacillus* (including *rhamnosus* and *casei*) may be the best choices for infectious diarrhea, for example, while some research points to *Bifidobacterium* strains as the best probiotic for irritable bowel syndrome. (Many yogurt-makers add several different strains of bacteria to their products.)

Eating yogurt may even boost your defenses against cancer and infections by strengthening immune cells in your gut. And people who are lactose intolerant often find that they can eat yogurt without digestive discomfort.

☐ DIETS

I initially lost weight on my diet, but then I stopped losing. Why?

It's the bane of many dieters: the dreaded weight-loss plateau. Why does it happen? For starters, rapid weight loss that often occurs early on in a diet inevitably slows down after a few weeks. That's because the body starts out by burning stored carbohydrate, in the form of glycogen, for energy. But when reserves of glycogen run dry, the body eventually shifts to burning fat. Carbs burn faster than fat; they also release more water as they are metabolized, which is why we sometimes say early weight loss is mostly "water weight."

It's also common for weight loss to hit a standstill after 6 months or so. For some people,

FACT OR FICTION

The Atkins Diet Is Easy to Stick To

Fiction. It might seem like eating lots of beef and other high-protein pleasures would make complying with this plan a snap. But many dieters miss their bread and bananas, it seems. Several studies show that most people can follow Atkins for only a few months. After 1 year, most dieters who try it are consuming twice as many carbs as the plan dictates.

the culprit is willpower: They slip and begin eating too much food or they get tired of working out. But what if you are still following your diet to the letter and exercising regularly? The problem may simply be that you have lost a significant amount of weight. Because your body has shrunk, you need fewer calories than you did. If you still need to lose more weight, you'll need to cut calories further and/or exercise more.

I lost weight on the Atkins diet. Can I stay on it?

Staying on the Atkins plan may be okay, though more research would be reassuring. On the original Atkins diet, you cut carbohydrates to a bare minimum in favor of protein and fat. For years, many physicians strongly suspected that eating too much fat and protein would endanger heart health. But studies lasting up to 2 years have mostly shown that the Atkins diet does not worsen most risk factors for heart

disease—with one possible exception. A 2007 study found that Atkins dieters experienced a small increase in LDL ("bad") cholesterol. That's worrisome, though the authors of that paper suspect that positive changes in the type of LDL particles in the blood may offset the rise in total LDL. Further study would help us know whether staying on a very low carb diet is safe for the long term. Worried about your kidneys? There's no good evidence that low-carb diets harm kidney function (though if you already have kidney disease, the Atkins diet may not be right for you).

☐ DIGESTIVE PROBLEMS

What foods should I avoid if I have an ulcer?

Spicy foods don't cause ulcers, but eating tacos or marinara sauce could make one feel worse. Likewise, acidic foods and beverages, such as citrus fruits and juice and coffee, may leave ulcer sufferers in pain. Avoiding these foods will spare you some anguish, but keep in mind that most ulcers are caused by bacteria that's easily wiped out with a course of antibiotics and Pepto-Bismol. Studies show that former ulcer sufferers often find that they can tolerate once-forbidden foods.

I can't bear prunes. Are there any other foods that will relieve constipation?

Plenty of them, including oat bran and other high-fiber foods. Fiber helps overcome constipation by making stools softer and easier to pass. In one recent study, 59 percent of people with severe, chronic constipation who increased their daily fiber intake by 5 grams by eating oat bran were able to quit using laxatives. Other good sources include fruits, vegetables, beans, and whole grains.

Do I have to give up nuts and popcorn if I have diverticulitis?

Probably not, though talk it over with your doctor. Diverticulitis is a condition that causes pain in the abdomen, cramps, nausea, and other gastrointestinal symptoms. It occurs when tiny pouches that form naturally in the intestines, known as divertic-

ula, become inflamed. For years, doctors thought the inflammation came from small bits of food that lodge in these pouches, so they ordered patients with diverticulitis to avoid nuts, corn, popcorn, and seeds (such as caraway or sesame). However, a 2008 study followed more than 47,000 men for 18 years and found that those who frequently ate nuts, seeds, and similar foods were *less* likely to develop diverticulitis. And men in the study who had diverticulitis but continued eating seeds and other previously forbidden foods did not have an increased risk for bleeding or other complications.

☐ ENERGY

I'm always exhausted. What foods will give me more pep?

Don't focus on specific foods for fighting fatigue; instead, rethink your overall eating habits.

DO THIS:

● *Start every day with breakfast.* You'll feel more alert and attentive, as a number of stud-

ies have found. Be sure to include some protein (from eggs, peanut butter, milk, or yogurt, for instance).

● *Refuel regularly.* Don't go more than 3 to 4 hours without a snack or meal, advises the American Dietetic Association.

● *Eat protein with every meal.* Many studies have shown that meals that include protein are less likely to leave you feeling drowsy. Protein provides amino acids necessary for forming the neurotransmitters dopamine and norepinephrine, which promote alertness and attention, according to Massachusetts Institute of Technology researcher Judith Wurtman.

● *Eat the right carbohydrates.* Lower-glycemic carbs are digested slowly, so they provide sustained energy. Swap out white bread for wheat, regular potatoes for sweet potatoes, and sugary cereals for high-fiber cereal, and don't forget to eat your peas, beans, and vegetables.

● *Be sure you get your Bs.* As in the various forms of vitamin B, which play a crucial role in converting food you eat into energy.

AVOID THIS MISTAKE

Adding Fiber Without Drinking More Water

Fiber fights constipation, but increasing your intake without drinking enough could make matters worse. Studies show that drinking eight glasses of water per day enhances the digestive benefits of fiber.

The B vitamins are found in many foods, but count this as another good reason to eat whole grains and lean meats.

DON'T DO THIS:

● *Rely on candy bars or sports drinks.* They may give you a jolt of energy, but the effects are fleeting and the empty calories will stretch your belt.

● *Drink too much caffeine.* A cup or two of coffee or tea can improve alertness, but too much caffeine can easily become counterproductive if it keeps you awake at night (and some people find it just makes them jittery).

● *Get dehydrated.* Your body needs water in order to keep your blood volume up and to help cells function effectively.

Keep in mind that chronic lack of energy is a symptom of many medical conditions, such as anemia and thyroid disease. If tweaking your fuel sources doesn't give you more pep, talk to your doctor.

□ FASTING

Will fasting for a few days "clean me out" and make me healthier?

There is no evidence that fasting for "internal cleansing" is beneficial. Proponents hold that abstaining from food for several days (or in some cases longer) helps to remove toxins such as pollutants, food addi-tives, preservatives, pesticides, and other chemicals that accumulate in the body. Some drink only water while fasting, but many others sip laxative teas, juice concoctions, or other fluids to "flush" their systems. Still others use enemas.

Surf the internet and you will find claims that fasting prevents heart attacks and even cures cancer. None has any scientific evidence. In fact, fasting could be harmful, since it can cause toxins—which are stored in fat tissue—to be released. Meanwhile, depriving your body of nutrients weakens your immune system's ability to destroy them. A prolonged fast could lead to muscle loss, irregular heart rhythm, kidney and liver damage, and even trigger a gout attack.

□ FIBER

I know fiber is healthy, but can I take it in a pill instead of eating all that roughage?

Yes, but it's not a great idea. Choosing fiber supplements means you'll miss out on the vitamins, minerals, and phytochemicals found in fruits, vegetables, and whole grains. Eating more of these foods helps prevent constipation, lowers cholesterol and blood sugar, and reduces the risk of cancer. Most people should aim for 25 to 30 grams every day, but the average person consumes only half as much. While you're working to bump up your intake of high-fiber foods, though, it's fine to take fiber capsules or powders to help fill a shortfall. Increase your dose slowly (to avoid gas) and drink plenty of fluids, or you could find yourself constipated.

□ FISH

What's the safest tuna, white or light?

Light tuna. All fish contains at least a trace of mercury, a contaminant found in both salt- and freshwater fish. Exposure to large amounts of mercury can damage developing brains, and some preliminary research suggests it may be bad for the heart, too. Light canned tuna comes from the skipjack species, which is small and short-lived. White canned tuna comes from the albacore, a large predator that lives for years, which means it absorbs lots of mercury from the smaller fish it eats. As a result, white tuna contains about three times more mercury than light tuna. The Food and Drug Administration recommends that women of childbearing age and small children eat no more than 6 ounces of white tuna per week.

Can I get parasites from eating sushi?

Yes. Sorry to spoil your appetite, sushi-lovers, but eating raw or undercooked fish can leave you with worms in your gut that cause severe pain, vomiting, and diarrhea. But the problem isn't exactly rampant: There have been about 150 reports of infections with the anisakis worm and its equally disgusting cousins worldwide since 2003, though that figure is probably low, since afflicted diners often don't seek medical attention. Sushi and sashimi (another Japanese dish that usually contains raw fish) aren't the only potential culprits: Any raw or undercooked freshwater fish such as mackerel, herring, cod, trout, striped bass, carp, pike, and freshwater eel can carry these squirmy parasites. That means you should beware of seviche (fish marinated in citrus juice), pickled herring, and salted fish, too.

There's no need to give up sushi (unless you're pregnant, in which case you should abstain). Just be sure to choose reputable, busy restaurants, where the stock turns over quickly. In the United States and Europe, by law, all fish used to make sushi must be frozen for at least 72 hours at a temperature between −4° and −31°F, which kills worms, so ask about the freezing practices at your favorite sushi bar. And adding flavor can help stave off other trouble: Studies show that wasabi and vinegar can kill any bacteria on sushi.

How Much Fish Is Safe to Eat?

Fish is nature's best source of omega-3 fatty acids, which have far-ranging health benefits. But some experts believe that the standard advice to eat fish twice a week may provide too little healthy fish oil—and expose some consumers to too much mercury. Toxicologist Gary Ginsberg, PhD, of the Connecticut Department of Public Health, and colleague Brian Toal, MSPH, assessed the risks and benefits of 16 common species of fish and came up with these recommendations. Choose fish listed in **bold** as often as possible; they're the top sources of omega-3's. There are many other fish in the sea; to find out if a variety not listed here is high in mercury, contact your local health department.

MOST ADULTS AND CHILDREN 6 AND OLDER	WOMEN OF CHILDBEARING AGE AND CHILDREN 5 AND YOUNGER
No limits	**No limits**
Cod, Flounder, **Herring**, Pollack, **Salmon (Pacific)**, Shrimp, Tilapia, **Trout**, Tuna (canned, light)	Flounder, **Herring**, Pollack, **Salmon (Pacific)**, Shrimp, Tilapia, **Trout**
Twice a week	**Twice a week**
Halibut, Lobster, Sea bass, Tuna (canned, white)	Cod, Tuna (canned, light)
Once a week	**Once a week**
Salmon (Atlantic)*, Tuna steak	**Halibut, Lobster, Salmon (Atlantic)*, Sea bass, Tuna (canned, white)**, Tuna steak
Never	**Never**
Shark, Swordfish, King Mackerel, Tilefish	Shark, Swordfish, King Mackerel, Tilefish

*Atlantic salmon is low in mercury but tends to have high levels of other toxins, including PCBs and dioxin.
Source: Environmental Health Perspectives, February 2009.

Will eating salmon get rid of my wrinkles?

Eating salmon and other oily fish may play a small role in keeping skin smooth. A popular antiwrinkle diet plan recommends eating a great deal of salmon on the theory that fish oil dampens skin-damaging inflammation triggered by sunlight, tobacco smoke, alcohol, and other influences. Studies have shown that fish oil protects skin, but subjects in this research took fish-oil supplements or applied skin preparations containing omega-3 fatty acids. It's not certain that eating salmon and other oily fish rejuvenates skin, but do so anyway; it will give your heart a nourishing dose of omega-3 fatty acids.

I just ate a dozen oysters, then realized we're not in an "R" month. Should I go to the ER?

Relax, there's little chance that the oysters will make you sick. There is some logic to the old adage that warns against eating oysters and other forms of shellfish from May through August, the only months spelled without an "R." Warm temperatures cause algae in seawater to bloom. Certain types of red-hued algae produce marine toxins that can contaminate oysters, clams, mussels, and other shellfish. Eating a bad bivalve can cause paralytic shellfish poisoning, sometimes within 15 minutes. Symptoms are usually mild, such as tingling or numb skin, a headache, and nausea, though, in rare cases, the condition can be fatal.

That said, most countries have large-scale monitoring programs that shut down shellfish beds tainted by so-called red tide.

These programs appear to be effective. For instance, between 1998 and 2002, only 13 people in the United States were hospitalized after eating tainted shellfish; none died.

□ FOOD ADDITIVES

Do food colorings and additives cause ADHD?

Not as far as experts know, but certain food colorings and additives may make a child with ADHD (attention deficit hyperactivity disorder) harder to handle. People with ADHD are fidgety, impulsive, and struggle to pay attention. A study published in the British medical journal *Lancet* found that kids become slightly more hyperactive after consuming beverages containing a common preservative (sodium benzoate) and certain red and yellow food colorings. British health authorities now advise parents to consider eliminating these ingredients from the diets of hyperactive children.

Does MSG make you sick?

Probably not. The flavor enhancer MSG, or monosodium glutamate, gets its bad reputation from several reports of diners who became ill after eating in Chinese restaurants way back in 1968. Worries arose that the culprit was MSG, which was soon blamed for causing headaches, asthma,

hives, and other bad reactions. Yet formal studies have failed to link MSG to any health problem. Nonetheless, doctors can't rule out the possibility that a small percentage of people are sensitive to MSG.

□ FOOD ALLERGIES

How can I tell if I'm allergic to something I ate?

The first clue will probably be itchiness in your mouth, nose, and eyes, and on your skin, which may break out in a rash. Your nose may become runny and your eyes may fill with tears. You may also vomit and develop diarrhea, or you might cough, wheeze, and find it hard to breathe. In severe cases, food allergies can cause a perilous drop in blood pressure, shock, unconsciousness, and other scary symptoms. If you don't get immediate help, a food allergy can be fatal.

The symptoms of a food allergy typically emerge within a few minutes to an hour or so after eating. Food allergies occur due to a glitch in the immune system, which mistakes a perfectly safe food for a toxin. However, having a bad reaction to a food doesn't necessarily mean you have a food allergy. For instance, if you lack the enzyme for digesting lactose, the sugar in dairy foods, you may feel gassy and bloated after drinking milk. But the inability to tolerate lactose isn't

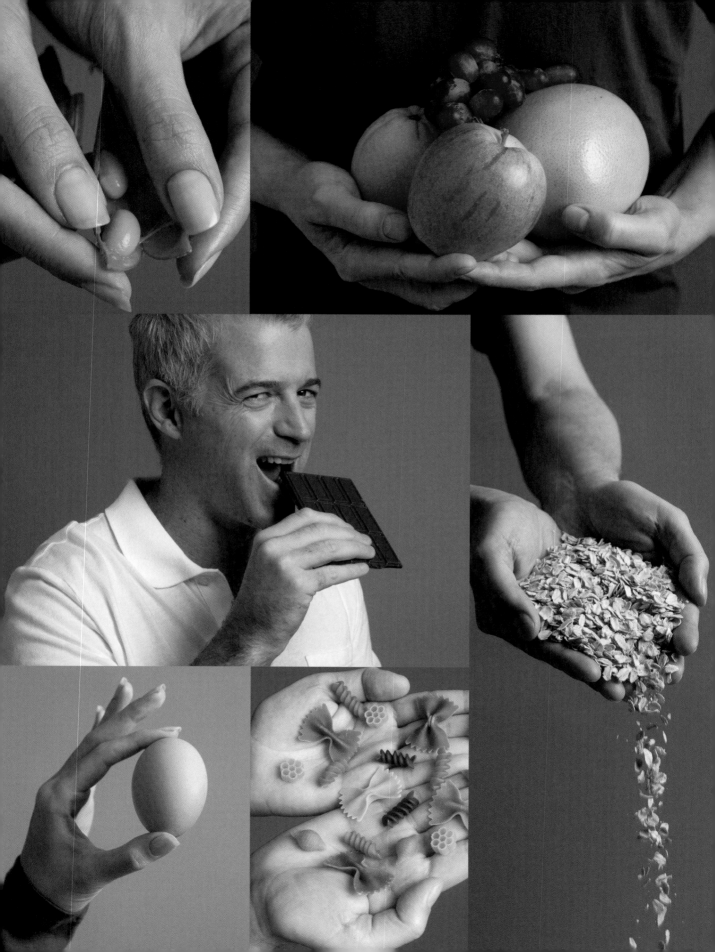

a true allergy because it isn't caused by a misguided immune system.

There are several medical tests that can help confirm whether or not you have a food allergy. In one, a doctor pricks your skin with a tiny liquid extract of a suspected food. Developing a small hive (called a wheal) within 20 minutes means you may have found the culprit. Blood tests that look for the presence of allergic antibodies are another option. Your doctor may also ask you to keep a food diary, in which you take notes about the food you eat and any symptoms you experience. If certain foods appear to trigger a reaction, eliminating them from your diet will help confirm the diagnosis.

Just a handful of foods account for most food allergies. The most common triggers in children are milk, eggs, peanuts, wheat, and soy. The most common triggers in adults are peanuts, tree nuts, fish, and shellfish.

What grains can I eat if I have gluten intolerance?

You can still get your fix of starchy foods. The names of some grains on lists of gluten-free foods may leave you scratching your head (amaranth or arrowroot, anyone?), but you'll also find more familiar offerings at your local supermarket or natural foods store, such as gluten-free breads and pasta made from flax, potato, rice, or corn. Ricelike quinoa is

MSG Occurs Naturally in Small Doses in Many Foods

These include milk, broccoli, peas, walnuts, grapefruit juice, and Parmesan cheese.

another alternative. Some old favorites are safe to eat, too, including cream of rice or grits for breakfast, as well as corn tacos and corn tortillas. You can find a list of foods to include and avoid at www.digestive.niddk.nih.gov/ddiseases/pubs/celiac_ez.

I ate something and now I'm swelling up. What do I do?

If the allergic reaction is mild and limited to a small patch of skin, it will likely pass soon. Taking an antihistamine may help with the discomfort. If the swelling is more widespread and you have been diagnosed with a food allergy, you should have injectable epinephrine on hand. If you don't, get to a hospital immediately, preferably by ambulance. If you do have it, inject the epinephrine, then go to the hospital.

☐ FOOD POISONING

How can I tell whether I have food poisoning? Should I go to the ER?

The symptoms of food poisoning vary depending on which type of

microbe has snuck into your system, but in most cases, you will develop stomach cramps, nausea, vomiting, and diarrhea. A bout with food poisoning usually lasts a day or so. The Centers for Disease Control and Prevention advise seeking medical care if you have diarrhea and:

- You have a temperature over 101.5°F
- There is blood in your stool
- You are vomiting frequently and can't hold down liquids
- You show any signs of dehydration, such as a decrease in urination, a dry mouth, or dizziness when you stand
- Your diarrhea lasts for more than 3 days

☐ FOOD SAFETY

How do you know when a raw egg is bad?

Place it in a pan of water. Old eggs have large air pockets, so if one floats, it's probably rotten. Or, crack the egg and examine the white. If it has a pinkish or rainbow-like hue, throw it out. That's evidence that the egg has spoiled. And of course, if the carton is past its expiration date, don't eat the eggs.

Is it okay to cut off the moldy parts of cheese and eat the rest?

There's no need to chuck the cheddar, but beware of mold on certain other cheeses. Follow these rules.

- *Eat it:* When mold develops on hard cheese such as cheddar, gouda, or Parmesan, cut 1 inch around and below the moldy spot. Mold can't penetrate deep below the surface of hard cheese, so the rest is safe to eat.

- *Toss it (in most cases):* Some cheeses, such as Roquefort, bleu, brie, and Camembert, are made with strains of mold. If you discover mold that grew on the product after you purchased it, throw the cheese away. Exceptions: Stilton and gorgonzola are hard cheeses, so you can trim away mold.

- *Don't even think about it:* Mold on any sliced cheese, grated cheese, or soft cheese (such as cottage cheese, cream cheese, or chèvre) is a signal to get rid of it.

I left the mayonnaise out all night. Should I toss it?

No. It's a common misconception that mayonnaise spoils rapidly, at least when it comes to the store-bought variety. When making mayonnaise, food processors use pasteurized eggs, which are bacteria-free. They also add plenty of vinegar and lemon juice, acidic ingredients that prevent or slow the growth of bacteria. That doesn't mean it's a good idea to eat a tuna salad sandwich left out in the hot sun all afternoon, however, and food-safety experts recommend returning mayonnaise to the fridge as soon as possible, if for no other reason than to preserve flavor. To be on the safe side, dispose of homemade mayo that's left out overnight.

☐ **FRUIT AND FRUIT JUICE**

I have diabetes. Can I drink fruit juice?

Fruit juice is not off-limits, but enjoy it in moderation. Juice is a concentrated source of carbohydrates in the form of sugar. Diabetes patients can safely consume carbohydrates, but controlling your intake is key for maintaining safe blood sugar levels. An 8-ounce glass of juice contains about 30 grams of carbohydrates. Filling up on juice could mean crowding out other, healthier foods such as whole fruit and whole grains.

Is it safe to drink grapefruit juice if I take medications?

It depends on what type of medications you take. Grapefruit interferes with an enzyme your body needs to process certain drugs. As a result, too much of the medication enters the bloodstream, which could result in side effects. Some people are more sensitive to grapefruit than others, but don't take a chance: Ask your doctor if it's okay to drink grapefruit juice if you're prescribed any drug, particularly medications for: anxiety, arrhythmia (irregular heartbeat), cancer, depression, high blood pressure, high cholesterol, HIV, insomnia, malaria, preventing rejection of organ transplants, seizures, or viral infections.

Will drinking cranberry juice clear up a urinary tract infection?

It won't clear up an existing urinary tract infection (UTI), but it could help you avoid another. Compounds in cranberries seem to prevent bacteria from attaching to cells in the urinary tract. Studies show that a daily glass of cranberry juice (as little as 6 ounces in some studies) could cut your risk for UTIs by up to 35 percent. Young and middle-aged women are most likely to benefit.

Can I count fruit juice as a serving of fruit?

Yes, according to the USDA. But aim to get most of your daily servings from whole or cut-up fruit. An 8-ounce glass of 100 percent fruit juice can provide you with a similar healthy dose of vitamins and minerals as you would get from eating an orange. But that glass of juice has about 40 calories more than the fruit and drives up your blood sugar faster, too. Meanwhile, orange juice has hardly any fiber, while eating an orange provides 3 to 4 grams of healthful roughage.

Should I wash fruit to get the chemicals off or is rinsing it good enough?

Rinsing fruit under cold running water will do the job. Don't wash it in soap or detergent; residue from these products could get absorbed into the fruit, so you could end up eating it. While rinsing, rub the fruit with your hands or use a produce brush. (Rinse berries thoroughly in a colander.) Also, rinse and scrub fruit that requires cutting, such as melon, so the knife won't transfer any bacteria on the skin into the flesh.

I feel a cold coming on. Will drinking orange juice help?

No. Orange juice is a tasty source of vitamin C, but upping your intake of this antioxidant won't stop your sneezing and sniffling. Research does show that consuming at least 200 milligrams of vitamin C daily (the amount in two to three tall glasses of OJ) *before* you develop a cold may make your

FACT OR FICTION

Apple Seeds Are Toxic

Fiction. Don't worry if you bite into an apple and swallow a few seeds. They do contain a substance called amygdalin, which is a natural source of the poison cyanide. But it would take massive amounts of apple seeds to make you sick.

symptoms vanish sooner. But not much: High doses of vitamin C cut the duration of a typical cold by about 8 percent.

☐ **GARLIC**

Will eating garlic lower my cholesterol?

The "stinking rose" may be good for you in other ways, but it won't lower your cholesterol. Scientists have examined this question in a number of studies and the overall consensus is that neither eating garlic nor taking garlic supplements lowers total cholesterol, LDL ("bad") cholesterol, or triglycerides, another fat in the blood.

☐ **GENETICALLY MODIFIED FOODS**

Is there any way to tell if a food has been genetically modified? Should I care?

There's no way to be sure if foods sold in the United States and certain other countries contain genetically modified (GM) ingredients; labeling of GM foods is mandatory in many other countries, however. GM products are plant (and, coming soon, animal) foods that have had genes from other species inserted into their genetic code to introduce some desirable trait, such as better taste, increased nutrients, or resistance to pests. The most common GM foods in your diet are probably ingredients in processed foods, such as corn syrup or soybean oil made from bioengineered crops.

Whether GM foods are dangerous remains a hotly debated question. Environmentalists have many concerns about GM foods. For example, they fear that genetically modified organisms will "escape" from farms and damage wild plants. Many doctors and scientists want more information about the safety of GM foods, too. However, there is currently no solid evidence that consuming GM foods has any ill effect on humans, according to the World Health Organization.

☐ **IMMUNITY**

Are there any foods that will boost my immune system?

Eating plenty of fruits and vegetables is a good start, but you should include fish and low-fat dairy, too. Vitamin D, found in fish as well as in milk and other fortified dairy foods, increases production of a certain germ-killing protein, and a 2009 study found that Americans who had the highest levels of vitamin D in their blood were significantly less likely to develop colds. (That was especially true for people with asthma; those with the lowest vitamin D were more than five times as likely to catch a cold.) While you're in the dairy aisle for milk, pick up some yogurt containing active cultures, another known immune-booster.

When it comes to vegetables, don't forget your carrots. Researchers recently discovered that the beta-carotene in carrots, sweet potatoes, cantaloupe, and other foods makes white blood cells more likely to focus on fighting infections and less likely to turn against the body to trigger autoimmune disorders such as rheumatoid arthritis and lupus.

Finally, a diet that's low in minerals, especially zinc, can weaken your immune system. Lean meats, breakfast cereals, and oysters are a few good sources of this important mineral.

☐ **MARGARINE**

Once and for all, which is better for me, butter or margarine?

Margarine, but only if you choose wisely. Margarine contains far less saturated fat than butter, and since it's made from vegetable oil, it contains no cholesterol. But the process that's used to convert vegetable oils to spreadable margarine, called hydrogenation, produces trans fats, which may be even deadlier than saturated fat. Stick margarine has the most trans fat, but even soft and liquid margarine contains too much. Fortunately, a growing number of food processors offer margarines that contain little or no trans fat. Check a product's Nutrition Facts label, which should list zero grams of trans fat (though that may mean it still contains up to 0.5 gram per serving). Then read the ingredient list. The first item should be a type of vegetable oil, such as canola, soybean, or olive oil. You should not see the word "hydrogenated" in the ingredients. If you do, the product contains trans fats.

Is it possible to eat too much of a cholesterol-reducing margarine?

It's no big deal if you eat more than the recommended servings (typically 2 to 3 tablespoons a day) now and then. But bear in mind that these spreads act like the prescription drug ezetimibe (Zetia), blocking the body's ability to absorb cholesterol. Although these margarines are generally considered safe, a few people who use them develop digestive side effects, such as nausea and diarrhea. Exceeding the recommended servings could raise your risk for these unpleasantries. Don't forget, every tablespoon of margarine contains about 80 calories.

☐ **MEAT**

What are the benefits of grass-fed beef?

A cow's natural diet is grass, but most cattle today are fed diets of grain. That's unfortunate because cows that graze in pastures produce beef that's richer in several important nutrients. For instance, grass-fed beef contains a higher concentration of conjugated linoleic acid (CLA), which lab studies show can block the growth of cancerous tumors. And grass-fed beef has about 60 percent more omega-3 fatty acids than grain-fed beef. What's more, beef from cattle raised eating grass contains less saturated fat and is less likely to have been treated with growth hormones and antibiotics.

Does organic beef contain hormones?

Beef labeled "organic" must not contain artificial hormones. In the United States and some other countries (but not in Europe), producers of nonorganic meat are permitted to treat cattle with hormones to make them grow faster. Nonorganic meat typically contains only traces of hormones and has not been proven to be a health threat. But if you want to play it safe, look for organic beef. (Note: Don't confuse "organic" and "grass-fed." Organic beef may come from cattle fed certified-organic grain.)

I look forward to cookouts every summer, but does grilled meat cause cancer?

There is some evidence that eating grilled meat raises the risk for certain cancers, but taking some simple steps can greatly reduce the threat. Substances called heterocyclic amines (HCAs) that form in most meats during cooking cause cancer in lab animals. (Organ meats, such as liver, are an exception.) Grilling or cooking with other high-temperature methods, such as broiling or frying, produces large amounts of HCAs. Population studies show that people who eat lots of meat cooked at high temperatures and who prefer well-done meat have a

greater risk for cancers of the colon, stomach, prostate, breast, and pancreas.

One way to minimize these threats is to marinate meat before grilling, which blocks the formation of HCAs. Studies have also shown that microwaving meat for 2 minutes before cooking reduces HCA content by up to 90 percent. Develop a taste for medium or medium-rare beef if you usually cook your meats all the way through; well-done meats contain more cancer-causing compounds. Finally, resist the urge to use pan drippings to make gravy; they are loaded with HCAs.

□ NUTS

I've heard nuts are good for the heart. But are all nuts good, even peanuts and cashews?

Eating a variety of nuts is your best bet. They are a great source of vitamins, minerals, fiber, and monounsaturated fat, the kind found in other healthy

foods such as olive oil that protects the heart. Nuts are also brimming with a variety of antioxidant-rich phytochemicals. Walnuts and pecans are the champs in total antioxidant content. Yet peanuts, which are relatively low overall, are a top source of resveratrol, a compound now widely studied for its antiaging properties.

Cashews' antioxidant content ranks them in the middle of the pack. But they're relatively high in saturated fat, which is bad for the heart, and low in fiber, so make them a rare treat. Major studies show that peanut butter–eaters have fewer heart attacks, so dig in, but limit yourself to 1 to 2 tablespoons per serving.

□ OLIVE OIL

Can I or can't I cook with olive oil?

Think twice before using olive oil to sauté or fry foods. High heat spoils its flavor and destroys antioxidants. One study found that at 350°F—just high enough for frying—olive oil loses 50 to 60 percent of valuable antioxidants in 10 minutes. To get the most health benefits from olive oil, use it to dress salads, and drizzle it over steamed vegetables. Buy extra-virgin olive oil, which has the most antioxidants.

Can olive oil lower my cholesterol?

Maybe a little. One study found that when 28 adults added 2 tablespoons of extra-virgin olive oil a day to their diets for 6 weeks, they experienced a 12 percent drop in total cholesterol. However, other studies have failed to show any such benefit. Include this emerald oil in your diet anyway; its real value lies in the ability to reduce inflammation in the blood vessels, which is strongly linked to heart disease and heart attacks.

□ PROTEIN

Will eating more protein help me lose belly flab?

Any low-calorie diet can help you trim inches from your waistline, but you may find that eating more protein speeds up your slimming. A few studies have found that high-protein diets shrink waistlines slightly more—by about ½ inch after 2 years, according to one 2009 study—if you stick closely to the diet. Keep in mind, though, that it's possible to lose weight on any low-calorie plan; the key is finding one that works for you.

□ SALT

I'm cutting back on sodium because I have high blood pressure. Can I use a salt substitute containing potassium?

Yes, unless you have kidney disease. If you do, consuming too much potassium could cause a life-threatening condition called hyperkalemia. People who have this condition are unable to remove excess potassium from the blood, so levels of the mineral could rise too high, resulting in irregular heartbeat and possibly cardiac arrest. If you have kidney disease and food tastes bland, try adding fresh herbs and spices.

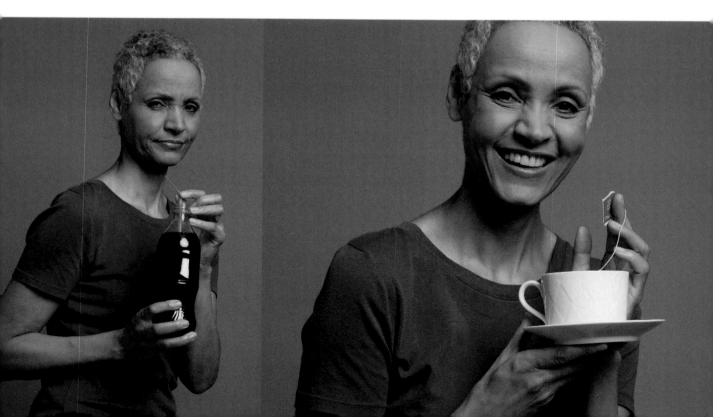

I have low blood pressure. Is salt okay for me?

There is no reason to avoid salt if you have low blood pressure. In fact, some people with this condition may even benefit from an extra shake or two. Also called hypotension, low blood pressure may occur naturally or can be a side effect of certain medications. Many people with low blood pressure never notice any symptoms, so there's little cause for concern. Others may feel dizzy and light-headed now and then upon rising from a seated position. A little dizziness from time to time is no big deal. But frequent bouts of unsteadiness could be a sign that you're dehydrated; drinking more water may help. If the problem persists, talk to your doctor. He or she may recommend sprinkling a little extra salt on food to increase the volume of your blood, which may minimize symptoms.

☐ SOFT DRINKS

Is cola bad for my bones? What if I switch to sugar-free?

Drinking too much soda, especially cola, may weaken your bones. Most soft drinks contain caffeine, which we know increases the risk for osteoporosis, or fragile bones. But cola packs a double whammy since it also contains phosphoric acid, an ingredient not found in most other carbonated drinks. Phosphoric acid lowers calcium, a building block of bone, and triggers hormonal changes that may harm your skeleton. A recent study by Tufts University researchers found that middle-aged women who drank cola every day had significantly lower bone density in their hips, even if they preferred sugar-free cola. Protecting your bones may be just one more reason to switch from soda to seltzer, water, or unsweetened tea.

☐ SOY

Is soy good for hot flashes?

Maybe. Soy is a rich source of compounds called phytoestrogens. Scientists have theorized that these plant hormones may help relieve hot flashes and other symptoms in women who have reached menopause, in whom estrogen levels drop.

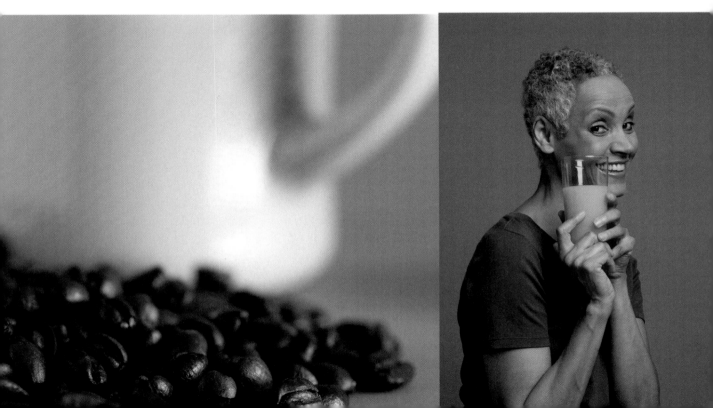

The results of studies have been mixed, however. In one 2007 experiment, women who took 250 milligrams of soy extract every day cut the frequency and severity of hot flashes in half. However, women in this study got their soy from supplements. Some experts say that women should avoid soy supplements, especially those who have had breast cancer.

Does soy cut my risk for cancer?

Eating soy may help prevent some common forms of cancer, but the evidence is limited. Rates of breast and prostate cancer are low in Asian countries where tofu and other soy foods are popular. Lab and animal studies show that plant estrogens called isoflavones can block the growth of some tumors. So far, though, studies have failed to show consistently that women in Western countries who consume large amounts of soy foods gain any defense against breast cancer (though young women who eat lots of soy may benefit later in life). In fact, getting soy from supplements and processed foods such as energy bars may backfire; animal research suggests that the refined soy used in these products behaves differently than soy in tofu and other whole foods—and could actually increase the risk of breast cancer.

 AVOID THIS MISTAKE

Counting on Soy Milk for Calcium

Unless you buy fortified soy milk, you may not be getting as much calcium in your diet as you think. Fortified soy milk typically has about as much calcium as dairy milk, around 300 milligrams per cup. But the same serving of unfortified soy milk contains only about 60 milligrams.

Studies have shown that soy extract slows rising prostate specific antigen (PSA), a marker for prostate cancer, but it's not certain that this legume prevents the disease. However, soy foods are a good source of lean protein, so including them as part of a balanced diet may be worthwhile.

☐ **SUGAR**

Is sugar better for me than high-fructose corn syrup?

No. High-fructose corn syrup (HFCS) is a sweetener derived from corn that food processors add to soft drinks, candy, bread, and a huge variety of other products. Most HFCS is little more than liquid sugar; it's made up of roughly equal parts of the simple sugars glucose and fructose—same as table sugar (which is usually extracted from sugar cane or sugar beet). Some researchers have pointed out that the glucose and fructose in HFCS break apart faster during digestion, but so far, there's no proof

that it poses a unique health threat. Of course, consuming too much HFCS or sugar can make you gain weight and raise your risk for diabetes, heart disease, and many other conditions. Enjoy sweets and sugary foods and drinks in moderation.

☐ **TEA**

Should I switch to green tea?

If you enjoy the mild, grassy flavor, why not? If not, keep sipping the black brew; it has important health benefits, too.

Green, black, and oolong tea all come from the same plant. (Leaves used to make green tea undergo lighter processing than those used for other varieties.) All tea is an excellent source of antioxidant compounds called catechins. Laboratory studies show that one catechin in particular—called epigallocatechin-3-gallate, or EGCG— has 25 to 100 times more antioxidant activity than vitamin C and appears to block the formation of cancer tumors. Green tea has up to 7 times more

EGCG than black tea, on average. Although research in humans has yielded mixed results, one preliminary study found that men who took 600 milligrams of green tea catechins (equal to several cups of green tea) a day for a year were 9 times less likely to develop prostate cancer.

Despite having less EGCG, black tea also appears to fight disease. For example, one analysis of 17 studies found that people who sip any sort of non-herbal tea up to three times a day enjoy an 11 percent drop in their risk for heart attacks. Scientists still have much to learn about tea, but it seems that sipping a few cups of green or black every day just might be a soothing way to improve your health.

□ TRANS FATS

How do I know if a food contains trans fat?

Read the label—carefully. Food processors in the United States can claim that a product has no trans fat as long as it contains less than 0.5 gram per serving of this dangerous stuff, which raises the risk for heart attacks.

You should consume less than 2 grams of trans fat daily, according to the American Heart Association. To spot hidden trans fat, scan ingredient lists for the words "partially hydrogenated" and "shortening."

If you're eating out, you may need to ask your server (and trust his or her word) to find out whether a menu item contains trans fat. French fries may be the most frequent offender, but a long list of other favorites at fast-food eateries and other restaurants can contain these fats, including onion rings, doughnuts, Buffalo wings, and fried seafood.

□ VEGETABLES

Are frozen and canned vegetables as good as fresh?

The fresh produce at your grocer is no healthier than frozen or canned, as a rule. That's largely because produce often travels thousands of miles to reach your supermarket, where it might continue to sit for days. So it's not that fresh after all. All that exposure to air and light robs produce of nutritional value. Fresh peas, for instance, lose 50 percent of their vitamin C within 2 days. By comparison, food processors pick vegetables at their peak of ripeness. They briefly blanch them in hot water, which leaches some vitamins, but freezing and canning halts the process and locks in nutrients. In fact, canned vegetables can sit in your cupboard for months and still retain 85 percent or more of their vitamin C.

So if frozen or canned veggies are cheaper or more convenient, don't worry about shortchanging your health. Of course, if you have access to a farm stand or green market where you can buy produce picked on the same day, that's your best bet. Once you get it home, lightly steam vegetables instead of boiling them to retain the most nutrients.

Do raw vegetables contain more nutrients than cooked ones?

It depends on the vegetable and the nutrient. Cooking actually boosts nutrient levels of some vegetables. For instance, cooked tomatoes contain far more of the antioxidant lycopene than raw tomatoes do. Likewise, cooked carrots contain significantly more beta-carotene than raw carrots do. On the other hand, heat does rob fresh produce of some nutrients, especially vitamins that dissolve in water, such as

AVOID THIS MISTAKE

Only Drinking Bottled Tea

Iced tea is nice, but studies show that hot brewed tea contains far more antioxidants than instant powders or bottled tea.

vitamin C, vitamin B₆, and folate.

The best strategy is probably to enjoy your vegetables both ways, eating baby carrots as snacks and cooking them as a dinner side dish, for example. Steaming or microwaving is a good way to cook vegetables and retain their nutrients.

Should I spend more for organic produce? Is it really better for me?

It's a personal choice. There's no clear evidence that organic fruit and vegetables are more nutritious than conventional produce. Some studies show that organic fruit and vegetables have higher levels of antioxidants, for example, but

many others have found no difference. Conventional produce does often have traces of herbicides and pesticides, which are not used in organic farming. But it's debatable whether minute amounts of these agricultural chemicals pose a major health threat. You may feel that organic fruits and vegetables taste better, but consumers can't tell the difference in side-by-side comparisons.

☐ WATER

What's healthier: tap water or bottled water?

It's a toss-up, though you may be better off going with the flow from your faucets. Companies that sell bottled water label their products with

images of pristine glaciers and mountain streams. Yet the Natural Resources Defense Council (an environmental watchdog group) tested 1,000 samples of bottled water and determined that their contents were no more pure or safe than tap water. In fact, they found that roughly one-quarter were simply bottled municipal water, which may or may not have been filtered.

Municipal water is generally safe, but occasionally contaminants find their way into the supply. The same is true of bottled water. Scientists at Texas Southern University analyzed the purity of 35 different brands of bottled water and found that four were laced with bacteria. On the other hand, bottled water is far less likely than tap water to contain added fluoride, which fights dental cavities. Another emerging area of concern may tip your preference to tap: Plastic bottles and caps contain substances known as phthalates, which disrupt healthy hormone function and have been linked to infertility, obesity, and a variety of health problems.

 WHAT YOU DON'T KNOW

Some Produce Is "Dirtier" Than Others

You may want to eat organic produce but balk at the prices. Solution: Be choosy. The Environmental Working Group (EWG), a watchdog agency, measured the pesticide residue on common conventionally grown fruits and vegetables and found that this "dirty dozen" carries the most contaminants:

Fruit: Peaches, apples, nectarines, strawberries, cherries, imported grapes, and pears

Vegetables: Sweet bell peppers, celery, kale, lettuce, and carrots

Buying organic versions of these fruits and vegetables could cut your exposure to pesticides by up to 80 percent, according to EWG.

☐ WEIGHT LOSS

Will eating breakfast every day help me lose weight?

Yes, eating the morning meal can actually help you shed pounds. People who have

FACT OR FICTION

Bedtime Snacks Make You Fat

Fiction. But that's not permission to nosh on cookies every night before turning in. Consuming more calories than you burn through physical activity produces belly rolls and flabby thighs no matter what time you overeat. A habit of snacking in front of the television every evening will lead to weight gain, but no more so than having a six-egg omelet for breakfast or vanquishing a bag of jelly beans at your desk every afternoon.

breakfast are less likely to eat diet-busting junk food and are more likely to exercise later in the day, studies show. People who skip breakfast, on the other hand, usually make up the calories—and then some—before day's end. Researchers found that 78 percent of the men and women included in the National Weight Control Registry—who have maintained an average weight loss of 66 pounds for more than 5 years—eat breakfast every day.

Is "grazing" really healthier than eating three square meals a day?

Eating many small meals throughout the day is probably no better for you than the traditional scheme of breakfast, lunch, and dinner. The idea that "grazing" is healthier comes from a few old studies showing that eating frequent meals throughout the day may burn more fat and lower insulin levels. But later studies have found no benefit to grazing. It's no healthier than eating three squares, according to the American Dietetic Association.

I've always eaten most of my calories at dinner. If I'm healthy, is there any reason not to keep doing this?

Hard to say. Intuitively, it sounds like a bad idea. Yet "one-mealers" tend to eat less food overall, scientists say, so your dining habit may actually help you stay trim. On the other hand, one small, brief study by USDA scientists found that eating just one daily meal may cause small increases in blood pressure, blood sugar, and cholesterol. If your annual blood tests show a rise in any key risk factors for heart disease or diabetes, you may want to reconsider your meal strategy.

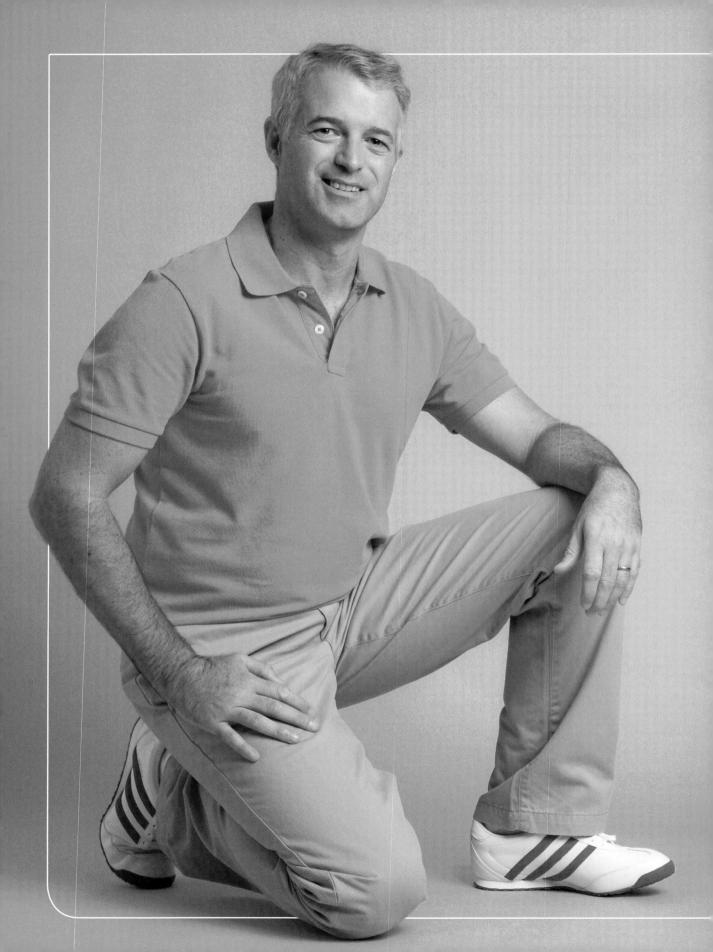

PART TWO

Drugs & Supplements

Over-the-Counter Drugs
From antacids to aspirin, cold medicines to cold sore creams, what to choose, warnings to heed, and when to save your money. Plus: Are store brands safe?

Prescription Drugs
Are sleeping pills addictive? Why do I need two different blood pressure medicines? How can I get off my antidepressant? Plus: Dangerous drugs for seniors.

Vitamins, Herbs, and Other Supplements
From beta-carotene to zinc: What works, what doesn't, and how to use it like the pros to get healthy and stay healthy.

FAQ Frequently Asked Questions
Over-the-Counter Drugs

Do I really have to throw out remedies that have passed their expiration date?

The date on the package shows how long the manufacturer can guarantee full potency. But if you've stored your over-the-counter (OTC) drugs in a cool, dry spot, they'll probably retain potency well past that date—at least 6 months and, in some cases, up to 15 years past, according to shelf-life tests conducted for the U.S. military. (If you store your meds in a hot and humid bathroom medicine cabinet, though, they'll deteriorate faster.) The biggest price you'll likely pay for using an expired over-the-counter drug is that it won't work quite as well.

If it's important to you that your medicine be at its full potency, toss the old stuff if it's more than a few months past the "use by" date and replace it. And outdated or not, toss a medicine if the color, texture, or consistency has changed (for example, if tablets begin to crumble); if it has a strong odor not present when you first bought it (outdated aspirin may have a strong vinegary smell); or if the appearance has changed in any other way (for example, if an ointment has separated or a liquid has crystallized or has particles floating in it).

Where is the best place to store my medicines?

In a cool, dark, dry spot such as the linen closet or a kitchen cabinet. Keep all over-the-counter meds in their original containers and be sure they're closed securely. Skip the bathroom medicine cabinet because steamy showers create heat and moisture that can degrade a drug's active ingredients. If kids or grand-kids frequent your house, be sure medicines are also out of reach and out of sight. Storing them in a box on a high shelf is a good idea in that case.

Are store brands as good as brand names?

Yes. Store brands and lower-priced, lesser-known brands don't get the prime spots on drugstore shelves that well-known brand-name products command, but they contain the same active ingredients and are just as tightly regulated to ensure safety and effectiveness. Consumer groups say there's little difference between them except the price. Some are even made in the same factories. If you're making the switch, compare big-name and store-brand or off-brand labels to be sure you're getting the same active ingredients at the same strength.

I find childproof caps impossible to open. What can I do?

Check the shelves for a version of the OTC products you use that doesn't have a child-resistant cap; the law allows one package size of every drugstore remedy to be sold with an easier-to-open lid. If you don't see it on the shelf, ask the pharmacist. And be smart about storing these drugs where kids can't see or reach them; medicines are the top cause of accidental poisonings in children.

Should I use my child's or grandchild's age or weight when deciding on the dose of an OTC drug?

Weight. Children of the same age can vary in body weight by 10, 20, 30 pounds or more, so using a child's age could lead you to give her too much or too little medicine. If there are no by-weight doses listed, call your doctor or check with your pharmacist before deciding on a dose.

I'm in my seventies. Do I have to be careful about which OTC meds I take?

Yes. Drugstore remedies for colds, allergies, insomnia, and heartburn can raise the risk for confusion, falls, blood pressure changes, and other problems in older people.

After about age 65, the body changes in ways that can alter how drugs affect you. For instance, your liver and kidneys, which process drugs, become less efficient; this can mean that drugs stay in your system longer. You lose muscle mass and gain body fat, which also makes some medicines hang around longer. You have less of a brain chemical called acetylcholine, and certain drugs, especially antihistamines and over-the-counter sleeping pills, depress these levels further. This can lead to slower reaction times, trouble paying attention, and some loss of short-term memory. It may also make you feel dizzy and cause blurred vision, dry mouth, constipation, and urinary problems.

If you've become more prone to gastrointestinal issues as you age, watch out for antacids, too. Those that contain aluminum or calcium may lead to constipation, while those that contain magnesium could trigger diarrhea and dehydration.

AVOID THIS MISTAKE

Taking an OTC Remedy Without Reading the Label

When it comes to over-the-counter drugs, many people have a blasé attitude, thinking "They can't really hurt me, right?" Wrong. Plenty of people end up with serious health problems from accidentally taking too much of an over-the-counter drug (such as a painkiller), overusing drugs such as laxatives or acid blockers, or taking something that interferes with another medication they're on. No matter how innocuous a drug may seem, it's *always* smart to read the label. It might surprise you.

Over-the-Counter Drugs

☐ ALERTNESS PILLS

Are "stay-awake" pills like NoDoz and Vivarin any more effective than a cup of coffee?

Most of these pills get their oomph from caffeine just like coffee and cola do. But with about 200 milligrams of caffeine per tablet, they contain almost twice as much as you'd get from a typical 8-ounce cup of brewed coffee and three times more than most instant coffees, teas, or cola drinks.

Don't make the mistake of washing these pills down with caffeinated soda or also drinking caffeinated coffee. Getting 300 milligrams or more of caffeine at one time, the amount in an OTC stimulant plus a cup of coffee, could induce "caffeine intoxication." A mild case will simply make you feel jittery and anxious, but you could also be in for a racing heart and a case of diarrhea, not to mention some killer insomnia.

☐ ALLERGY MEDICINES

Do nondrowsy allergy medicines work as well as the older kinds?

They're safer because they don't make you as sleepy, but alas, they're not as effective. Research suggests that the older antihistamines such as brompheniramine (Dimetapp) and diphenhydramine (Benadryl) dry up runny noses and stop sneezes better than newer drugs. But up to 35 percent of people who use older antihistamines become sleepy and can't concentrate after taking one—a situation that could be dangerous if you're driving or operating any kind of machinery. In one study, people who took one of these drugs and then took a simulated driving test drove as if they were drunk; newer nondrowsy antihistamines had little or no effect.

Most allergists recommend using nondrowsy antihistamines

such as loratadine (Claritin), fexofenadine (Allegra), or cetirizine HCl (Zyrtec) first. Take them before you're exposed to allergens—such as just before visiting a home with a pet that makes you sneeze—for best effect. If you need more relief, use the older, stronger drugs only if you won't put yourself or others in danger should you become drowsy.

Do OTC antihistamines work as well as prescription ones?

Yes. In fact, several OTC antihistamines, including loratadine (Claritin) and cetirizine HCl (Zyrtec), started out as prescription drugs. If you have frequent allergy symptoms and an antihistamine isn't enough, however, it may be time for a prescription drug such as a steroid nasal spray. Used on an ongoing basis, these sprays reduce inflammation and are the most effective fix for five major allergy symptoms: sneezing, runny nose, congestion, itchy nasal passages, and itchy, watery eyes, according to researchers from the University of Sydney, Australia, who recently reviewed dozens of drug studies.

I'm pregnant. Is it okay to take an antihistamine?

Talk with your doctor before taking any antihistamines during pregnancy, and try drug-free allergy fixes first, such as doing all you can to avoid your allergy triggers and using a saltwater nasal rinse. While animal studies suggest that some antihistamines may not be risky for a developing fetus, there are virtually no human studies of the effects these drugs may have on a baby, or mother, during pregnancy.

According to the American College of Asthma, Allergy, and Immunology, the over-the-counter antihistamines chlorpheniramine (Chlor-Trimeton) and diphenhydramine (Benadryl) have been used during pregnancy "with reassuring animal studies" but can cause drowsiness. The newer, less-sedating antihistamines loratadine (Claritin) and cetirizine HCl (Zyrtec) may be a better choice because they're less sedating and also don't seem to trigger fetal problems in animal studies.

□ ANTACIDS
How often can I safely take antacids?

If you follow the package directions, it's generally safe to take an OTC antacid for up to 2 weeks. If the burning pain persists, it's time to talk with your doctor about lifestyle changes and other medications to help control and stop the causes of heartburn.

In the meantime, there are a few caveats about OTC antacids. If you use a calcium carbonate–based antacid, such as Tums, be sure your total daily calcium intake from supplements is close to the 1,000 to 1,200 milligrams recommended for bone health; don't exceed a safe upper limit of 2,500 milligrams a day. A single antacid tablet may contain 400 milligrams of calcium, so you may have to skip or cut down on any calcium supplements you're taking. Getting too much calcium from supplements can, over time, lead to

WHAT YOU DON'T KNOW
Certain Antacids Work Better Than Others

You'll get better results if you choose an antacid that contains an ingredient called alginic acid. It creates a foamy barrier in your stomach that can prevent stomach acid from backwashing. Baylor College of Medicine researchers who reviewed ten clinical trials report that antacids with this ingredient eased mild heartburn by 60 percent, while antacids without it reduced symptoms by just 11 percent.

an overdose condition called hypercalcemia that can harm your kidneys.

Check the sodium content, too. Some antacids contain 500 milligrams or more of sodium in each dose, nearly one-fourth of the total sodium you should get in a day. If you're trying to control your sodium intake, choose low-sodium versions.

Are newer acid-stopping drugs better than regular antacids?

They're more effective—but they aren't risk-free. Taken a half-hour before a meal, acid-stopping H2 blockers such as cimetidine (Tagamet HB), famotidine (Pepcid AC), nizatidine (Axid AR), and ranitidine (Zantac 75) help about half of all people with heartburn symptoms. These drugs are good for immediate relief of symptoms, but for longer-term control, acid suppressors called proton-pump inhibitors (PPIs) work better. They include over-the-counter omeprazole (Prilosec OTC). PPIs completely shut down production of stomach acid and are often prescribed in the treatment of serious heartburn, called gastroesophageal reflux disease, so that tissue in your throat, damaged by stomach acids, can heal.

Don't use H2 blockers or proton-pump inhibitors for more

Taking Sedatives if You Have Heartburn

People who took prescription drugs called benzodiazepines (Valium, Xanax, Halcion) to fall asleep were 50 percent more likely to have heartburn at night than those who didn't in one large survey. Other research has shown that these prescription antianxiety drugs loosen up the lower esophageal sphincter, the ring of muscle that keeps stomach acid where it belongs.

than 14 days without talking with your doctor. Even over-the-counter versions can cause serious side effects. For example, in one study, H2 blockers increased the risk for dementia 2.4 times in people over age 65 who used the drugs continuously for at least 2 years. Users of H2 blockers and of PPIs were 4.5 times more likely to have a vitamin B_6 deficiency than nonusers, presumably because decreasing stomach acid lowers absorption. (Vitamin B_6 is necessary for the formation of red blood cells, which deliver oxygen to every cell in your body.) Long-term use of PPIs can raise your risk for pneumonia. And in one recent study, risk for hip fractures was 30 percent higher in people who used PPIs for 2 years or more and 18 percent higher for those who used H2 blockers for 2 years or more. Research suggests that PPIs may interfere with the ability of bones to absorb calcium.

☐ **ANTIBIOTIC OINTMENTS**

I have a cut. Should I use an antibiotic ointment on it?

Yes. Antibiotic ointments prevent bacteria that are always present on the surface of your skin from infecting a cut or wound. Research suggests that bacteria-fighting ingredients in the ointments, plus the presence of the ointment itself, both seem to help. In one study, just 5 percent of wounds treated with an antibiotic ointment became infected compared to 18 percent that were covered with petroleum jelly. It's possible that ointments (but not creams or gels) help in another way, too, by protecting broken skin so that cells can more easily form connections necessary for growing new skin.

☐ ATHLETE'S FOOT ANTIFUNGAL PRODUCTS

Does it matter whether I use a powder, cream, gel, or spray for my athlete's foot?

No. In the battle against tinea, the family of stubborn fungi responsible for athlete's foot as well as jock itch, the active ingredient in your antifungal product seems to make a bigger difference than the form that the product takes. When researchers reviewed 72 studies of the effectiveness of creams, gels, sprays, powders, and lotions, they found that all were effective, but some seemed to work better than others. Those containing the active ingredient terbinafine (Lamisil AT) cured about 70 percent of athlete's foot infections; products containing tolnaftate (Tinactin, Aftate) knocked out about 64 percent;

and those containing miconazole (Micatin) cleared up about 47 percent.

How long should I use an athlete's foot product?

As long as the label directions tell you to, if not longer. The shortest-acting over-the-counter antifungal ingredient, terbinafine (Lamisil AT) can clear up an infection in as little as 1 week. Other types may require 2 to 4 weeks. But you might want to use them longer to prevent a repeat infection because athlete's foot comes back about 70 percent of the time. (Remember, the fungus responsible for athlete's foot thrives not only on the floors of locker rooms but also on the decks around pools, on your bathroom floor and tub or shower if someone in your house has athlete's foot—and even in your shoes if you've

had an infection.) In one small study of 16 athletes who used miconazole (Micadin) spray powder on one foot daily for 3 weeks, researchers found that their untreated feet showed significantly more fungus than the treated feet. There doesn't seem to be any harm in using these products long-term.

Using an antifungal on your feet daily is also a good idea if you have a toenail infection, which is usually caused by the same type of fungi that causes athlete's foot. In a study of 2,761 people with nail fungus, researchers found that 1 in 3 also had athlete's foot.

☐ COLD SORE CREAMS

Do drugstore cold sore creams work?

Whether over-the-counter or prescription, topical cold sore products just don't work very well. You're much better off with a prescription antiviral tablet such as valacyclovir (Valtrex), which can prevent a cold sore from forming if you take one as soon as you get that tingly, burning feeling that means one is on the way. (If you frequently get cold sores, your doctor might have you use one of these drugs daily for prevention).

If you feel a cold sore coming on and don't have a prescription pill on hand, an OTC cream may

FACT OR FICTION

Cuts Should Be Washed with Hydrogen Peroxide

Fiction. Leave that brown bottle on the shelf and clean cuts and scrapes with running water instead, then apply an antibiotic ointment. Peroxide does kill bacteria that may have invaded a cut, but it also knocks off cells working hard to knit your skin back together. In one study, wounds treated with hydrogen peroxide healed more slowly than those treated with an antibiotic ointment or with an ointment that didn't contain any germ-fighting ingredients.

continued on page 104

Drug Interactions to Watch For

Your best protection against OTC drug reactions and interactions is simply to read the label—carefully. Note any warnings that apply to you, and take the drug as directed. Stick with the right dose at the right time, and follow any advice on whether you should take it with or without food or should avoid the drug at certain times of day. Don't exceed the maximum daily dose recommended on the bottle unless your doctor explicitly tells you to. It's also wise to be aware of some common interactions between frequently used OTC medications and other drugs, food, alcohol, and supplements. Below are some examples.

ALERTNESS DRUGS

Drug: Energy and stay-awake remedies containing caffeine

Interactions

Can cause jitteriness, insomnia, irritability, and rapid heartbeat if taken along with coffee, tea, or other drinks containing caffeine. The antibiotics ciprofloxacin (Cipro) and norfloxacin (Noroxin) can magnify caffeine's effects by interfering with its breakdown in your body. Caffeine can increase levels of the bronchodilator drug theophylline (Theo-24, Uniphyl) in your bloodstream and lead to nausea, vomiting, and heart palpitations.

ANTIHISTAMINES

Drug: Brompheniramine, chlorpheniramine, dimenhydrinate, diphenhydramine, doxylamine

Interactions

Increases the sedating effects of sleeping pills, sedatives, muscle relaxants, and antianxiety drugs, such as alprazolam (Xanax), diazepam (Valium), lorazepam (Ativan), and temazepam (Restoril).

COUGH MEDICINES

Drug: Dextromethorphan

Interactions

Do not take within 2 weeks of using antidepressants called monoamine oxidase (MAO) inhibitors such as isocarboxazid (Marplan), phenelzine sulfate (Nardil), or tranylcypromine sulfate (Parnate). The combination can cause "serotonin syndrome," which involves agitation, fever, and sweating. Can make you dangerously drowsy if you also drink alcohol. Boosts the sedative effect of tranquilizers, sedatives, and sleeping pills.

DECONGESTANTS

Drug: Pseudoephedrine

Interactions

Do not take within 2 weeks of using antidepressants called monoamine oxidase (MAO) inhibitors such as isocarboxazid (Marplan), phenelzine sulfate (Nardil), or tranylcypromine sulfate (Parnate). The combination can increase blood pressure to dangerous levels. Reduces the effectiveness of blood pressure–lowering drugs. Can increase anxiety, nervousness, and insomnia if you're taking stimulant diet pills.

HEARTBURN MEDICATIONS

Drug: Calcium carbonate antacids

Interactions

Don't take within 1 to 2 hours of other medicines, especially some antibiotics like tetracycline and quinolones, osteoporosis drugs called bisphosphonates (Fosamax, Boniva, Actonel, Reclast), and the thyroid hormone drug levothyroxine (Synthroid).

Drug: H2 blockers

Interactions

These drugs, including cimetidine (Tagamet), ranitidine (Zantac), and famotidine (Pepcid), may increase or decrease levels of many drugs in your bloodstream. Talk to your doctor if you take antifungal drugs such as ketoconazole (Nizoral), the antibiotic amoxicillin (Augmentin), benzodiazepine tranquilizers, beta blockers such as propranolol (Inderal), calcium channel blockers such as diltiazem (Cardizem CD), the heart drug digoxin (Lanoxin, Digitek), morphine-based pain relievers, the antiseizure drug phenytoin (Dilantin), the antimalaria drug quinine, the asthma drug theophylline, or the blood thinner warfarin (Coumadin). May also decrease the absorption of calcium.

Drug: Proton-pump inhibitors

Interactions
Can increase levels of the blood thinner warfarin (Coumadin), the antianxiety drug diazepam (Valium), the immune-suppressing drug tacrolimus (Prograf). Can reduce levels of atazanavir (Reyataz) and reduce absorption of oral antifungal drugs ketoconazole (Nizoral) and itraconazole (Sporanox).

MOTION SICKNESS DRUGS

Drug: Dimenhydrinate, diphenhydramine, mezicline

Interactions
Drinking alcohol could increase these drugs' sedative effects. Taking antihistamines could reduce absorption of the drugs.

NICOTINE REPLACEMENT PRODUCTS

Drug: Nicotine

Interactions
Nicotine in gums, patches, or sprays may alter the way your body metabolizes some antidepressants or asthma drugs. Ask your doctor if your dose of those drugs needs to be adjusted.

PAIN RELIEVERS

Drug: Acetaminophen

Interactions
Can lead to liver damage or liver failure if you also drink 3 or more alcoholic drinks per day. Can increase risk for liver damage if you also take the antibiotics rifampin (Rifadin, Rimactane) or isoniazid (INH).

Drug: Nonsteroidal anti-inflammatory drugs (NSAIDs) including aspirin, ibuprofen, ketoprofen, and naproxen

Interactions
Taking more than one type of NSAID or an NSAID plus a corticosteroid can increase your risk for gastrointestinal bleeding and ulcers. Using aspirin plus ibuprofen or naproxen can cancel out the clot-reducing benefits of aspirin. Can increase blood-thinning effect of warfarin (Coumadin). Can increase levels of drugs to suppress the immune system, such as cyclosporine (Neoral, Sandimmune), heart medications such as digoxin (Lanoxin, Digitek), and the anticancer drug methotrexate (Trexall). Can decrease the effectiveness of diuretics used to treat water retention and high blood pressure, as well as other high blood pressure drugs, including beta blockers, ACE inhibitors, vasodilators, central alpha-2 agonists, peripheral alpha-1 blockers, and angiotensin receptor blockers. Aspirin can increase levels of the antiseizure drugs phenytoin (Dilantin) and valproic acid (Depakene).

If you take lithium, talk to your doctor before using NSAIDs; they can increase lithium levels in the bloodstream.

be slightly better than doing nothing. Products containing docosanol (Abreva) healed cold sores about 18 hours sooner than a cream with no active ingredients in one study—but the users had to apply the cream five times a day. Docosanol seems to work by preventing the herpes virus responsible for cold sores from fusing with cell walls, which stops it from entering cells and replicating.

Creams containing an extract of the herb *Melissa officinalis*, also known as lemon balm, may also help a little, but again, this means just a little. In one German study, lemon balm speeded healing and eased stinging and itching slightly when compared to a placebo cream. Skip creams containing salicylic acid, which can damage your skin and slow healing.

☐ COUGH AND COLD MEDICINES

There are so many different cough medicines on the shelf. How do I know which one to take?

It might not matter, since it turns out that these elixirs really don't offer much relief anyway. Classic cough-suppressing ingredients such as dextromethorphan and diphenhydramine have little power to squelch the hacking, it turns

DRUG-FREE FIX

Lip Balm with Sunscreen

Ultraviolet (UV) rays from the sun can trigger a new cold sore by activating herpes virus particles. Using a lip balm with a sunscreen can solve the problem. In one study of 38 cold sore–prone people, those who wore a sun-blocking lip balm had no outbreaks after exposure to UV light; 71 percent of those who used a fake cream got cold sores.

out. British scientists who reviewed 15 studies of cough remedies concluded in 2002 that "there is no good evidence for their effectiveness." And when the American College of Chest Physicians reviewed studies of nearly a dozen cough medicine ingredients in 2006, the group recommended against their use for coughs due to colds and upper respiratory tract infections for the same reason—they don't really work.

If your cough is caused by postnasal drip, consider taking a decongestant and an antihistamine to dry things up, which should help.

Which cough medicines can I give my child?

None. Very serious side effects of an overdose, though rare, include convulsions, rapid heart rate, loss of consciousness, and even death. In the United States, cough and cold remedies now carry warnings that children under age 4 should not

take them, but experts suggest that parents skip these medications in children under the age of 6. The American College of Chest Physicians recommends avoiding using them in kids younger than age 14.

The medicines aren't worth the risk, especially since they don't work very well. "No medication available in the United States has been shown to effectively treat cough in children," noted doctors who reviewed 38 studies of cough and cold remedies. In one study of 100 kids ages 2 to 18 with upper respiratory infections, remedies with the active ingredients dextromethorphan and diphenhydramine were no better than a placebo at stopping nighttime coughing.

When I have a bad cold with lots of symptoms, don't I want a product that contains the whole works?

Multi-symptom products pack lots of active ingredients into a

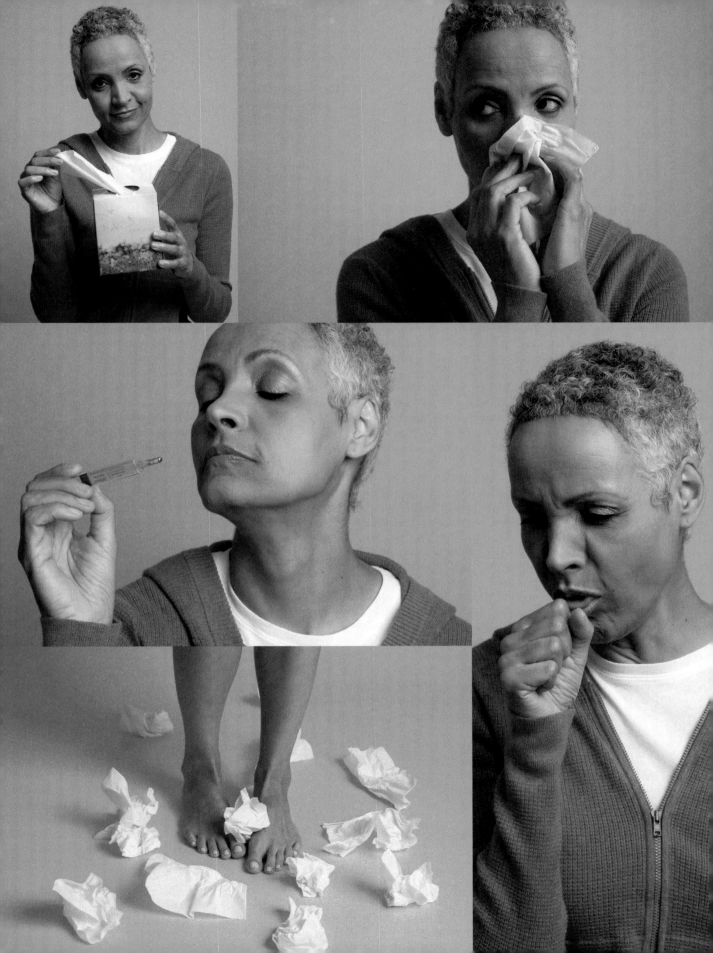

single dose in order to dry up congestion, open clogged sinuses, cool off a fever, soothe a sore throat, and stop coughs. One problem with the products is that they contain ingredients you don't need if you don't have all the symptoms. A bigger problem is that unless you read the ingredient list, you may accidentally overdose on certain ingredients. For instance, if you don't realize that a remedy contains acetaminophen, you'll overdose if you also take acetaminophen separately. Getting even a little too much of this pain reliever raises your risk for liver damage.

You might also swallow ingredients that you shouldn't take. For instance, the product may contain a decongestant, which you should avoid if you have high blood pressure or heart disease, or an expectorant, which could worsen asthma or emphysema.

Focus instead on taking exactly what you need for your symptoms. A decongestant can help you breathe easier, and if your throat is sore, take a separate pain reliever. If you do choose a combination product, make sure its intended only for the symptoms you have, and don't take additional remedies along with it.

I heard you can get high on cough syrup. How do I know if my teen is doing it?

Taking high doses of cough syrups containing dextromethorphan (DXM for short) is a form of drug abuse sometimes called robotripping or dexing. Overdose can cause blurred vision, itching, sweating, fever, high blood pressure, diarrhea, hallucinations, seizures, coma, and death. Abusers may become violent or disoriented—one teen high on DXM died when he tried to cross a busy highway.

DXM is found in more than 100 over-the-counter cough and cold remedies. While some states and counties have banned the sale of these products to people under the age of 18, an estimated one in ten teens has used DXM to get high. And cough syrups containing it, such as some Robitussin, Sudafed, and Tylenol products, are among the top five drugs teens steal from their parents according to the Partnership for a Drug-Free America.

Be on the lookout for any symptoms of overdose as well as empty cough medicine boxes or bottles in the trash, boxes or bottles missing from the medicine cabinet, signs that your child is visiting pro-DXM websites with information on how to abuse this drug, declining grades, a change in behavior and attitude, missing household money, and unusual chemical or medicinal smells in his or her room. You may also hear your child talking with friends about the drug using names such as CCC (triple C), Dex, DM, Red Devils, Drex, Robo, Skittles, Velvet, and Vitamin D.

Can I take a decongestant if I have high blood pressure, glaucoma, or an enlarged prostate?

If you have high blood pressure or an enlarged prostate,

DRUG-FREE FIX

A Spoonful of Honey

One teaspoon at bedtime made coughs less severe, less frequent, and less bothersome in one study of 105 kids and teens, ages 2 to 18. The American Academy of Pediatrics recommends ½ teaspoon of honey for children ages 2 to 5 years, 1 teaspoon for children ages 6 to 11 years, and 2 teaspoons for children 12 years and older. Honey not only coats and soothes the throat but also discourages the growth of bacteria. Caution: Never give honey to a child under the age of 1; it may contain botulism spores that young digestive systems can't destroy.

no. Pills, syrups, and even nasal sprays containing the decongestants pseudoephedrine, phenylephrine, or oxymetazoline work by constricting blood vessels, which is great for relieving a stuffy nose but also temporarily increases your blood pressure. You should avoid them if you have high blood pressure or a heart arrhythmia or have had a heart attack or stroke. Because they may cause water retention, also avoid them if you're having trouble with an enlarged prostate.

In addition to constricting blood vessels, decongestants also increase the pressure of the fluid within the eyes. They appear safe for people with the most common type of glaucoma, called primary open-angle glaucoma, but avoid them if you have narrow-angle glaucoma, in which the pressure of fluid in the eyes can rise dramatically, causing pain and even blindness if not treated immediately.

Talk with your doctor before using decongestants if you have diabetes because these remedies may raise blood sugar. The same applies if you get migraines (tightening blood vessels may trigger a headache) or have hyperthroidism, in which the body produces too much thyroid hormone (the active ingredients may raise your blood pressure, which may already be elevated). There's also some evidence that people with underactive

DRUG-FREE FIX

A Homemade Saline Solution

When researchers from England's Royal National Throat, Nose, and Ear Hospital reviewed eight studies on methods of preventing sinus infections, they concluded that a daily saline rinse cuts risk for chronic sinus infections by up to 72 percent. You can buy ready-made saline or make your own by mixing ½ teaspoon salt, ½ teaspoon baking soda, and 16 ounces warm tap water. Fill a clean ear bulb syringe, a neti pot (available in health food stores), or a Waterpik fitted with a special nasal adaptor. Lean over a sink with your head turned to the right and gently flush your left nostril with 8 ounces of saline. The water will drain out your right nostril. Gently blow your nose, then repeat with the other nostril.

thyroid (hypothyroidism) may become extra-sensitive to the stimulating effects of some decongestants.

Which decongestants will keep me awake at night and which won't?

Pills containing pseudoephedrine (found in Sudafed, Drixoral, Triaminic AM Decongestant Syrup) work best for fighting congestion but are also the most likely to keep you awake. If you use one, try to do it early in the day so that the effects can wear off before bedtime. (You'll have to ask for drugs containing pseudoephedrine at the pharmacy counter; by law they must be kept behind the counter to stop their use in the production of the illegal drug

methamphetamine.) While "nighttime" decongestants in pill form promise a good night's sleep, they contain a less effective decongestant called phenylephrine (found in Sudafed PE and others), that keeps noses open for only a few hours. If you need something before bed, you're better off with a decongestant nasal spray containing oxymetazoline (Afrin). These are less likely than oral drugs to keep you awake because very little of the drug is absorbed into your bloodstream.

If I have a runny nose from a cold, am I better off drying it up or letting it go?

Go ahead and make yourself comfortable. Congestion and a

runny nose are side effects of your body's efforts to fight off the viral infections that cause colds and flu. Reversing them with a decongestant won't slow down healing and may in fact help you avoid complications like a sinus infection.

To unstuff your nose, decongestants containing pseudoephedrine are more effective than those containing phenylephrine. A British study of 283 women and men with stuffy noses found that those who took 60 milligrams of pseudoephedrine reported a 30 percent drop in congestion after just one dose. Products containing phenylephrine, which can't be used to make illegal stimulants, are available on drugstore shelves but aren't worth the money. At 10 milligrams, the legal U.S. dose, this ingredient simply won't open up a congested nose.

How long can I use a nasal spray to unstuff my nose?

Two to 3 days. Over-the-counter sprays containing phenylephrine (Neo-Synephrine) or oxymetazoline (Afrin, Dristan) shrink swollen blood vessels in the lining of your nose, allowing trapped mucus to drain. The good thing about the sprays is that they work almost instantaneously, and they won't keep you awake at night or cause other side effects typical of oral decon-

Single-Symptom Products Work Best

If you're going to use a decongestant, buy a product that's *just* a decongestant, not a multi-symptom remedy. Combination cold products for adults often contain less than 60 milligrams of pseudoephedrine, the recommended adult dose.

gestants. The downside is that, after 3 to 5 days, they can cause rebound congestion— the more you use them, the faster your nose gets stuffed up again after each spray, leading you to use more and more. To avoid this problem, some experts recommend using a spray for no more than 2 to 3 days at a time. Then stop for 3 days. If you're still congested, it's okay to use it again for 2 to 3 days.

☐ DIARRHEA REMEDIES

Is it better to use a diarrhea remedy or to let my body, um, "flush out" the problem?

Most of the time, it's better to simply drink lots of fluids to replenish what you're losing and otherwise let Nature take its course. Diarrhea medicines provide relief, but they can interfere with your body's efforts to rid itself of viruses and contaminated food, the two biggest reasons for sprints to the bathroom. Turning diarrhea off could trap the

organism causing it in your intestines, prolonging your discomfort. That said, if you're also suffering from cramps, you might opt for the relief. Be sure to call your doctor if diarrhea lasts for more than 2 days.

Use caution when giving diarrhea remedies to kids. Don't give remedies containing bismuth subsalicylate (Pepto-Bismol) to children under age 12 without consulting a doctor first, and check with a doctor before giving remedies containing loperamide (such as Imodium) to children under 6 or those who weigh less than 47 pounds.

Can taking Pepto-Bismol really prevent traveler's diarrhea?

It can reduce your risk dramatically. When you arrive at your destination, start taking two 262-milligram tablets or 2 ounces of a liquid antidiarrhea remedy containing bismuth subsalicylate (the stuff in Pepto-Bismol) four times a day. Doing so can lower your odds for developing Montezuma's Revenge by 60 to 85 percent.

The drug seems to work by preventing the bacteria from attaching to the lining of the intestines and by decreasing the amount of fluid in your intestines.

Note that bismuth subsalicylate can turn your tongue and your bowel movements black, and taking too much could cause ringing in your ears. Skip the pink stuff if you're pregnant, are allergic to aspirin, or if you take blood thinners such as warfarin (Coumadin), methotrexate (Rheumatrex, Trexall), or the gout drug probenecid (Benuryl).

Even if you use Pepto on the road, you'll still want to avoid contaminated water and food. Don't drink or brush your teeth with tap water, skip ice cubes in drinks, and stick with foods that are "peelable, packaged, purified, or piping hot."

☐ **DIET PILLS**

Do drugstore diet pills work? Are they safe?

There is only one FDA-approved over-the-counter weight-loss pill: Alli, a lower-strength version of the prescription drug orlistat (Xenical). Alli could help you lose a tiny bit of extra weight: Studies show that in a year, you could drop 3 more pounds than you would through diet and exercise alone. People who take it must also cut calories and get more exercise, the same recipe for weight loss that works without adding a drug.

Orlistat works by blocking the absorption of some of the fat you eat. The OTC version seems to stop about 25 percent of fat from being taken up. Thanks to all of that undigested fat moving through your digestive system, though, you may have side effects such as urgent bowel movements, diarrhea, and gas with oily spotting. In 2009, the FDA announced it would review reports of serious liver damage in 32 people taking orlistat.

Be very wary of other over-the-counter "diet pills." The FDA has found that many products hyped as "herbal" or "all natural" were illegally laced with hidden and potentially dangerous prescription drugs, such as sibutramine, an ingredient in a prescription-only weight-loss drug Meridia that can cause high blood pressure, seizures, fast heart rate, heart attacks, and strokes; rimonabant (found in Accompli), a drug not approved for sale in the United States that can cause depression, anxiety, and nausea; the antiseizure medicine phenytoin (found in Dilantin); the laxative compound phenolphthalein, a suspected cancer-causing substance; and the potent diuretic bumetanide (found in Bumex), which can increase the risk for depression and suicidal thoughts. Still other pills may contain the amphetamine fenproporex, which can cause chest pain, heart palpitations, headaches, and insomnia.

It's wise to avoid any OTC diet pill that promises easy weight loss, claims to be a miracle cure or a scientific breakthrough, uses impressive terms like *thermogenesis* or *hunger stimulation point*, or implies it's safe because it's "natural" or "herbal."

☐ **EYE DROPS**

I have eye allergies and OTC "allergy" eye drops barely work. What does?

Look for a brand that contains ketotifen (Zaditor, Alaway). Once sold only in prescription eye drops, ketotifen products became available over-the-counter in 2007. This ingredient acts as both an antihistamine, which quickly blocks the release

AVOID THIS MISTAKE

Taking an Antidiarrheal if You Have a Fever

Never treat yourself at home with a diarrhea remedy if you also have a fever or if there's blood or mucus in your bowel movements. These are signs of an infection and warrant a call to your doctor.

of itchy chemicals called histamines during an allergy attack, as well as a mast cell stabilizer, which prevents release of histamines for several hours. In a Harvard Medical School study of 89 allergy-sufferers with itchy eyes, drops containing ketotifen relieved itchiness in 15 minutes, and the effects lasted for 8 hours.

If newer OTC eye drops aren't helping, ask your doctor about a prescription version. These generally contain higher doses of active ingredients and are often more effective.

Avoid eye drops that contain decongestants. After 2 to 3 days, they can cause rebound redness that may continue even after you stop using them.

I have dry eyes, but the drops I tried only lasted a minute. Which last the longest?

Thicker eye drops, such as Systane, Liquigel, or Celluvisc. In research studies, these drops, which contain ingredients such as polyethylene glycol, propylene glycol, and carboxymethyl cellulose sodium, lasted on the eye for 20 to 30 minutes or longer before beginning to disintegrate. In contrast, thinner drops lasted for just a few minutes at most. Even thicker drops or gels are available for overnight use.

If you find yourself reaching for eye drops more than four times a day, consult your doctor. Dry eyes may simply be the result of staring at a computer screen for too long and not blinking often enough to replace your eyes' natural film of moistening, cleansing tears, but it could also be a sign of a medical problem such as rosacea or Sjögren's syndrome. Medications such as hormone replacement therapy and some blood pressure drugs, decongestants, and antidepressants can also be the cause. If dry eye won't quit, your doctor may recommend the prescription drug cyclosporine (Restasis), which decreases inflamma-

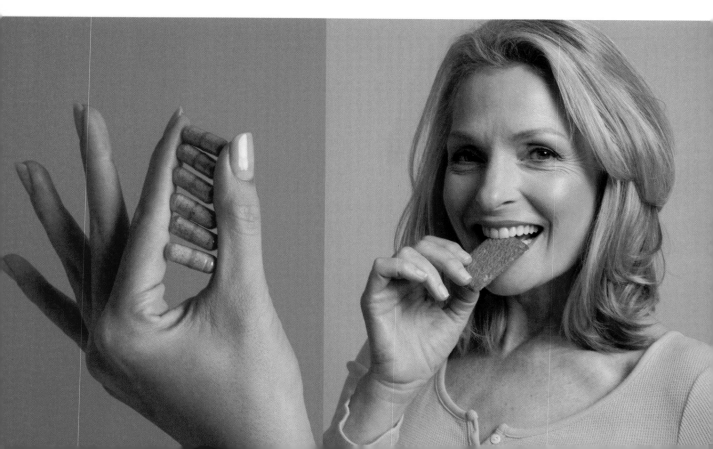

tion and can increase tear production. She may also suggest using tiny silicone plugs to block your tear ducts, so that the tears on the surface of your eyes don't drain away as quickly.

What form of fiber supplement is best—pills, wafers, or the type you mix with water?

They all work equally well—as long as you're also drinking enough water. Without water, fiber can't do its job, which is to help form larger, softer stools that are easier to pass. Taking fiber without drinking enough water may even do more harm than good by making you more constipated.

Note that "bulk-forming" laxative pills can get stuck in your throat or esophagus and begin to swell if you don't wash them down with enough water. If you have swallowing problems, opt for a powdered fiber supplement that you can mix with water.

Can I take a fiber supplement instead of eating a high-fiber diet?

If you do, you're shortchanging your health. A supplement will win you some of the fiber's benefits, such as better bowel regularity and healthier cholesterol levels. But getting fiber solely from supplements robs your body of hundreds of beneficial vitamins, minerals, and other nutrients found in high-fiber foods, like whole grains, fruits and vegetables, and beans, that reduce your risk of cancer, heart disease, and diabetes, among other diseases. Adding more of these foods to your diet also helps you cut your intake of saturated fat, which the body uses to make "bad" LDL cholesterol.

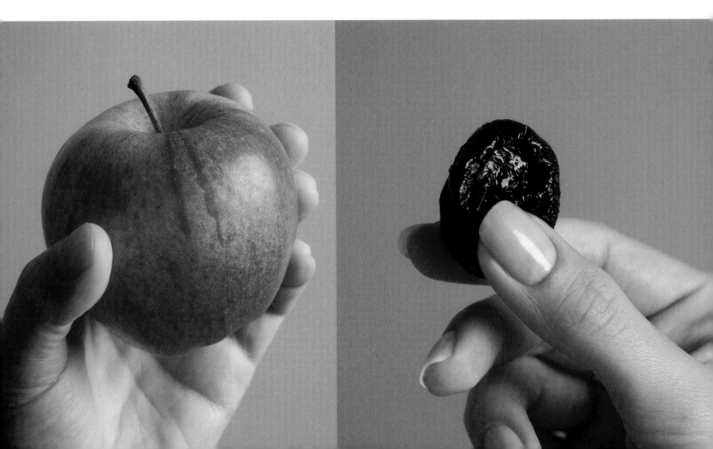

Will fiber supplements interfere with my medications?

It's possible. They can reduce or slow the absorption of many prescription drugs, including tricyclic antidepressants such as amitriptyline (Elavil), doxepin (Sinequan), and imipramine (Tofranil); diabetes medications such as glyburide (Diabeta) and metformin (Glucophage); the heart drug digoxin (Lanoxin, Digitek); cholesterol-lowering statins; lithium; and penicillin. To avoid potential problems, take any medications 1 to 2 hours before or 2 to 3 hours after you take a fiber supplement. Fiber does not seem to interfere with the absorption of multivitamins or calcium supplements.

☐ GAS REMEDIES

I get terrible flatulence. Do gas remedies work?

The problem with gas is that by the time you have it, it's too late to do anything about it. Once the gas bubbles are in your intestines, they need to come out. The only strategy that works is to stop the gas bubbles from forming, either by avoiding gas-producing foods like beans and cabbage (and any dairy foods if you are lactose intolerant) or by taking Beano, an enzyme you sprinkle on your first bite of food or take as a tablet before you dig in. This enzyme breaks down indigestible sugars in gassy foods so your body can digest them without embarrassing side effects.

Most other anti-gas remedies contain the active ingredients simethicone or activated charcoal. Simethicone (Gas-X, Mylanta Gas) can relieve abdominal pain due to gas but doesn't reduce gas production. And in one study, people who took activated charcoal after eating a gas-producing meal had the same quantity of intestinal gas as those who didn't.

☐ LAXATIVES

How often can I safely use a laxative?

"Bulk-forming" fiber supplements such as Citrucel, FiberCon, or Metamucil are the only laxatives that most people can safely use daily for weeks, months, or years. These laxatives contain soluble fiber that acts like a sponge in your intestines, soaking up water and increasing the size of your stools.

Bigger stools stimulate the muscular walls of your intestines to contract and move the stools along and out.

All of the other types of laxatives crowding drugstore shelves, including stimulants (Correctol, Dulcolax, Purge, Senokot), lubricants (Fleet, Zymenol), osmotics (such as Cephulac, Sorbitol, Miralax), stool softeners (Colace, Surfak), and saline laxatives or milk of magnesia (Phillips' Milk of Magnesia), should be used only once in awhile for, as the commercials say, "occasional irregularity."

Overuse of stimulant laxatives can make constipation worse by interfering with your colon's natural muscle contractions and essentially making them reliant on the medicine. You may find that you need larger and larger doses to get the same results.

If you've been using laxatives for a long time, you can retrain your body to have bowel movements naturally by increasing the fiber in your diet, using a bulk-forming laxative, drinking plenty of water, getting more physical activity, and creating a

 WHAT YOU DON'T KNOW

Gut Bacteria Can Cause Gas

If you have irritable bowel syndrome (IBS) and intestinal gas that won't quit, your gas may be due to an overgrowth of bacteria in your intestinal tract. In one Lebanese study of 124 people with IBS who took the antibiotic rifaximin for 10 days, 42 percent said they had significantly less gas.

DRUG-FREE FIX

Prunes

Prunes are a great source of fiber, but that's not the only reason they get your bowels moving. Some unidentified substance in these dried plums and in their juice stimulates contractions of the intestinal walls and seems to make stool heavier, wetter, and more slippery, all of which makes it easier to pass. In one study, prunes stimulated the bowels more than any other food.

regular bathroom schedule so that your body knows when it's time to go.

☐ MOTION SICKNESS REMEDIES

Which motion sickness drugs work best?

There are three major drugstore motion sickness remedies: cyclizine (Marezine), meclizine (Bonine, Antivert, Dramamine Less Drowsy), and dimenhydrinate (Dramamine). All of them can prevent queasiness when you're traveling if you take them before you begin your journey. Choosing the right one depends on how much you want to stay awake. While all will make you somewhat drowsy, meclizine products claim to be less sedating, and one small study suggests that cyclizine won't make you feel as sleepy as dimenhydrinate.

If you've tried one and aren't happy with the results, experiment with the others. According to the U.S. Coast Guard, the different active ingredients in these drugs work better for different people. Trial and error is the way to find the best one for you.

☐ PAIN RELIEVERS

If I take low-dose aspirin for my heart, what should I take for pain?

You can safely use ibuprofen, if you time it right and if you take uncoated aspirin instead of enteric-coated tablets. Otherwise, the ibuprofen can block aspirin's heart-protecting ability to reduce the risk for blood clots.

Both drugs attach to the same binding sites inside platelets, the component of blood that forms clots. If aspirin gets there first, your platelets are protected against clotting and your risk for a heart attack declines by about 30 percent with regular use. If ibuprofen gets there first, aspirin can't get in—and you lose protection against heart attacks and, a recent study shows, strokes, too.

For best results, take your daily low-dose aspirin in the morning, then wait 1 to 2 hours before taking up to 400 milligrams of ibuprofen for pain. If needed, take another ibuprofen dose of up to 400 milligrams before bed in the evening. Make sure there's at least an 8-hour gap before you take your aspirin again the next morning.

If you can't be bothered with a complicated pill schedule or if you use an enteric-coated

DRUG-FREE FIX

Acupressure

If you forgot your Dramamine and you unexpectedly feel sick while traveling, use the pad of your thumb to press hard on the center of your inner wrist at a spot three finger-width's below your palm. This spot, known as P6, is said to keep motion sickness at bay. You may have to keep pressing until your trip ends, but several studies suggest that this technique does work. You can also use a wristband with a plastic knob that applies pressure when tightened. Sea-Band, sold in pharmacies, is one brand.

aspirin, which takes longer to dissolve and be absorbed into your bloodstream, you're better off using acetaminophen (Tylenol) or naproxen (Aleve) for pain. Or ask your doctor about stronger, prescription-strength pain relievers.

Is it true that ibuprofen can increase the risk of heart attacks?

There's some evidence that taking ibuprofen (Advil, Motrin) regularly for more than 4 weeks can raise your blood pressure. But unless you're already at high risk for a heart attack, this translates into a very small added heart attack risk. When Danish researchers checked the health records of one million healthy people, they found that, compared to those who took virtually no pain relievers, those who used ibuprofen raised their heart attack risk by 1 percent. Those who used a prescription nonsteroidal anti-inflammatory such as rofecoxib (Vioxx, now off the market due to heart risks) or celecoxib (Celebrex) nearly doubled their heart attack risk. Those who used naproxen were 3 percent *less* likely to have a heart attack.

The same researchers found that among people who'd already had a heart attack, ibuprofen may be more dangerous. In an earlier study involving heart attack survivors, those who took large doses of ibuprofen for several weeks (about 1,800 milligrams a day for 37 days) boosted their risk for a second heart attack by about 50 percent.

If you have heart disease, are a heart attack survivor, or are at high risk for heart disease, it's smart to ask your doctor about alternatives to ibuprofen if you tend to use it regularly.

I've heard that too much Tylenol is dangerous. What's a safe dose?

Acetaminophen, the key ingredient in Tylenol, Excedrin, and dozens of multi-symptom cold and flu remedies, is generally safe. Unlike aspirin and ibuprofen, it won't irritate the lining of your stomach. But thanks to what experts call a narrow safety margin, this painkiller also causes more liver damage than any other drug. Taking just a little too much can cause liver damage or even liver failure, and in fact, liver problems caused by acetaminophen send tens of thousands of people to emergency rooms each year.

Growing concerns about acetaminophen prompted an expert panel of doctors to recommend that the FDA reduce the recommended daily limit and to cap the safe level of a single dose at 650 milligrams. The currently accepted daily limit is 4,000 milligrams, but some experts suggest a safer daily total might be 2,600 milligrams. Be very careful not to accidentally overdose by taking acetaminophen and a multi-symptom product that also contains the drug. Read recommended dosages on products for children carefully. Avoid alcohol while you're using acetaminophen. And stay well under the daily limit if you regularly have three or more alcoholic drinks per day.

AVOID THIS MISTAKE

Taking a Daily Aspirin without Asking Your Doctor

Some people shouldn't take aspirin every day, especially since it can cause stomach bleeding. Doctors usually recommend it only for people who have an increased risk of heart attack and stroke. Women may not benefit as much from aspirin therapy as men. And some people appear to be resistant to aspirin's anticlotting effects. (Tests are available to check for aspirin resistance, though some doctors question their accuracy).

Will taking aspirin or ibuprofen often give me an ulcer or make my stomach bleed?

Side effects of nonsteroidal anti-inflammatory drugs (NSAIDs) such as bleeding and ulcers send hundreds of thousands of people to emergency rooms each year and cause thousands of deaths. That's because all NSAIDs—aspirin, ibuprofen, ketoprofen (Actron, Orudis, Oruvail), and naproxen —block a compound in the body that protects the stomach lining from the corrosive effects of stomach acid.

You can cut your risk of stomach problems by taking NSAIDs as directed. Don't take the next dose sooner than you should; don't take more than your doctor or the label recommends; don't take it more often than recommended (even if you don't exceed the maximum daily dose); and don't take more than one medication that contains NSAIDs at the same time.

Certain people should talk with their doctors before taking an NSAID on a regular basis. These include people over age 60, those who've had a stomach ulcer, and people who take steroids or blood thinners.

Signs that your NSAID is causing stomach bleeding or an ulcer include stomach pain, dark black or tarry or bloody stools, or vomiting up blood or a substance resembling coffee grounds. Get emergency help if you're vomiting blood.

Are some pain relievers better at relieving certain types of pain than others?

Yes. Acetaminophen, aspirin, ibuprofen, ketoprofen, and naproxen can all cool off a fever and ease a headache, but there are situations when it's smart to choose one over the others.

● *For a headache, start with acetaminophen.* Taken as directed, this pain reliever is as effective as an NSAID for the occasional headache and won't irritate the stomach lining the way aspirin or other NSAIDs may. If pain won't quit, move on to ibuprofen, naproxen, or ketoprofen. In one study, all three were equally effective at relieving tension headaches.

● *For muscle strains and sprains, choose ibuprofen, naproxen, or ketoprofen.* All reduce inflammation as well as relieve pain.

● *For menstrual pain, take ibuprofen or naproxen.* These drugs short-circuit cramp-producing substances called prostaglandins released at the start of menstruation.

● *If you have asthma, think twice about aspirin.* One in five people with asthma is sensitive to aspirin, which can trigger an asthma attack. If you're allergic to aspirin, avoid ibuprofen, too. Stick with acetaminophen.

☐ **SLEEPING PILLS**

Are over-the-counter sleeping pills addictive?

They aren't physically addictive, but using them every night could lead to psychological dependence. If you use one for more than a few nights, you could have trouble sleeping once you stop. The other disadvantage to these pills: The effects might not fully wear off for 16 to 20 hours. That's well into tomorrow, when you want to feel bright-eyed and alert. Over-the-counter sleep aids can also cause side effects such as dry mouth, constipation, and urine retention and, in older people, may cloud thinking or even trigger delirium. Studies show that they're not very effective when it comes to helping people get more sleep anyway.

A lot of sleeping pills are for pain, too. What if I don't have pain, just insomnia?

It's always wise to use only the medication you really need, so if you really need a sleeping pill for a night or two but don't have pain, look for a regular version without pain relievers. The pain medication found in "PM" sleep tablets is usually acetaminophen, aspirin, or ibuprofen. All are effective for pain, but none is risk-free. If you're not in pain and you want a sleeping pill, find one that skips the extra ingredients.

FAQ Frequently Asked Questions
Prescription Drugs

Are generic drugs really as good as brand-name drugs?

In most cases, yes. Generic drugs contain the same active ingredient in the same amount as the branded drug. They're much cheaper only because they don't require the years of intense clinical testing that brand-name drugs go through, since that testing has already been done. Generic drugs can contain different amounts or types of inactive ingredients such as lactose or gluten. These variations from the brand-name drug can change the way your body reacts to the medication, though this is rare.

There have been anecdotal reports of problems with a few generic drugs, particularly anti-epileptic drugs, the anticlotting drug warfarin (Coumadin), and some immunosuppressants used to prevent rejection after organ transplants. A study comparing patients taking the generic warfarin with those taking Coumadin, however, found no differences. No such studies have been conducted with antiepileptic or immuno-suppressant drugs.

If you have concerns, talk with your doctor. If he wants you to take a branded drug and your state allows pharmacists to switch to a generic, your doctor should write "Do not substitute" on the prescription. It doesn't guarantee that your insurance company will cover the extra cost, but it does guarantee that you'll get the drug your doctor prescribed.

I save money by taking my medicine every other day or less often. Is that okay?

Definitely not. You should take your medicine exactly as prescribed to get the maximum benefit—and for your own personal safety. Patients who stop taking prescription medications are far more likely to die than those who continue their medications. You may not feel sick right away if you fail to take your medication every day, but eventually you're likely to pay a steep price as your health condition spirals out of control (at which point it may cost you *more* money, especially if you land in the hospital).

If you have trouble paying for the medicine, tell your doctor. He might be able to switch you to a lower-cost generic, a different type of medication, or a higher dose pill that can be split in half, giving you twice the medication for the same price (the cost of a pill is often the same regardless of the dosage). Your doctor may also be able to provide you with free samples if there are no generic or less-expensive branded drugs available in that category, but this isn't a good long-term solution. Also, many drug companies offer discount cards or even free drugs to patients who can't afford them, though they often require you and/or your doctor to complete a significant amount of paperwork. Another way to save money is to use a mail-order pharmacy. Mail-order pharmacies typically charge a 1-month co-payment for 3 months of medication.

I just heard a scary news report about my drug; should I stop taking it?

No. Abruptly stopping a medication could be very dangerous and may lead to some nasty symptoms. Instead, make an appointment with your doctor to discuss your concerns or call your pharmacist, who may be able to tell you whether the report applies to you and what you should do in the short run. One report does not necessarily mean a drug is unsafe.

I just saw a TV commercial about a new drug for my condition. Should I ask my doc for it?

You saw one of the hundreds of "direct-to-consumer" advertisements that drug companies run every year. They are designed to get people to do exactly what you're thinking of doing: Ask their doctors for a prescription. And it works—research shows that up to 10 percent of people who viewed such ads asked their doctors for the medication. And nearly half the doctors did prescribe it, but often because

they felt pressured to, not because they thought it was a better choice for the patient.

Keep in mind that newer drugs have shorter track records than older ones, and therefore may be riskier. About 10 percent of prescription drugs that hit the market are later discovered to cause serious side effects that didn't turn up in clinical trials. Remember the painkiller Vioxx? It was heavily advertised on TV and was later removed from the market due to safety concerns that came to light when millions of people started using it. What's more, newer drugs, though more expensive, may not work any better than older drugs already on the market.

If you're unhappy with your current treatment, talk to your doctor about a switch. But if you don't have a problem with it, stay the course. It is usually safer, easier, and cheaper to stick with what you're already using.

I'm having a reaction to a new drug I started. Should I stop taking it right away?

It depends on how serious the reaction is. If you are having trouble breathing or otherwise functioning then, yes, stop taking it and get to an emergency room immediately. Otherwise, call your doctor but keep taking the drug until your doctor decides on an appropriate course of action.

I take multiple medicines and can't remember what to take, when. What should I do?

This is a common problem but one you can easily overcome. Here's how:

- *Use a pill dispenser.* Choose a type that works best for you and your pill regimen. Some have one compartment for every day of the week or the month; some have multiple compartments for each day. Load it up with the appropriate pills, and you'll be able to see at a glance whether you took your pill or not. Some pillboxes even vibrate, flash, or sound an alarm when it's time to take your next dose.

- *Set an alarm.* You can buy medication reminder watches that you can set with up to 12 alarms to remind you when to take your medicine. One manufacturer is Cadex.

- *Get into a routine.* Most medicines need to be taken first thing in the morning or last thing at night, or just before, during, or after meals. Use memory triggers that relate to the time you take the medicine. For instance, if you need to take it in the morning or at bedtime, keep the medicine by your alarm clock. Need to take it with breakfast? Put it by the coffeepot.

- *Make a chart on the computer.* Put the time you should take the pill at the top and the pill name along the side. Print enough charts for the week and check off each pill as you take it.

- *Hire a call service.* Yes, there are services that will call you when it's time to take your next pill. Some are even free. Make sure they have your cell phone number and keep your cell with you at all times.

I take several drugs prescribed by more than one doctor. How can I find out if they'll interact with each other?

Use the same pharmacy to fill all your prescriptions. The pharmacist will watch out for potentially dangerous interactions. You can also call or visit the pharmacy and ask the pharmacist to double-check your prescriptions for any interactions. Don't forget to also tell her about any nonprescription drugs and dietary supplements you take. It's smart to make sure that all your doctors have a list of every medication you take, why you take it, the dosage, and the doctor who prescribed it.

Is it safe to buy drugs online?

It is safe to buy drugs online from a reputable provider. The FDA recommends you look for an online pharmacy that:

- Is located in the United States
- Is licensed by the state board of pharmacy in the state in which the website operates (www.nabp.info provides a list of state boards)
- Requires a prescription
- Has a licensed pharmacist available to answer questions over the phone
- Displays the National Association of Boards of Pharmacy's Verified Internet Pharmacy Practice Sites (VIPPS) seal
- Offers a secure site for credit card purchases

Signs that a site might be unsafe include offering prices that are dramatically lower than the competition; failing to protect your personal information (for instance, the site is not encrypted); asking for a social security number; offering no way to contact the site by phone; or sending you the wrong drug or dosage or drugs of unclear origin. To ensure that you're getting the right drug, take them into your local pharmacy and ask the pharmacist to check. You can also type the drug's imprint code (letters or numbers listed on the medication) into a website such as RxList's Pill Identification Tool (www.rxlist.com/pill-identification-tool/article.htm) or the federal government's site, pillbox.nlm.nih.gov, designed to help identify unknown medications.

Is it safe to buy drugs from another country?

Drugs produced and sold in other countries are not subject to the same oversight and restrictions as those purchased in the United States. The FDA has found counterfeit drugs and medications with dangerous additives sold in other countries. One FDA operation found that nearly half the drugs intercepted from India, Israel, Costa Rica, and Vanuatu were shipped to consumers in the United States who believed the drugs were from Canada. Many were not labeled properly, and some were fake. Finally, the drugs you're ordering may be more expensive than generic versions available in the United States.

Why would I need a prescription for a drug that's available over-the-counter?

Generally, if the same drug is available with and without a prescription, the prescription version comes in a higher dose. In some cases, though, the over-the-counter (OTC) and prescription strengths are the same. If you can't afford an over-the-counter drug, sometimes a doctor will write a prescription for it so that it will be at least partially covered by insurance. If you don't have prescription drug insurance, you will likely find it much cheaper to use the OTC version, even if you have to take more than recommended on the label to get the dose your doctor wants you to have.

How can I be sure the pharmacist gives me the right drug?

By checking. Before you leave the counter, pull the medicine out of the bag and open the bottle. If it is a refill, make sure it looks like the medicine you've been taking. If it doesn't, ask why. Also compare the name and dose of the drug to the bottle you're refilling. If it's a new medication, hold out a pill and ask the pharmacist to double-check the dosage and medication. Another option is to wait until you get home and look it up on the Internet on a pill identification website such www.rxlist.com/pill-identification-tool/article.htm or pillbox.nlm.nih.gov.

As an older woman, do I need a lower dosage of drugs than other people need?

You may. As you age, your body becomes less efficient at breaking down and eliminating the drugs, so they often remain in your system longer than they would in someone younger. If you take the same dosage as a younger person, this could lead to dangerous levels of the drug in your bloodstream. Doctors should consider a person's age as well as their kidney and liver functions when writing prescriptions, but not all of them do. It couldn't hurt to ask your doctor if you could benefit from a lower dosage when he writes a prescription, or ask the pharmacist when you get the prescription filled.

When I'm traveling across time zones, how do I know when to take my medicines?

Most medicines that are taken once a day can be taken any time of the day. So if you took it at 8 a.m. at home, you can take it at 8 a.m. in your new location. If you normally take your medication just before or after meals, such as thyroid medication, which is typically taken before breakfast, continue doing so. One medication that may need adjusting, however, is insulin. If you travel across fewer than five time zones, you should be fine. However, if you travel across more than five time zones going east, which shortens the day, you may need to reduce the amount of insulin you take on the day you travel; if traveling west, which lengthens the day, you may require more insulin. No matter what medicine you take, check with your doctor about any necessary adjustments.

Is an "off-label" use of a drug safe?

Generally, yes. Drugs are approved for specific conditions, but once they've hit the market, doctors are legally free to prescribe them for any purpose. Off-label use is particularly prevalent in children and in cancer treatment. Doctors also use some medications off-label to treat chronic pain, prescribing antiepileptic medications like gabapentin (Neurontin) or certain antidepressants like amitriptyline (Elavil). Sometimes there is good evidence supporting the off-label use of a drug, but in many cases, there isn't. If your doctor prescribes a drug for you off-label, ask why and what proof there is that it will work for your condition.

How can I tell if someone is abusing a prescription drug?

Prescription drug abuse can be just as dangerous as abusing illegal drugs like heroin or cocaine. The most commonly abused prescription drugs are narcotics like hydrocodone, oxycodone (OxyContin), and morphine. Signs that someone is abusing the drug include rapid increases in the amount of drugs needed and early refills. Sometimes people "doctor shop," switching from one doctor to another to get new prescriptions. Other signs include slurred speech, flushed skin, and constricted pupils.

Prescription Drugs

☐ ADHD MEDICINES

My son is taking a stimulant medication for his attention deficit disorder. Is it okay to give him a drug "holiday" during the summer?

The nice thing about stimulants is that they are short-acting, meaning they don't stay in the body very long. So you can stop and start them with no problem. Some parents want to take their children off stimulants when school is out, thinking that since the kid doesn't have to sit in a classroom all day, he doesn't need the focus and concentration the medicine affords. Also, because the drugs can suppress growth in the short-term, doctors used to recommend such drug "holidays" on weekends and vacations. Today, however, we know that stimulants have no long-term effect on growth.

The thing to remember is that ADHD doesn't go away when school ends. Many children have symptoms beyond attention deficits, such as social skill and behavior problems, that their medications help. So any decision to take your son off the medication depends on the severity of his symptoms and side effects of his medication.

The most common side effects from stimulant medication are reduced appetite and weight loss, insomnia, and moodiness or irritability when the medicine wears off. If side effects are the problem, consider giving him weekends off. There is some evidence that this reduces side effects without significantly affecting symptoms.

My granddaughter is now taking medication for ADHD. I heard it can lead to sudden death. Is this true?

There is some evidence that children taking stimulant

medications like methylpheni-date (Ritalin) for ADHD may have a slightly higher risk of sudden cardiac death, in which the heart stops beat-ing. However, the data is not conclusive. Even if there *were* a link, the risk of sudden car-diac death is extremely rare. However, your granddaughter should have had a thorough medical examination before she started taking the drug.

Is it normal to lose your appetite when taking medi-cation for ADHD?

Yes. About 80 percent of people taking ADHD medica-tions report some loss of appetite, though only 10 to 15 percent lose weight. To avoid appetite loss, talk to your doctor about lowering the dose you take, taking the medicine with a meal, changing from a short-acting formula that you take several times a day to one that lasts for 8 hours or more, or changing to a different stimu-lant or even a different type of medication. You can also take weekends off from the medi-cation without causing any major problems.

WHAT YOU DON'T KNOW

Steroids Take Time to Work

Don't expect instant relief from a steroidal nasal spray. They can take up to 2 weeks to be fully effective, so be patient.

☐ ALLERGY MEDICINES

I have really bad allergies to cats. Now my doctor wants to put me on a steroid. Aren't they dangerous?

The steroid your doctor wants you take is likely a glucocorti-coid nasal spray, such as beclomethasone (Beconase), budesonide (Rhinocort), or flu-ticasone propionate (Flonase), used to relieve allergy symp-toms. Unlike oral steroids such as prednisone, the long-term use of which can lead to seri-ous side effects such as bone loss and diabetes, nasal spray steroids are much safer, caus-ing few side effects when taken as directed.

If I'm using a nasal steroid spray, is it okay to also take an oral antihista-mine?

You can take both if your doctor says it's okay. While a steroid spray is designed for long-term use to prevent allergy symp-toms, an antihistamine provides quick relief for symptoms that

do develop, like itchy eyes, stuffy nose, and hives.

☐ ALZHEIMER'S DISEASE MEDICINES

Why would my doctor prescribe an antipsychotic medication for my mother's dementia?

These medications, which include olanzapine (Zyprexa), risperidone (Risperdal), and quetiapine (Seroquel), are often prescribed to calm the agitation and combative behavior that may occur with dementia. They are not approved for this use, but doctors can legally pre-scribe them "off-label." It might not be a good idea, though. A University of South-ern California study found that these drugs offer little benefit when prescribed for dementia, and they could increase the risk for sudden death.

Researchers followed 421 people with Alzheimer's disease who took Zyprexa, Risperdal, Seroquel, or placebo capsules for up to 36 weeks to ease prob-lems like aggression, agitation, delusions, and hallucinations. The result: Psychotic symptoms improved by 26 to 32 percent for people on the drugs—scarcely better than the 21 percent improvement in the placebo group. More troubling is that

continued on page 125

Dangerous Drugs for Seniors

If you're 65 or older and your doctor prescribes any of these drugs, you run the risk of serious side effects. This list, known as the Beers List, was developed by a panel of geriatric experts to provide guidance about which drugs are potentially inappropriate to prescribe to seniors, whose bodies generally take longer to break down drugs and who therefore may end up with dangerous levels of the drugs in their bloodstreams. If your doctor prescribes any of these medications, ask if they are safe for you to take or if you should consider an alternative.

ALLERGY MEDICATIONS

chlorpheniramine (Aller-Chlor, Chlor-Trimeton, Polaramine, Teldrin); diphenhydramine (Benadryl, Excedrin PM, Nytol, Sominex, Unisom, and some prescription products)	May cause confusion, blurred vision, constipation, dry mouth, light-headedness, and bladder problems

ANTIBIOTICS

nitrofurantoin (Macrobid, Macrodantin)	May cause lung damage

ANTIDEPRESSANTS

amitriptyline (Elavil); chlordiazepoxide amitriptyline (Limbitrol); perphenazine amitriptyline (Triavil); imipramine (Tofranil); nortriptyline (Aventyl)	May cause confusion, blurred vision, constipation, dry mouth, light-headedness, and bladder problems
fluoxetine (Prozac)	May cause agitation and insomnia

ANTIPSYCHOTICS

chlorpromazine (Thorazine)	Increased risk of death in older adults with dementia
mesoridazine (Serentil); thioridazine (Mellaril)	May cause tremors and other central nervous system changes

BLOOD PRESSURE MEDICATIONS

guanethidine (Ismelin); guanadrel (Hylorel); clonidine (Catapres)	May cause very low blood pressure upon standing, leading to dizziness and falls

DIABETES MEDICATION

chlorpropamide (Diabinese)	May cause prolonged low blood sugar (hypoglycemia)

HEART MEDICATIONS

amiodarone (Cordarone)	May cause irregular heartbeat; there is no evidence of efficacy in the elderly
cyclandelate (Cyclospasmol); isoxsuprine (Vasodilan)	There is no evidence of efficacy in the elderly
nifedipine (Procardia, Adalat)	Short-acting versions can cause dangerously low blood pressure and constipation
ethacrynic acid (Edecrin)	May cause high blood pressure/fluid imbalance

MUSCLE RELAXERS

disopyramide (Norpace)	May cause heart failure; strongly sedating
dipyridamole (Persantine), short- and long-acting	May cause low blood pressure upon standing, leading to dizziness and falls
methyldopa (Aldomet); methyldopa-hydrochlorothiazide (Aldoril)	May slow heart rhythm and worsen depression
ticlopidine (Ticlid)	No more effective than aspirin at preventing
carisoprodol (Soma); chlorzoxazone (Paraflex); cyclobenzaprine (Flexeril); metaxalone (Skelaxin); methocarbamol (Robaxin); oxybutynin (Ditropan); orphenadrine (Norflex)	May cause confusion, blurred vision, constipation, dry mouth, light-headedness, and bladder problems

PAIN RELIEVERS

propoxyphene (Darvon)	No advantage over acetaminophen (Tylenol) for pain relief but all the disadvantages of a narcotic (constipation, dizziness, nausea, risk of dependence)
indomethacin (Indocin)	Risk of fatal gastrointestinal bleeding, confusion, psychosis, and kidney damage
pentazocine (Talwin)	Confusion and hallucinations
meperidine (Demerol)	Not effective pain reliever in doses used; may cause confusion
ketorolac (Toradol)	Significant risk of stomach bleeding
naproxen (Naprosyn, Aleve, Avaprox); oxaprozin (Daypro); piroxicam (Feldene)	Long-term use can cause gastrointestinal bleeding, kidney failure, high blood pressure, and heart failure

PARKINSON'S DISEASE MEDICATION

trihexyphenidyl (Artane)	May cause confusion, blurred vision, constipation, dry mouth, light-headedness, and bladder problems

SLEEP AIDS AND SEDATIVES (also prescribed for anxiety and depression in the elderly)

diazepam (Valium); alprazolam (Xanax); buspirone (Buspar); hydroxyzine (Vistaril, Atarax); lorazepam (Ativan); oxazepam (Serax); temazepam (Restoril); triazolam (Halcion); zopiclone (Imovane); zolpidem (Ambien)	Linked to nearly fourfold increased risk of suicide; older people are more sensitive to benzodiazepines such as Valium and Ativan so they should receive very low doses; higher doses could result in dizziness and falls

continued

SLEEP AIDS AND SEDATIVES (continued)

diphenhydramine (found in over-the-counter medications such as Excedrin PM, Nytol, Sominex, Unisom, and in numerous prescription medications)	May cause confusion, blurred vision, constipation, dry mouth, light-headedness, and bladder problems
chlordiazepoxide (Librium); doxepin (Adapin, Sinequan); flurazepam (Dalmane); meprobamate (Miltown); quazepam (Doral); clorazepate (Tranxene)	Mood changes or drowsiness; dizziness; increased risk of falls
All barbiturates (except phenobarbital), unless used to control seizures	Highly addictive and cause more side effects than other sedatives or hypnotics

STOMACH MEDICATIONS

atropine; scopolamine (Scopace); dicyclomine (Bentyl); hyoscyamine (Levsin, Levsinex); propantheline (Pro-Banthine); belladonna alkaloids (Donnatal and others); clidinium-chlordiazepoxide (Librax); cimetidine (Tagamet)	May cause confusion, blurred vision, constipation, dry mouth, light-headedness, and bladder problems
trimethobenzamide (Tigan)	Tremors
Stimulant laxatives such as bisacodyl (Dulcolax), cascara sagrada, and castor oil	Long-term use (unless taking an opioid pain reliever) could make bowel problems worse
Mineral oil	Older people may have trouble swallowing this thick liquid, which could be accidentally sucked into the lungs

TESTOSTERONE

methyltestosterone (Android, Virilon, Testred)	May cause overgrowth of prostate cells; heart problems

THYROID MEDICATION

desiccated thyroid (Armour, Naturethroid, Westhroid, Qualitest)	May cause cardiovascular problems such as irregular heartbeat or even heart attack

URINARY MEDICATIONS

tolterodine (Detrol)	May cause poor memory and lower decision-making ability
doxazosin (Cardura)	May cause low blood pressure, dry mouth, and urinary problems

taking the drugs may raise death risk by 50 percent.

Is it worth taking drugs for Alzheimer's disease?

Maybe. It depends in part on how far the disease has progressed. It is best to start treatment as early as possible, and most of the drugs currently available appear to have little or no benefit in treating advanced Alzheimer's.

The medications, which include the cholinesterase inhibitors donepezil (Aricept), rivastigmine (Exelon), and galantamine (Razadyne) and the glutamate regulator memantine (Namenda), don't cure the disease, but if they're taken early on, they can slow its progression. In the first long-term study of the drugs taken in the "real world" (not as part of a research study), people with Alzheimer's disease who took either a cholinesterase inhibitor or memantine had much less memory loss than those who didn't receive either drug.

Those who received both drugs declined the least. Researchers predicted that the longer the patients received both drugs, the slower their memory and other cognitive losses would be, suggesting that the treatment might actually help protect brain cells typically destroyed as part of the disease.

The primary side effects of these drugs are nausea, vomiting, and appetite loss. They are generally mild and can be reduced by taking the medication with food. Exelon is also available in a patch form, which has far fewer side effects than the oral form. Only Aricept appears to have any benefit in advanced Alzheimer's.

☐ ANTIANXIETY DRUGS

My doctor prescribed Ativan for my panic disorder. I heard it's addictive; is this true?

Antianxiety medications like lorazepam (Ativan), clonazepam (Klonopin), alprazolam (Xanax), and diazepam (Valium) belong to the benzodiazepine class of drugs. They are typically prescribed for anxiety, insomnia, and muscle pain, among other uses. Although safe when taken as directed for immediate relief of short-term anxiety, they can be quite habit-forming if taken on a regular basis for weeks or months. Over time, you may build up a tolerance to the drug, meaning you need higher and higher doses to get the same effect, or you may develop a physical

and psychological addiction, in which you experience severe withdrawal symptoms if you can't get your regular dose. Such symptoms include anxiety, increased heart rate and blood pressure, insomnia, and sensitivity to noise and light. In more severe cases, people hallucinate and experience seizures.

My doctor just prescribed a beta-blocker for my anxiety. My husband takes one for his high blood pressure. Did the doctor give me the wrong prescription?

No. Beta-blockers, which include the drugs propranolol (Inderal) and metoprolol (Lopressor), commonly prescribed for high blood pressure and angina (chest pain caused by clogged arteries) work by blocking the effects of hormones, such as adrenaline and norepinephrine, that increase blood pressure. These are the same hormones that are released when you're under

 AVOID THIS MISTAKE

Quitting an Antianxiety Med Cold Turkey

If you've been taking an antianxiety medicine for a long time, do *not* quit abruptly. Talk to your doctor about how to gradually taper the dose. Otherwise, you could experience very serious complications such as seizures.

stress, triggering the pounding heart, sweating, and hyperventilation of anxiety. Blocking the effects of those hormones reduces blood pressure and slows your heart rate, relieving these symptoms. One caveat: Don't take beta-blockers if you have asthma or circulation problems. Never stop taking a beta-blocker suddenly. Doing so can lead to dangerous heart-related side effects. Work with your doctor to taper off the medicine.

☐ ANTIBIOTICS

I've been on an antibiotic for 3 days now. Is it okay to go out in the sun?

It depends what type of antibiotic you're taking. The ones most likely to make your skin extra-sensitive to the sun include

tigecycline (Tygacil), sulfa drugs such as mafenide (Sulfamylon) and sulfacetamide (Klaron), and tetracyclines such as doxycycline (Periostat) and minocycline (Minocin). If you're taking one of these, limit your time in the sun, and when you must be out in it, cover up well with clothing, a hat, sunglasses, and sunscreen. This goes for the entire time you're on the drug.

I'm on an antibiotic for a vaginal infection, and now I have a splitting headache. Could it be related?

Yes. Most people think of tummy troubles when they think of antibiotic side effects, but certain antibiotics can trigger other unwanted problems, too. For instance:

- *Metronidazole (Flagyl).* Prescribed for vaginal, pelvic, and

abdominal infections. It can cause a wicked headache if you drink alcohol while taking it.

- *Telithromycin (Ketek).* Prescribed for mild pneumonia. It can cause temporary vision changes.

- *Fosfomycin (Monurol).* Used to treat bladder infections. It can cause diarrhea.

My antibiotic is making me nauseated. What can I do?

Take it with plenty of food unless your doctor tells you otherwise.

Every time my doctor gives me an antibiotic, I get diarrhea. Is there anything I can do to prevent that?

Because antibiotics can wipe out good as well as bad bacteria, including the beneficial bacteria that help maintain normal digestion, some people experience diarrhea and other digestive problems when taking antibiotics. You can get around this problem by restoring your gut's supply of good bacteria by eating plenty of yogurt that contains live, active cultures or by taking probiotic (live bacteria) supplements. Studies found that volunteers who took a dietary supplement containing the probiotics *bifidobacterium* and *lactobacilli*

FACT OR FICTION

Antibiotics Make Birth Control Pills Less Effective

Fiction. The only antibiotic proven to interact with oral contraceptives is rifampin (Rifadin), which is prescribed for tuberculosis and leprosy. If you take this medication, you will need to use a backup form of birth control such as condoms. Although there have been some reports of women getting pregnant while taking penicillin and tetracycline while taking the Pill, there is no scientific evidence that either drug interferes with the action of birth control pills. More likely, the women weren't taking the contraceptive as directed. That said, using a condom for extra insurance never hurts.

AVOID THIS MISTAKE

Using Old Antibiotics for a New Infection

First, you should have finished the entire prescription the first time around. Second, many antibiotics are specific to the type of infection you have. Taking the wrong antibiotic might not work and can lead to antibiotic-resistant bacteria, making treatment for that type of infection more difficult the next time.

during and after treatment with the antibiotic amoxicillin had far less diarrhea than those who received a placebo.

☐ ANTIDEPRESSANTS

I've been on an antidepressant for a week now, and I don't feel much better. Should I ask for a higher dose or a different drug?

Finding the right antidepressant is a little bit like buying shoes: It may take a while to find the right fit. That's the conclusion of the nation's largest-ever study of depression treatments. Ultimately, 67 percent of the 3,671 volunteers found relief, but some tried four different treatment methods before finding the right one, including antidepressants, therapy, or a combination of both. Just 37 percent were symptom-free after up to 16 weeks on the first drug their doctors prescribed. Generally, you

should wait at least 2 weeks before increasing the dose or switching antidepressants. However, it's worth a call to your doctor to see if you should be switched or the dosage increased sooner.

Do antidepressants really increase the risk of suicide?

It appears that they do increase the risk of suicidal thoughts and actions in young adults ages 18 to 24. However, there doesn't appear to be any increased risk in adults older than 24, and there is actually a reduced risk in adults 65 and older, according to the FDA. Warnings about the increased risk in young adults are included on the labels of all antidepressants, no matter

what type. If someone you know in this vulnerable age group is taking an antidepressant and the depression gets worse, or that person starts talking about suicide, call the doctor or 911 immediately. Do not have the person stop taking the medicine without first checking with the doctor.

I'm feeling much better, and I want to stop taking my antidepressant. Can I just quit tomorrow?

No. Suddenly stopping some antidepressants can lead to what's called antidepressant discontinuation syndrome. Although it's not dangerous, it can make you feel pretty lousy for a week or so. Symptoms include anxiety, headache, fatigue, nausea and vomiting, insomnia, diarrhea, and, in some cases, tingling in your arms and legs. The syndrome is most common with the selective serotonin reuptake inhibitors (SSRIs) paroxetine (Paxil) and sertraline (Zoloft). Other antidepressants associated with discontinuation

WHAT YOU DON'T KNOW

It Takes Time to Adjust to Antidepressants

The side effects of antidepressants, which may include nervousness, nausea, and headache, often disappear within the first days or weeks as your body gets used to the drug.

syndrome include tricyclic antidepressants such as amitriptyline (Elavil), desipramine (Norpramin) and doxepin (Sinequan), and venlafaxine (Effexor), mirtazapine (Remeron), trazodone (Desyrel), and duloxetine (Cymbalta). Abruptly halting a monoamine oxidase (MAO) inhibitor antidepressant, such as phenelzine (Nardil) or tranylcypromine sulfate (Parnate), can also lead to balance problems, agitation, and even psychosis.

Talk to your doctor about how to gradually wean yourself off your medication over a period of anywhere from a week to several months, depending on the drug you take.

□ ANTIFUNGALS

I'm taking liquid nystatin (Bio-Statin) for thrush. Can I keep my dentures in while I use this medicine?

Actually, dentures are often the source of fungal infections in the mouth, which occur up to three times as often in people with dentures than in people without. Not only should you take your dentures out when you take the medicine but also you should apply antifungal powder or cream to them. To avoid future fungal infections, soak your dentures every night in a solution of 10 drops of bleach to 1 cup of water or immerse non-metal dentures in water with denture cleaner or the water/bleach combination and microwave on high for 2 minutes.

I finished my antifungal drug for my toenail fungus, but the nail doesn't look much better. Why not?

Fungal nail infections are notoriously hard to treat. Antifungal creams and lotions are worthless against nail infections, also called onychomycosis. Even oral treatments have high rates of treatment failure and recurrence, and may need to be taken for weeks, even months. The best options appear to be terbinafine (Lamisil) and itraconazole (Sporanox), which are more likely to cure the condition than older medications such as griseofulvin (Grisovin). It may take a few months after you finish the drug to see the full results, since the new nail takes time to grow in.

Not all nail infections necessarily need to be treated. But it's important to treat a nail infection if you have diabetes or a history of cellulitis of the legs, a bacterial infection affecting the skin and underlying tissue.

□ ANTIPSYCHOTICS

My 32-year-old daughter has schizophrenia and her doctor prescribed an antipsychotic. I heard they can increase the risk of a stroke; is that true?

There doesn't appear to be any increased risk of stroke in young people without dementia. There is some evidence that antipsychotics can increase the risk of stroke in elderly people, for whom they are often prescribed to reduce the agitation and psy-

WHAT YOU DON'T KNOW

Not All Nail Problems Are Fungal Infections

Fungal infections are responsible for only 50 to 60 percent of nail abnormalities (other causes include the skin conditions psoriasis and lichen planus). That's why it is important to see a doctor and receive a definitive diagnosis with a KOH test, in which the doctor scrapes some of the nail area onto a slide, covers it with potassium hydroxide, and examines it under a microscope. Many insurance companies now require this test before approving antifungal medications.

chosis that accompanies dementia. A study published in the *British Medical Journal* in 2008 found that the risk of stroke was 69 percent higher in people between the ages of 71 and 87 who took typical antipsychotics such as phenothiazines (Compazine), butyrophenones (Haloperidol), and thioxanthenes (Navane) than in people not taking an antipsychotic. The risk was 132 percent higher in people taking atypical antipsychotics, which include olanzapine (Zyprexa), risperidone (Risperdal), and quetiapine (Seroquel). In people with dementia, typical antipsychotics doubled the risk, while atypical antipsychotics increased the risk nearly fivefold. The results of that study led the authors to conclude that the risks of antipsychotics in people with dementia outweighed the benefits and should be avoided whenever possible.

☐ **ANTISEIZURE MEDICINES**

Can the antiepileptic medicine Dilantin cause heart problems?

Maybe. In a study published in the *Annals of Neurology*, researchers switched people who had been taking the most widely prescribed anticonvulsants, phenytoin (Dilantin) and carbamazepine (Carbatrol), to two newer antiseizure drugs, lamotrigine (Lamictal) or levetiracetam (Keppra). After

 AVOID THIS MISTAKE

Taking an Antipsychotic Without Asking Why You Need It

Don't accept a prescription for an antipsychotic drug if you don't have schizophrenia or other severe mental illnesses like psychosis without asking your doctor "why this drug?" A study published in the *Journal of Clinical Psychiatry* and sponsored by the National Institutes of Health found that the majority of people prescribed these drugs didn't have schizophrenia or other severe mental disorders for which the drugs are approved. Instead, they had conditions like depression, anxiety, or post-traumatic stress disorder that could be managed with safer, less-expensive medications. Although some antipsychotics are labeled for use in depression, they should be used as a last resort if typical antidepressants don't work.

6 weeks on the new drugs, participants' total cholesterol, "bad" cholesterol, and triglyceride levels plummeted, as did levels of C-reactive protein, a marker for inflammation. Such changes substantially reduce the risk of heart disease. Unlike the older drugs, the newer drugs do not affect enzymes involved in metabolism, which accounts for the differences seen in these cardiovascular risk factors when people switched to a different drug.

If your seizures are well-controlled on your current drug, there may not be any clear reason to switch, but if you're concerned about your own risk of heart disease, or you have other heart disease risk factors, talk to your doctor about whether the drug you're taking is still the best.

☐ **ASTHMA MEDICINES**

Why do I have to use my Flovent inhaler when I'm breathing fine?

Fluticasone (Flovent), along with other inhaled corticosteroids such as beclomethasone (QVAR) and budesonide (Pulmicort), are designed to prevent the inflammation in your lungs that can lead to an asthma attack. They are long-term control medications; you take them every day no matter how you feel. By contrast, quick-relief medications or rescue medications such as albuterol (Proventil, Ventolin) are short-acting bronchodilators designed to open your lungs when you have an attack so you can breathe easier. They're used only when you have symptoms.

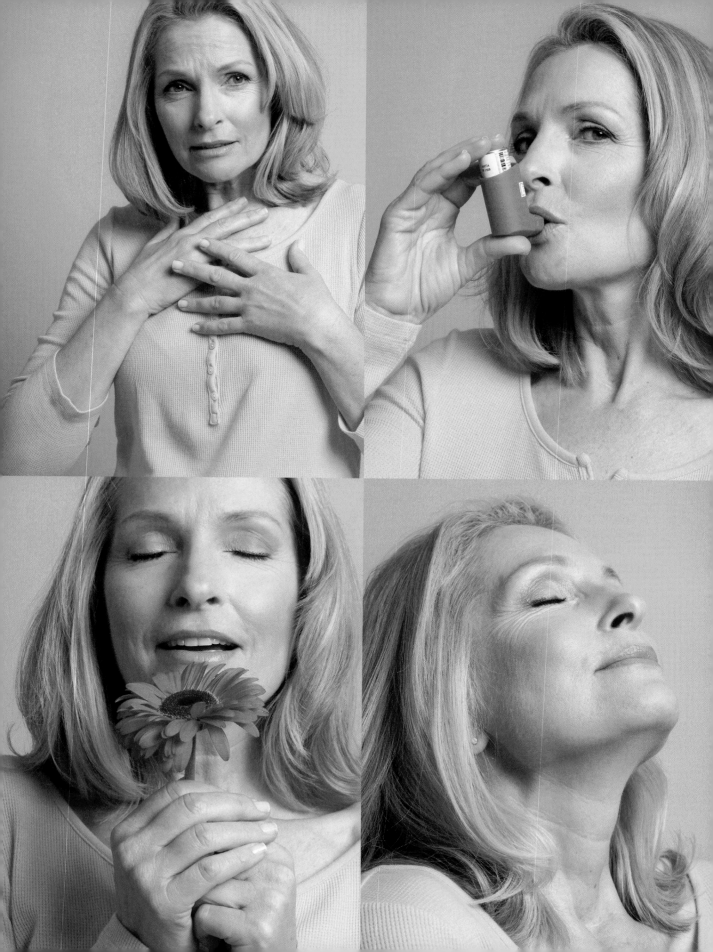

The reason you don't have any symptoms now is because your controller medicine is doing its job. So don't stop taking it. One study found that children who took these medications for years and then stopped saw their asthma symptoms return.

Why has my voice gotten so hoarse since I started using my steroid inhaler?

Although inhaled steroids are much safer than oral steroids, they can have some unwanted effects, such as hoarseness and other voice changes. In your case, it appears the steroid has weakened the muscles in your larynx, or voice box, causing steroid inhaler–induced laryngitis. Once you stop using the inhaler, your voice should return to normal. Don't quit the inhaler without first talking to your doctor, however.

I've been using my albuterol inhaler about four times a day lately. Is that too much?

Yes. If your asthma is properly managed, you shouldn't need a short-acting bronchodilator like albuterol (Proventil, Ventolin) more than twice a week. If you're using yours as often as you say, talk to your doctor about how to get your asthma under better control.

Why did my doctor prescribe a heartburn medication for my asthma?

For years, doctors thought that people with poorly controlled asthma had so-called silent heartburn, when stomach acid backs up, or refluxes, into the esophagus and throat but only causes coughing, wheezing, and breathlessness—no stomach pain or burning. So, doctors routinely prescribed drugs called proton-pump inhibitors (PPIs) to reduce the amount of acid their stomachs produced. But a study conducted at 20 medical centers found no benefit to the drugs for poorly controlled asthma. The message: It's time to ask your doctor why you're still on the medication.

☐ **BIRTH CONTROL PILLS**

I've been on birth control pills for 5 years, and now I want to get pregnant. How long do I have to be off them before my husband and I can start trying?

Women used to be advised to wait at least a month after halting the Pill before getting pregnant because of fears that residual hormones could trigger a miscarriage. No more. Now doctors know that you can safely start trying to get pregnant the day you stop taking the Pill. You should ovulate within 2 weeks and have your first period 2 to 4 weeks later unless, of course, you're already pregnant!

I heard that birth control pills can cause cancer. Is that true?

It is pretty clear that taking oral contraceptives for 5 or more years increases the risk of cervical cancer by 90 percent (almost double). The good news is that the risk drops as soon as you stop taking the Pill. After 10 years post-Pill, the risk of cervical cancer is identical to that of women who never took the pill.

The evidence is less clear when it comes to breast cancer. A 1996 analysis of 54 studies involving more than 150,000 women found that those taking oral contraceptives had a 24 percent increased risk of breast cancer 1 to 4 years after they quit taking the Pill. That risk dropped each year, and by 10 years post-Pill, their risk was the same as that of women who never took birth control pills. A later analysis found no increased risk of breast cancer in women who took oral contraceptives. The difference between the two reports is likely related to the lower doses of estrogen used in today's pills. Estrogen stimulates the development and growth of breast tumors, so the less estrogen, the less risk.

On the plus side, numerous studies find that oral contraceptives can slash the risk of ovarian and endometrial cancer by half and the risk of colon cancer by about a fifth after at least 5 years of use.

☐ **CANCER MEDICINES**

I'm getting chemotherapy for lung cancer. Is it okay to take antioxidant supplements like vitamin C and beta-carotene?

No. Studies in mice and in cells show that high doses of vitamin C can actually prevent chemotherapy from destroying cancer cells, somehow protecting the cell from destruction. In one of the few studies in humans, researchers gave 90 women with breast cancer megadoses of vitamins, minerals, and antioxidants and compared their outcomes to 180 women who did not receive the supplements. There was some evidence that the women taking the supplements had worse rates of survival than those who didn't. Bottom line: Don't take any over-the-counter supplements or medications without first checking with your oncologist.

I just finished chemotherapy for breast cancer and everything looks great. But my doctor wants me to take Herceptin for at least a year. Why?

Because it will cut your risk of a recurrence. Experts say trastuzumab (Herceptin) should be standard therapy for at least a year after cancer treatment for all women who have HER2 positive tumors, which account for about 20 percent of breast cancers. In three landmark studies, Herceptin cut the risk of a killer cancer recurrence by 50 percent.

If you're over age 50 or have risks for heart failure (such as a previous heart attack or diabetes), talk with your doctor about the drug's heart risks; it can increase the risk of congestive heart failure by 2 to 16 percent.

My family rolls their eyes when I say I have "chemo brain." But it's real, isn't it?

You bet. The fogginess, loss of concentration, and forgetfulness, following chemotherapy was dismissed for decades, but recent research finds that it is a very real condition that can last for years after the final chemo treatment. There are some ways to attack it, how-

ever. Researchers found that the drug modafinil (Provigil), which improves wakefulness in people with sleep disorders, can also improve memory and concentration in people with chemo brain. Other options include a type of therapy called memory and attention adaptation training, in which you literally talk yourself through various tasks like a play-by-play spiel from a radio sports announcer. Even meditation and exercise may have some benefit. So, if you're suffering from chemo brain or, as some experts would like to rename it, cancer brain, don't ignore it. Talk to your doctor about options to restore your clear thinking.

Why do some people lose their hair when they undergo chemo and others don't?

It depends on the type of drug they receive and for how long they receive it. The hair loss occurs because chemotherapy targets rapidly dividing cells—which includes hair cells. Some drugs lead to hair loss all over your body including your eyelashes; others just on your head or under your arms or on your legs. The chemo drugs most likely to lead to hair loss include doxorubicin (Adriamycin), methotrexate (Trexall), cyclophosphamide (Cytoxan), 5-fluorouracil (Adrucil, Efudex, Fluoroplex), and paclitaxel

(Taxol). The good news is that the hair loss is temporary; when the drugs end, the hair returns.

I'm about to start my first course of chemotherapy. Am I really going to throw up as much as people in the movies?

The nausea and vomiting of chemotherapy is nearly a thing of the past, thanks to treatment with antinausea drugs that often begins even before your first dose of chemo and continues after the final drop. The most effective medications are the 5-HT3 receptor antagonists ondansetron (Zofran), granisetron (Kytril), dolasetron (Anzemet), and palonosetron (Aloxi). These drugs are to nausea and vomiting what water is to fire. They prevent the actions of the neurotransmitter 5-HT, a chemical that acts on the brain and gut to trigger nausea. The best part is that they have very few side effects beyond mild headache and constipation.

The newest antinausea medication on the market is the neurokinin-1 receptor antagonist Emend—aprepitant in pill form and fosaprepitant as an injection. This drug interferes with other vomit-inducing chemicals. Finally, your doctor may prescribe a corticosteroid such as dexamethasone or methylprednisolone. Ideally, you should get either of these in combination with a 5-HT receptor antagonist or neurokinin-1 receptor antagonist.

☐ CHOLESTEROL MEDICINES

Why did my doctor put me on Lipitor even though my cholesterol levels are normal?

There are many reasons your doctor could have prescribed atorvastatin (Lipitor), a drug that belongs to the class of medications called statins. These drugs help prevent heart attacks and stroke by blocking production of a liver enzyme that makes cholesterol. No matter what your cholesterol level, if you have heart disease, clogged arteries, or diabetes, your doctor may want you to take a statin. The same applies if you have significant risk factors for heart disease, such as a family history of the disease or high blood pressure. A major trial found that by taking a statin, people with healthy cholesterol levels but high levels of a protein linked with inflammation could slash their risk of a heart attack by more than half and their risk of stroke or surgery to open clogged arteries by nearly half.

I have high triglycerides but my LDL and HDL levels are normal. Will a statin help?

It should. Triglycerides are a form of fat found in blood and stored in fat cells. High levels are linked to heart disease. Studies find that statins, best known for lowering "bad" LDL cholesterol levels, can also cut triglyceride levels up to 28 percent. The higher your starting level of triglycerides, the greater the drop you should see.

What can I do to survive the flushes I get with the niacin my doctor prescribed to improve my cholesterol?

Prescription-strength niacin, a B vitamin, is a powerful, multitasking cholesterol drug. It is the only cholesterol drug that not only reduces artery-clogging

 DRUG-FREE FIX

Hazelnuts

Instead of medication for high triglycerides, try hazelnuts. Just 1.5 ounces a day for 4 weeks shaved triglyceride levels about a third in 15 men with high levels.

LDL cholesterol but also improves "good" HDL cholesterol, the type that acts as a kind of garbage truck to remove the bad stuff. An added bonus: Niacin also reduces triglyceride levels. While very safe, its annoying side effect of flushing leads many people to stop taking it, even though most flushes last less than an hour. However, there are ways to reduce the flushing:

- Take an aspirin 30 minutes before or at the same time you take the niacin.

- Take the niacin with meals or at bedtime.

- Avoid alcohol, hot drinks, spicy foods, and hot baths or showers after taking the niacin.

- Take extended-release niacin; taken once a day at bedtime, it significantly reduces flushing.

The good news is that a combination drug of extended-release niacin and a drug designed to prevent flushing called laropiprant (Cordaptive) has been approved in Europe and is being investigated in the United States.

Ever since I started taking a statin, I've been feeling a little tired and my memory has gotten fuzzy. Is there a connection?

Possibly. Cholesterol-lowering drugs called statins may reduce levels of an enzyme called co-enzyme Q10 (CoQ10). Found in every cell in the body, it plays an important role in energy production. Some doctors believe that low levels could lead to fatigue, muscle pain and damage, and liver damage. They could also make congestive heart failure worse. Talk to your doctor about supplementing with 30 to 60 milligrams of CoQ10 while taking a statin.

☐ CHRONIC FATIGUE SYNDROME MEDICINES

I've read that drugs for ADHD help with chronic fatigue syndrome. Is that true?

It might be. Stimulant medications such as methylphenidate (Ritalin, Concerta), typically prescribed for people with attention deficit disorders, are thought to work by increasing levels of the neurotransmitter dopamine in the brain, particularly in the part of the brain responsible for complex thinking. They also improve fine motor movement as well as concentration and focus. Ritalin has been used to improve fatigue in people with cancer and HIV, and has traditionally been used for people with sleep disorders such as narcolepsy. Now these drugs are being investigated for their benefits in chronic fatigue syndrome (CFS).

Studies in people with CFS show some benefit. One study of 60 people with CFS who received either 10 milligrams of Ritalin twice a day or a placebo found that the Ritalin group had lower scores on a scale that assesses fatigue and improved on a scale that assesses concentration. The main side effect was dry mouth. These drugs may work best for a small percentage of CFS patients known as responders.

☐ CONSTIPATION MEDICINES

I have chronic constipation and over-the-counter options like milk of magnesia and Colace don't help. Neither do fiber supplements. Are there prescription options?

There are three main options: lubiprostone (Amitiza), lactulose (Enulose, Generlac, Kristalose), or polyethylene glycol (MiraLax, GlycoLax). Amitiza is approved to treat chronic constipation with no obvious cause and to treat constipation-related irritable bowel syndrome in women (it hasn't been tested in enough men). The most common side effects are nausea, diarrhea, and headache, although you may also feel some tightness in your chest or shortness of

⚠ WHAT YOU DON'T KNOW

Certain Diabetes Drugs Can Trigger Heart Failure

The oral diabetes drugs rosiglitazone (Avandia) and pioglitazone (Actos) can lead to heart failure in people with diabetes regardless of their age or whether they take insulin. While both drugs are implicated, the risk with Avandia appears to be higher. Researchers evaluating nearly 40,000 people age 66 or older who took either drug found that those taking Actos during a 6-year period were 23 percent less likely to be hospitalized for heart failure and 14 percent less likely to die than those taking Avandia. If you have risk factors for heart failure such as high blood pressure or a previous heart attack, talk to your doctor before taking these medications.

breath about an hour after taking a dose. Lactulose attracts water into the bowel to soften and loosen stool so it's easier to pass. The main concern with this drug is gas, diarrhea, and cramps. Polyethylene glycol works by keeping water in the intestine to trigger a bowel movement. Only take it once a day, and let your doctor know if you haven't had a bowel movement within 3 days.

☐ COUGH MEDICINES

Why did my doc give me a prescription for cough syrup? Can't I just buy it over-the-counter?

First, you should know that there is very little benefit to over-the-counter cough medicines (see "Cough and Cold Medicines" beginning on page 104). The difference is that prescription cough medicine usually contains hydrocodone, a narcotic that suppresses the urge to cough. It doesn't cure the cough, but it can help you (and your partner) get a good night's sleep until your cold or bronchitis improves. Never take more than the recommended dose of prescription cough syrup; doing so can have serious side effects.

☐ DIABETES MEDICINES

I started taking Januvia and now I'm getting headaches and diarrhea. Is this normal?

Sitagliptin (Januvia), one of the newest oral diabetes drugs to hit the market, works by super-

charging a digestive hormone called GLP-1 that tells the pancreas to make more insulin and prevents the liver from creating glucose, thus lowering blood sugar levels. The most common side effects include coldlike symptoms and headache, although some people get stomach upset and diarrhea. These effects should diminish as your body gets used to the medicine, but tell your doctor if they don't.

Watch out for allergic symptoms such as rash, hives, or trouble breathing. If any of these symptoms occurs, stop taking the medicine and call your doctor right away. If your doctor has prescribed both Januvia and a sulfonylurea such as glipizide (Glucotrol), watch out for dangerously low blood sugar levels and tell your doctor right away if you experience them.

What are the advantages of an insulin pen over a syringe?

The advantage of insulin pens is that everything is self-contained—you simply insert a prefilled insulin cartridge into the pen. The cartridge typically has enough insulin for several days. You don't have to worry about drawing up the correct amount of insulin from a vial into a syringe; you simply dial up your dose, making the pens more accurate than syringes. Some pens even come prefilled—finish the insulin and toss the pen.

☐ **DIARRHEA MEDICINES**

Why did my doctor prescribe the pain reliever Lomotil for my chronic diarrhea?

Because Lomotil (diphenoxylate with atropine) is a version of Demerol, an opioid that causes constipation. Doctors sometimes prescribe Lomotil, morphine, codeine, or opium tincture (Paregoric) for people with severe diarrhea if over-the-counter drugs haven't worked. Make sure you drink plenty of water and other fluids to prevent dehydration.

I have a serious illness that often causes chronic diarrhea. My doctor wants to give me injections of Sandostatin. What should I know about this drug?

Octreotide (Sandostatin) is used to treat chronic diarrhea and some types of gastrointestinal tumors. It's not an easy drug to take—it is either injected or infused into your body through an IV. You may experience some pain or burning at the injection or infusion site, but that should go away in about 15 minutes. Serious side effects that require an immediate call to your doctor include increased urination and thirst, problems breathing, and feeling feverish.

I have irritable bowel syndrome (IBS) and my doctor wants to start me on Lotronex. Is it safe?

Alosetron (Lotronex) is a very powerful drug that interferes with actions of a chemical called 5-HT3. This compound plays a role in stomach pain, the movement of digested food through the intestines, and various secretions throughout the gut, all of which are involved in the pain and bathroom problems of IBS. Lotronex is very effective in women who have severe IBS-related diarrhea that doesn't respond to other therapies (it hasn't been tested enough in men or children). However, it can have some very serious side effects, including severe constipation or ischemic colitis (impaired blood flow to the colon that causes sudden swelling, pain, and severe diarrhea). That's why doctors have to enroll in a special educational program about the drug and its side effects before they can prescribe Lotronex, and they must affix a sticker to the prescription indicating that they have done so. If you feel a new or worse pain in your stomach area or see blood in your bowel movements after taking Lotronex, call your doctor immediately.

☐ **ERECTILE DYSFUNCTION MEDICINES**

Are all the different ED drugs more or less the same?

Three oral medications are currently approved for use in men with ED (erectile dysfunction): sildenafil (Viagra), tadalafil (Cialis), and vardenafil (Levitra). All work in much the

WHAT YOU DON'T KNOW

Antacids May Be Linked to Severe Diarrhea

If you have chronic diarrhea and you've been taking the proton-pump inhibitor lansoprazole (Prevacid), it might be time to stop the medication. Recent reports in medical journals reveal a connection between the drug and changes in the lining of the colon that can cause severe diarrhea. People had been taking the drug for 3 to 6 months before their problems started. When they stopped taking it, the diarrhea vanished.

10 Ways to Use Prescription Drugs More Safely and Effectively

1. ASK QUESTIONS

Before leaving the doctor's office with a new prescription, make sure you understand why the medicine is being prescribed, how long it will take before it starts working, how you should take it, what side effects you should expect, and whether you should change any of your normal activities (such as driving or spending time in the sun) while taking it.

2. KEEP A LIST OF THE MEDICATIONS YOU TAKE

For each medication, include the drug's generic and brand name, the dosage, the name of the doctor who prescribed it, when to take it, and any special instructions (such as taking it with food or first thing in the morning).

3. READ THE LEAFLET PROVIDED BY THE PHARMACIST

Most of us just throw this piece of paper away, but it contains valuable information about side effects and drug interactions. These days, they're even written in plain English!

4. STICK WITH ONE PHARMACY

Most pharmacies today have electronic databases that can instantly tell if a newly prescribed medication will interact with one you're already taking. They can also track any drug-related allergies. If you fill your medications at different drugstores, there's no way to track this information.

5. TALK TO THE PHARMACIST

Pharmacists are founts of information when it comes to medications. When you are prescribed a new medicine, ask the pharmacist about any dangerous side effects or warning signs, and let him know about any other medical problems you have. Some medications can make certain conditions worse, something your doctor may miss.

6. REQUEST A "BROWN BAG REVIEW"

When visiting a new doctor, and at least once a year with your regular doctor, schedule an appointment for a review of your medications. Put everything you take (including vitamins, supplements, herbs, and over-the-counter medications) into a bag and bring them with you to the appointment. The doctor can make sure that you still need all the drugs and also identify any interactions or overlaps—different drugs that perform the same function.

7. TAKE AS DIRECTED

Even if you're feeling fine, take the medicine as your doctor prescribed.

8. STAY IN TOUCH

Call your doctor if you experience bothersome side effects, don't feel better after the medication is supposed to have started working, or have trouble taking the medicine. Don't wait for your next visit.

9. CHECK THE EXPIRATION DATE

If your doctor prescribed a sleeping pill 4 years ago and you're now experiencing another bout of insomnia, check the expiration date. Some medications may lose some of their potency starting a few months after the expiration date has passed. If the drug is expired, it's probably time for a visit to your doctor anyway to make sure the medication is still appropriate for you.

10. STORE IT RIGHT

Some medicines should be stored in the refrigerator, others on a cool shelf. The worst place to keep your meds is in a humid, steamy bathroom.

same way, by increasing the amount of a chemical in the penis that relaxes smooth muscle cells, enabling more blood to fill the penis to create an erection. All work just as well with similar side effects, including headache, flushing, and stomach upset. Men taking Viagra also have a higher risk of temporary vision changes.

Perhaps the biggest difference between the three is how soon you need to take them before the romance starts. One form of Cialis (Cialis 36) works for 36 hours, while another version can safely be taken every day, no matter what your bedroom plans. Viagra lasts up to 4 hours, and Levitra is designed to be taken an hour before sex. Don't expect miracles, however. Studies find that the drugs are worthless in about half of all men with erection problems.

I tried Viagra but it made me very dizzy. Is this normal?

Are you also taking an alpha blocker, such as doxazosin (Cardura), prazosin (Minipress), or tamsulosin (Flomax) for an enlarged prostate or high blood pressure? If so, that could be your problem. The combination can cause dangerously low blood pressure. To reduce the risk, avoid taking Viagra within 4 hours of taking an alpha blocker.

I'm taking an antibiotic for a sinus infection. Is it okay to still use Cialis?

It depends on the antibiotic. If it's erythromycin, then you should skip the tadalafil (Cialis)—and either of the other two erectile dysfunction (ED) drugs, (Viagra, Levitra)—until you finish the prescription. Erythromycin interferes with the action of an enzyme needed to metabolize the ED drugs which could lead to a dangerous buildup in your bloodstream.

☐ FLU MEDICINES

Why didn't the Tamiflu my doctor prescribed make me feel better?

Oseltamivir (Tamiflu) is one of two antiviral medicines used to treat the most common forms of influenza. The other is zanamivir (Relenza). While these drugs can be a blessing, cutting the flu short by about a day, they work only if you take

them within 48 hours of your first symptom. And some influenza viruses have become resistant to the drugs, making the drugs less effective than an aspirin when it comes to making you feel better. Your best bet when it comes to flu is prevention: Get vaccinated.

Why would the nursing home where my mother lives prescribe antiviral medication when she's not sick?

Thanks to close living quarters and lots of elderly people with weakened immune systems, nursing homes are hotbeds of infection in the winter. In people age 65 and older, a case of the flu can be especially dangerous, potentially leading to deadly secondary infections such as pneumonia. Nursing home residents and workers may be given an antiviral drug even if they're not sick just to help prevent the flu (and therefore prevent the spread of the virus to other people).

DRUG-FREE FIX

Lifestyle Changes for ED

Instead of popping an expensive pill for your erection problem, try changing your lifestyle. An Italian study of 209 men found that 58 percent of those who lost weight, improved their diets, and exercised more cured their erectile dysfunction in 2 years without any other treatments, compared with 38 percent of a control group.

You Can Ask Your Doctor for a Flu Drug if You're Not Sick

If someone in your household has the flu, you can ask your doctor to prescribe an antiflu drug so that you don't get sick. Doctors are most likely to prescribe the drugs for people at high risk of complications, such as those over 65, people with chronic medical conditions such as heart or lung disease or diabetes, and pregnant women.

My 7-year-old has the flu. Should I ask his doctor for Tamiflu?

You could, though it's not necessary. Kids are usually able to fight the flu on their own. And one study found that kids taking Tamiflu were more likely to throw up than kids not taking it. Tamiflu is approved to treat children 1 year and older. The other major flu drug, zanamivir (Relenza), is approved to treat children age 7 and older.

□ **GLAUCOMA MEDICINES**

Can I drive at night after taking pilocarpine for my glaucoma?

No. Pilocarpine (Salagen) treats high pressure in the eye that causes glaucoma. However, it makes your pupils constrict and can cause blurring, affecting your vision and depth perception. So either have a designated driver take the wheel or call a taxi.

What is the best way to get my glaucoma drops into my eye instead of on my face?

You're not alone in your struggle. A recent study found that while more than 9 in 10 people using eye medications said they thought they were pretty good at getting the drops in their eyes, only about a third really knew what they were doing. If you're not careful, you could miss your eye, put too many drops in your eye, or, most dangerous, touch the tip of the applicator to your eye, risking infection. Here is the best way to apply eye drops:

1. Wash your hands with soap and hot water.

2. Sit or lie in a comfortable position and lean your head back while looking up.

3. With one finger, gently pull down the lower lid of your eye to form a small pocket.

4. Apply the drop into this "pocket."

5. Close your eyes for a couple of minutes and block your tear ducts (they are on the side of your eye closest to your nose) with your thumb or index finger. Don't blink! Blinking can make the medicine move from the eye to the tear duct and into your nose instead of remaining in your eye.

□ **HEARTBURN MEDICINES**

I heard that taking a lot of medicine for my sour stomach could harm my bones. Is that true?

It depends what type of medicine you're taking. Medications often used to treat serious heartburn, called gastroesophageal reflux disease (GERD), are proton-pump inhibitors (PPIs) such as esomeprazole (Nexium), lansoprazole (Prevacid), and omeprazole (Prilosec). They work by reducing the amount of acid your stomach produces. But that acid is needed to help your digestive system absorb calcium. Without calcium, bone breaks down. Studies find that taking a PPI for 7 or more years nearly doubles the risk of an osteoporosis-related fracture. It increases the risk of hip fracture even more: by 62 percent after 5 years and more than 350 percent after 7 or more years. Talk to your doctor about your risk for osteoporosis and about alternatives to PPIs if you need to take them long-term.

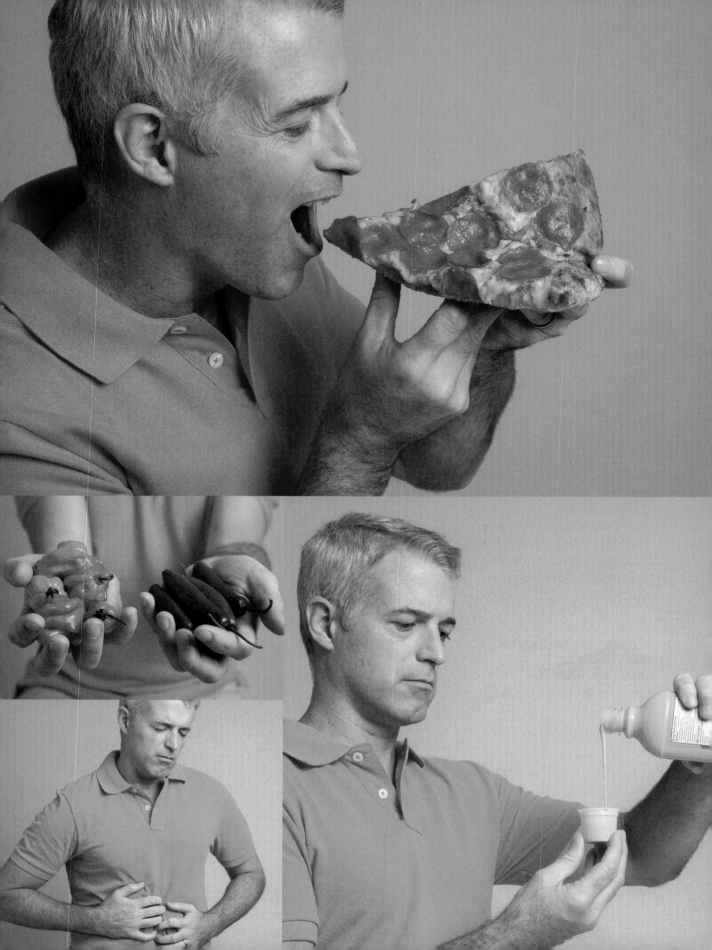

Is there anything I can take for the terrible heartburn and nausea I get when I'm pregnant?

Although it's not specifically approved for pregnancy-related heartburn, the drug metoclopramide (Reglan) is often used for that purpose in Europe. It works by speeding up stomach muscle contractions so the food you eat reaches your intestines faster. In the United States, Reglan has typically been used only for the most serious cases of pregnancy-related nausea, usually when a woman is hospitalized. But a large study published in *The New England Journal of Medicine* in 2009 found the drug was safe for both developing baby and mom when used in the first 3 months of pregnancy. One caveat: Using Reglan for more than 3 months could cause a serious movement disorder called tardive dyskinesia.

Can I still take an antacid if I'm taking an H2 blocker?

While antacids provide faster relief for heartburn (they neutralize the acid in your stomach), H2 blockers like cimetidine (Tagamet) or famotidine (Pepcid) provide longer-lasting relief. But they can take a while to work (they reduce the amount of acid your stomach produces). That's why many people opt to continue using their antacid, too.

That's okay—for a while. Once the H2 blocker begins working, you should stop taking the antacid. And don't take them both at the same time, since the antacid could prevent your stomach from absorbing the H2 blocker.

Why am I supposed to stop taking Tagamet after two weeks?

If you're taking it for two weeks and you still have significant heartburn, then something else more serious than a sour stomach may be going on. Before you start another course of Tagamet, see your doctor. He may want to switch you to a stronger acid reducer, likely a proton pump inhibitor such as lansoprazole (Prevacid), pantoprazole (Protonix), or esomeprazole (Nexium).

☐ HEART DISEASE MEDICINES

I am on medication for heart failure and, lately, I've been feeling very dizzy. Could it be the medicine?

It could. All medications for heart failure are also used to reduce blood pressure. If you already have normal or low blood pressure, these drugs can make your blood pressure drop too low, leading to dizziness. Ironically, even though high blood pressure

can cause heart failure, low blood pressure often makes it worse. An option for people with heart failure and low blood pressure is valsartan (Diovan). One major study found that it increased blood pressure as well as reduced the risk of heart attack and other medical problems or death in these people.

Why did my doctor tell me to go easy on lettuce and spinach since I started taking a blood thinner?

Leafy green vegetables like lettuce and spinach are rich in vitamin K, which helps blood to clot. They could reduce the anticlotting effects of drugs such as warfarin (Coumadin). Other foods high in vitamin K that you should eat sparingly include kiwifruit, blueberries, cranberries, broccoli, cabbage, Brussels sprouts, asparagus, cauliflower, and kale. You should also avoid supplements of vitamin E, fenugreek, ginkgo, and glucosamine, all of which act as anticlotting agents that can increase the effects of warfarin, possibly causing excessive bleeding.

Why did my doctor take me off Avapro for my congestive heart failure?

Because it doesn't work. Your doctor probably started you on irbesartan (Avapro), which is typically used to reduce high blood pressure, because small studies showed some benefit in treating heart failure. However, a large study published in *The New England Journal of Medicine* in 2008 showed that, while the drug worked well at controlling blood pressure, in people with heart failure, it didn't reduce the risk of hospitalization or death from heart-related causes or stroke. It also didn't improve people's quality of life.

I've been taking Coumadin and recently my gums have been bleeding. Is this normal?

Warfarin (Coumadin) is used to prevent blood clots. It works well, but it can be difficult to achieve the ideal dose. Take too little and you could get clots; take too much and you could experience bleeding. That's why blood levels of the drug are tested often when you first start, less often after you've been on it a while. Even if the dosage is correct, you may still experience a little bleeding, resulting in bruises or gum bleeding or even the occasional nosebleed or heavier-than-usual menstrual period. You should mention your gum bleeding to your doctor, but it's probably not a cause for concern.

However, if you notice red, dark, coffee or cola-colored urine, red or tarlike bowel movements, bleeding from the gums or nose that you can't stop on your own, or coffee-colored or bright red vomit, call your doctor immediately and, if you can't reach your doctor, go to the nearest emergency room. Other signs of major bleeding include severe headache or stomachache; sudden, unexplained bruising; a cut that doesn't stop bleeding within 10 minutes; and dizziness or weakness.

☐ **HERPES MEDICINES**

I'm confused. When my regular doctor gave me a Valtrex prescription for cold sores, the dosage and timing was different than when my gynecologist prescribed it. Why?

The dosage and timing can be different depending on whether you get sores on your mouth or your genital region—and which drug you're using. If you get both types of outbreaks, and you're confused as to how much to take and when, call your doctor for clarification. Sometimes herpes medications are prescribed to prevent outbreaks, in which case you'll take it daily.

Can I spread genital herpes to my partner if I'm taking medication for it?

Yes, it's possible. Even when you're not having an outbreak, the virus could still be active on the surface of the skin. If you're taking valacyclovir (Valtrex) to prevent outbreaks, you'll significantly lower the chances of spreading herpes to your partner. But you should still practice safe sex by using condoms and avoiding sex during an outbreak.

☐ **HIGH BLOOD PRESSURE MEDICINES**

Why were my husband and I prescribed different blood pressure medicines?

Doctors have a huge arsenal of medicines at their disposal to treat high blood pressure, including diuretics, angiotensin-converting enzyme (ACE) inhibitors, angiotensin receptor blockers (ARBs), beta-blockers, calcium channel blockers, and others. The best drug for you depends on your personal medical history and condition. For example, a newly diagnosed diabetic patient with high blood pressure might be best treated with an ACE inhibitor.

That said, one type of high blood pressure drug, known as

thiazide diuretics, is among the most effective and also has the advantage of being time-tested (it's one of the oldest class of drugs) and cheap. Thiazides and other diuretics work by increasing the amount of urine you excrete to reduce overall blood volume. This, in turn, reduces the pressure placed on blood vessels. The drugs include hydrochlorothiazide (Microzide, HydroDiuril, and others), chlorothiazide (Diuril), and chlorthalidone (Thalitone).

A major review of the benefits of all high blood pressure drugs found that low doses of thiazides worked best at reducing blood pressure, resulting in an average reduction of 13/5 mmHg points. They reduced the risk of death from hypertension-related conditions by 11 percent, stroke by 32 percent, heart disease by 28 percent, and heart attack or angina (chest pain caused by clogged arteries) by 30 percent.

Why does my doctor want me to take two blood pressure medications?

Studies find that most people with high blood pressure will need at least two blood pressure medications, often three, to bring their blood pressures under control. The good news is that new "combination" drugs that combine two or, in at least one case, three classes of high blood pressure drugs into one pill are now

 WHAT YOU DON'T KNOW

Beta-Blockers May Not Be the Best Choice

Skip the beta-blockers for your high blood pressure unless you have other heart problems. In an analysis of 13 studies involving more than 105,000 people, Swedish doctors found that the drugs could increase the risk of stroke by 16 percent compared with other hypertension medications. Beta-blockers also carried a 3 percent higher risk for death even though they didn't raise the odds for heart problems. Behind the risk: Experts suspect that beta-blockers don't lower blood pressure near the heart as well as pressure-taming meds like diuretics, ACE inhibitors, calcium antagonists, and angiotensin-receptor blockers.

available. This makes it much easier to take your medicine as directed, making it more likely that you'll get your blood pressure under control. Currently available drugs combine a diuretic with an angiotensin II antagonist (Diovan HCT, Hyzaar), a calcium channel blocker and an angiotensin II antagonist (Exforge), an ACE inhibitor and calcium channel blocker (Lexxel, Lotrel, Tarka), and a calcium channel blocker, ARB, and diuretic (Exforge HCT).

I am African-American. Is it true that some drugs for high blood pressure don't work as well in black people?

Experts don't exactly know why some drugs work differ-

ently in blacks, but they do know that high blood pressure tends to be more severe and occur more often in black people than in white people, and is less likely to respond to treatment. It's clear, for instance, that beta-blockers work less well in black people than in people of other ethnicities. Blood pressure medicines may even pose greater risks in blacks. For instance, one large study comparing the ACE inhibitor lisinopril (Prinivil, Zestril) with the diuretic chlorthalidone (Thalitone) revealed a higher risk of stroke in black people taking lisinopril than in other ethnicities taking either drug.

A review of clinical trials involving African-Americans with high blood pressure concluded that calcium channel blockers, which include amlodipine (Norvasc), Verapamil (Calan, Isoptin), and diltiazem (Cardizem), were most effective.

I have diabetes *and* high blood pressure and my doctor has me on three different blood pressure drugs. Isn't that crazy?

No. The combination of diabetes and high blood pressure (which often go hand in hand) sends your risk of heart disease and kidney disease skyrocketing. That's why you need to get your blood pressure even lower than most people with hypertension (130/80 mmHg or lower) to reduce your risk of complications. Expect to need at least two, possibly three, medications to achieve that goal.

Nearly all classes of antihypertensives work well in people with diabetes, but if you're taking a beta-blocker or a thiazide diuretic, watch your blood sugar levels carefully as these drugs can increase them. Thiazide diuretics include hydrochlorothiazide (Microzide, HydroDiuril, and others), chlorothiazide (Diuril), and chlorthalidone (Thalitone). Beta-blockers include atenolol (Tenormin), felodipine (Plendil), and ramipril (Altace). If your doctor recommends a calcium channel blocker, he should skip nitrendipine; a large study comparing the drug with the ACE inhibitor lisinopril found the ACE inhibitor worked best at reducing the number of heart attacks.

☐ HORMONES

I've been hearing a lot about bioidentical hormones. What's the difference between that type of hormone and the kind my doctor prescribes?

The phrase "bioidentical hormone" typically refers to estrogen- and/or progesterone-based medications created in a compounding pharmacy. These pharmacies custom-make drugs, individualizing the dosage and sometimes creating mixtures of products that aren't otherwise available. Some compounding pharmacies use saliva tests to measure a woman's hormone levels to determine an "appropriate" dosage, though these tests haven't been FDA-approved for this purpose. Most compounded estrogen therapy products contain synthetic estradiol, one of three forms of estrogen your body naturally produces. But you can get this very same form of estrogen in commercially available drugs, including the oral estrogens Estrace, Ortho-Est, and Climara; the skin patches Vivelle-Dot, Climara, Estraderm, and Alora; the vaginal ring Femring; and the skin cream and gel Estrasorb and Estrogel.

Bioidentical hormone drugs require a prescription, just as regular hormone drugs do. And despite claims to the contrary, there is no evidence that bioidentical or compounded products are any safer or more effective than manufactured drugs or that they have any fewer side effects. In fact,

DRUG-FREE FIX

Red Clover

Most studies show that red clover isn't effective for hot flashes. That said, if you really believe it will work, it's worth a try. That's because hot flashes are incredibly susceptible to suggestion. In other words, if you take something that you *think* might work to cool you off, chances are it will. A recent well-designed study comparing red clover to a placebo found that the herb reduced symptoms by 57 percent—and the placebo reduced them by 63 percent! This led the researchers to conclude that red clover doesn't work, but that the placebo effect sure is strong. After all, a 57 percent improvement is nothing to sneeze at.

compounded drugs are not approved by the FDA, which doesn't regulate drug production in compounding pharmacies as it does in manufacturing plants. So there's no guarantee that the dose you receive is safe or that the drug hasn't become contaminated during manufacturing.

My doctor wants me to take estrogen therapy for my hot flashes, but I heard it causes breast cancer. Does it?

Maybe. The Women's Health Initiative was the seminal study on the risk of breast cancer in women taking hormone replacement therapy. This study involved more than 27,000 women taking Premarin, an estrogen-only hormone therapy, or Prempro, an estrogen/progestin therapy. The risk of breast cancer increased in women who took Prempro for at least 5 years, though the increase was relatively small (8 additional cases of breast cancer for every 10,000 women each year). Women taking the estrogen-only preparation (Premarin) actually developed fewer breast cancers over the 7-year study than women taking a placebo, though they had 50 percent more abnormal mammograms and underwent a third more breast biopsies than women taking a placebo.

The decision to take hormone therapy to help with hot flashes is one that can only be determined with the help of your doctor and a careful assessment of your medical history and other risk factors for breast cancer. If you do decide to take hormone replacement therapy, experts advise using the lowest effective dose for the shortest time possible.

My sex drive is nil and my husband is getting frustrated. Would testosterone help?

Probably—but the dangers of using it long-term aren't known. While testosterone is often thought of as a male hormone, women make it, too. About half of their testosterone is produced in the ovaries (the rest in the adrenal glands), so when menopause hits and the ovaries go into retirement, the flow of testosterone slows to a trickle. Since testosterone appears to play a role in women's sexual desire, some experts think that low levels after menopause and, sometimes, before, may be related to the loss of sex drive some women experience.

For years, some doctors have prescribed low doses of testosterone in creams or patches "off-label" to women with low libidos, with most studies finding that the supplemental testosterone helped in the bedroom. The downside: Testosterone in

women can have some annoying side effects, including hair growth where you don't want it (such as on your face), weight gain, and acne. These effects are less likely at lower doses. There are also concerns about the risks of using testosterone for a year or more that aren't well-understood.

Nevertheless, several pharmaceutical companies are racing to get a testosterone product for women to market. One company developed a patch for women only to have the FDA deny approval several years ago, saying that more long-term study was needed. That patch has since been approved in Europe, and other patches and a testosterone gel are in late-stage trials in the United States. The only way to know if testosterone therapy may be right for you is to talk with your doctor.

☐ INSOMNIA MEDICINES

How long can I take sleeping pills before I become addicted?

It depends what type of pill you're using. Most sleeping pills are designed for short-term use. The popular drugs ezopiclone (Lunesta), zaleplon (Sonata), and zolpidem (Ambien), known as nonbenzo-diazepine sedatives, are not physically addictive, though they can be psychologically addictive. Only Lunesta has been tested for long-term

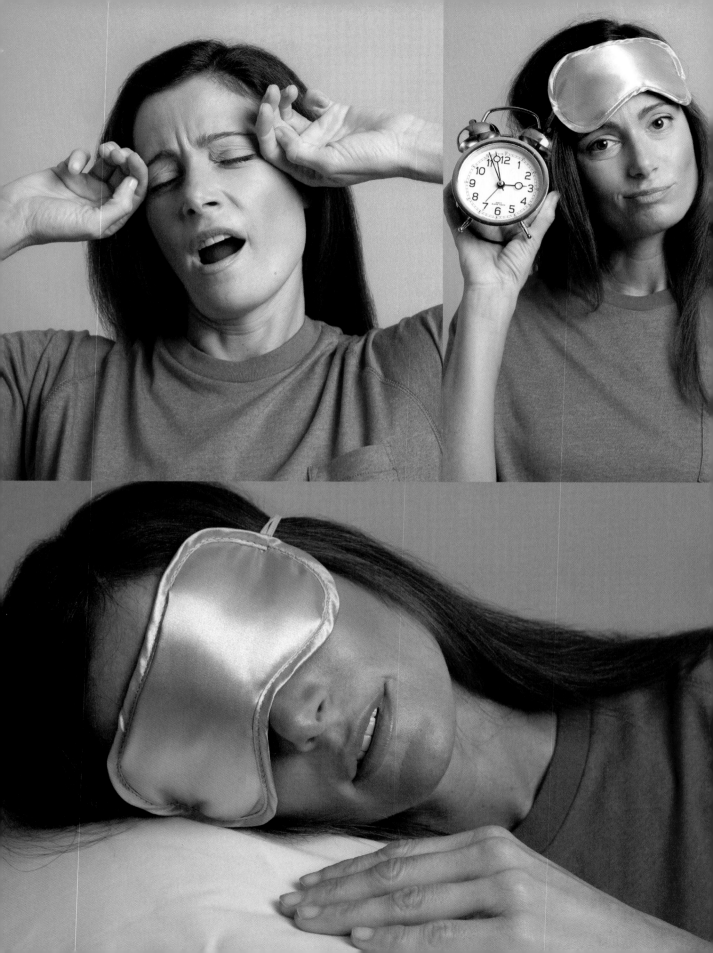

use—and then only for 6 months. The other two are only approved for short-term use, 2 weeks or less.

Certain other drugs do carry a risk of dependence. These include the benzodiazepine sedatives flurazepam (Dalmane), temazepam (Restoril), estazolam (ProSom), and quazepam (Doral). They should only be used for the occasional night of insomnia, not for weeks at a time. Another medication, ramelteon (Rozerem), mimics the sleep hormone melatonin. It only works for people who have trouble falling asleep, not for those who have trouble staying asleep. It can be taken for as long as your doctor recommends with no worries about dependence.

Why did my doctor prescribe an antidepressant for my insomnia when I'm not depressed?

Believe it or not, the antidepressant trazodone (Desyrel) is one of the most commonly prescribed medications for insomnia, even though it's not officially approved for that use. A side effect of this drug is sleepiness, which explains why it's prescribed for insomnia, in much lower doses than you'd get for depression. Unlike other sleeping pills, trazodone can be used long-term. It's rarely pre-

Sleeping Pills Don't Work As Well As You Think

Pop a pill and fall blissfully into a deep, lasting sleep. That's what you'd imagine happens when you take a sleeping pill. But the reality is far less impressive. A study conducted by the National Institutes of Health found that people who took prescription sleep aids received very little objective benefit. On average, they fell asleep only about 13 minutes faster than those who took placebo pills and slept only 11 to 32 minutes longer, though most people thought they'd slept much better. It could be that, because of the pill's effects on short-term memory, people just didn't remember tossing and turning.

scribed for men because it can cause painful or long-lasting erections. Other side effects can include flulike symptoms, problems with urinating, and blood pressure changes. Other antidepressants often prescribed for insomnia include doxepin (Sinequan), amitriptyline (Elavil), and mirtazapine (Remeron).

I've heard about people doing weird things while taking sleeping pills, like driving while asleep. Which drugs cause this strange behavior?

Ever had that dream where a cop stops you and when you get out of the car, you realize that you're wearing your nightgown or, worse, you're naked? Well, for some people

taking one of the newer, supposedly safer sleeping pills—eszopiclone (Lunesta), zaleplon (Sonata), and zolpidem (Ambien)—that was no dream. As more people started taking these drugs in the first decade of the 2000s, the FDA began receiving reports of people sleepwalking, eating while sleeping, having violent outbursts and, yes, driving while asleep (their eyes were open). Some even developed nighttime eating disorders. One woman woke up and found she'd painted her front door.

Drinking alcohol while taking the medicine seems to increase the risk of these behaviors which are, overall, quite rare. Such problems were seen only with these newer drugs, but the FDA now requires that all sleep aids carry a warning about them.

☐ **MIGRAINE MEDICINES**

I take Imitrex for my migraines, but how do I know if I should take medicine to *prevent* migraines?

Doctors generally prescribe preventive, or prophylactic, medication for migraine if your headaches significantly interfere with your daily routine, you have two or more debilitating migraines a month, you use medication to stop a migraine more than twice a week, or if you simply want to stop having as many migraines. The first-choice drugs are beta-blockers, which are also used to reduce blood pressure. The most studied and most often prescribed are propranolol (Inderal) and timolol (Blocadren). Although other options are available, beta-blockers are the safest and most effective, with between 50 and 80 percent of people taking them having fewer migraines or none at all. The only downside? Beta-blockers can leave you tired and lethargic.

Other preventive drugs include the antidepressant amitriptyline (Vanatrip, Elavil), the calcium channel blocker verapamil (Calan, Isoptin, Verelan, and others), the anticonvulsant divalproex sodium (Depakote), and the angiotensin II blockers irbesartan (Avapro) and candesartan (Atacand). None except divalproex is specifically approved for preventing migraines, but over the years, doctors have learned that these drugs prevent the pain, so today they prescribe them "off-label."

The only other FDA-approved medication for migraine prevention is the anticonvulsant topiramate (Topamax). While effective, it has more side effects than many of the other options, so it's not usually a first choice.

I have heart disease. Can I still take Imitrex for my migraines?

Sumatriptan (Imitrex) is one of several drugs known as trip-

tans. They revolutionized migraine treatment when they were introduced in 1992 because they are so effective. Triptans work in one of three ways: constricting blood vessels in the head, reducing inflammation around these blood vessels, or reducing the amount of pain you feel in your head. However, they also constrict coronary blood vessels. Thus, some people complain of tightness, pressure, and pain in their chests, necks, or throats, and there have been reports of people experiencing increased blood pressure, angina (chest pain caused by clogged arteries), heart attacks, and heart rhythm changes after taking a triptan. So if you have heart disease or any risks for heart disease, talk with your doctor about other migraine options.

☐ **OBESITY DRUGS**

Can I still eat hamburgers if I'm taking Xenical?

Orlistat (Xenical) works in your gut to prevent your body from absorbing some of the fat you eat. Coupled with diet and exercise, it can help you lose up to 50 percent more weight than diet and exercise alone. But if you ignore warnings to avoid fatty foods while taking Xenical, you will suffer the consequences: cramps, gas, and stool leakage.

?? FACT OR FICTION

A Prescription Migraine Medicine Is Always Best

Fiction. Over-the-counter "migraine formulas" that combine acetaminophen, aspirin, and caffeine, such as Excedrin Migraine, may be all you need if your migraines are mild and don't involve nausea or vomiting. One study found that for such people, these drugs worked as well as low doses (50 milligrams) of Imitrex.

WHAT YOU DON'T KNOW

Xenical Can Reduce Cholesterol

Because it blocks the absorption of some of the fat you eat, it also lowers levels of LDL or "bad" cholesterol and blood fats known as triglycerides.

Is Xenical safe?

Generally speaking, the drug is thought to be safe. But in 2009, the FDA received reports of 32 cases of serious liver injury in people taking prescription-strength Xenical or the half-strength over-the-counter version called Alli. The issue is still being investigated. But if you have any risk for liver disease, such as hepatitis C or heavy drinking, talk with your doctor about whether Xenical is right for you.

Will I become addicted if I take phentermine to help me lose weight?

You shouldn't. Phentermine (Adipex-P, Pro-Fast) is a cousin of amphetamine, a stimulant that reduces appetite but is highly addictive. Phentermine also reduces appetite, but it doesn't have any effect on brain areas related to addiction. If you take it as directed for weight loss, you should be fine. Note that taking too much of this medication can cause serious, life-threatening side effects.

I'm taking Prozac for depression, and I want to take Meridia for weight loss. Is that okay?

No. Selective serotonin reuptake inhibitors (SSRIs) such as fluoxetine (Prozac) increase levels of serotonin, a neurotransmitter that plays a role in mood and appetite. So does sibutramine (Meridia). Too much serotonin in your system can cause a potentially life-threatening condition called serotonin syndrome. Symptoms include agitation, rapid heartbeat, hallucinations, diarrhea, and nausea.

☐ OSTEOPOROSIS MEDICINES

Why do I have to sit after I take Fosamax for my osteoporosis?

You don't. You can stand or walk and generally carry on with your normal activities—as long as you don't lie down for at least 30 minutes, or 60 minutes if you take ibandronate (Boniva). Otherwise you might experience heartburn or irritation of the esophagus, which can make swallowing painful or difficult. It's important to take alendronate (Fosamax) on an

WHAT YOU DON'T KNOW

Osteoporosis Drugs Can Affect the Jawbone

Very rarely, some people who take a bisphosphonate drug such as alendronate (Fosamax), zoledronic acid (Reclast), and risedronate (Actonel) experience osteonecrosis, a condition in which the jawbone literally crumbles as its cells die off. The risk is highest in people receiving high doses of an IV bisphosphonate for cancer-related bone loss or rheumatic diseases, particularly if they also receive chemotherapy or immunotherapy. Other risk factors include smoking and dental problems such as abscesses, gum disease, and dentures that don't fit right. If you're taking a bisphosphonate, take good care of your teeth and mouth (brush and floss at least twice a day), see your dentist at least twice a year, and tell your dentist that you take a bisphosphonate.

empty stomach; otherwise the drug won't work. That's why you should take it first thing in the morning, with a full glass of water (again to prevent irritation of the esophagus).

Since I'm taking medication for my osteoporosis, do I still have to take vitamin D and calcium?

Yes. It's important that you get enough vitamin D (at least 1,000 IU a day) and calcium (1,000 milligrams or 1,200 milligrams a day, depending on your age) from diet or supplements when you're taking a bisphosphonate drug such as alendronate (Fosamax) or ibandronate (Boniva). While bisphosphonates slow bone loss, you still need calcium and vitamin D to build bone. Calcium is a major component of bone, and vitamin D enables you to absorb calcium from food or supplements. Low levels of either could interfere with the drugs' ability to slow bone breakdown. At least one study found that people with low vitamin D levels while taking bisphosphonates had lower bone mineral density at the hip than those with higher levels of vitamin D.

Most people, particularly those age 65 and older, need to supplement with vitamin D because it is so difficult to get it from food or even sunshine (if you always wear sunscreen or you live in a Northern climate). One way to get enough vitamin D with your bisphosphonate is to take Fosamax Plus D, which combines the once-a-week Fosamax dosage with 5,600 IU of the vitamin (equal to 800 IU a day).

☐ **OVERACTIVE BLADDER MEDICINES**

I've heard of Botox for wrinkles, but now my neighbor says her doctor is using it for her overactive bladder. Why?

Botox (botulinum toxin type A) is a bacterial poison. Injected into the face, it reduces muscle contractions by blocking the nerve signals to those muscles, resulting in reduced wrinkles. The fact that Botox can reduce muscle contractions also makes it useful in cases of overactive bladder, in which twitchy bladder muscles cause the frequent urge to urinate. Several studies find that Botox is very effective for overactive bladder, with a single dose providing relief for up to 24 weeks. It's not easy getting the Botox where it needs to go, however. The drug is administered through a needle at the end of a cysto-scope, a long tube inserted into the bladder. Another downside is that some people retain urine in their bladder after receiving the injections and need catheterization to remove the fluid.

Why does my vision become blurry when I take Ditropan for my overactive bladder?

Oxybutynin (Ditropan) belongs to a class of drugs called antimuscarinics. They work by preventing bladder contractions that make you feel as if you have to go to the bathroom all the time. Unfortunately, the same mechanism used to relax the bladder muscle also relaxes muscle fibers in the eye, leading to blurry vision. Other common side effects from these medications include constipation, hives, fatigue, nausea, dry mouth, and vomiting. If the side effects bother you, ask your doctor about taking a lower dose or switching to another medicine in this class. One of the newer drugs in this class, trospium (Sanctura), appears to have fewer and less-intense side effects than its cousins, while the one you're taking, Ditropan, tends to have the greatest risk of side effects. Don't use alcohol while taking these drugs, as it can make the blurred vision worse.

☐ PAIN RELIEVERS

I'm taking Celebrex for arthritis. Will it damage my heart?

Celecoxib (Celebrex) belongs to the COX-2 inhibitor class of drugs. These nonsteroidal anti-inflammatory drugs (NSAIDs) were widely prescribed as pain relievers in the 1990s and early 2000s because it was thought that they didn't harm the stomach lining and cause as much gastrointestinal bleeding as NSAIDs like ibuprofen and aspirin. But in 2004, a clinical trial evaluating the use of Celebrex to prevent precancerous polyps in the colon was stopped when researchers learned that people taking the drug had a 3.4 times greater risk of heart attacks, unstable angina (sudden and increasing chest pain), stroke, or other heart problems than those not taking it. In addition, it turned out that COX-2 inhibitors didn't prevent gastro-intestinal bleeding.

After careful evaluation, the FDA determined that, for some patients, the benefits of Celebrex outweighed the risks, so the drug remained on the

AVOID THIS MISTAKE

Waiting Out the Pain

It is much easier to stop pain from getting worse than it is to reduce pain once it maxes out. So, for instance, if you feel a bad headache coming on, don't wait until you're lying curled in a fetal position in a dark room to take something. Take it the minute you feel the first throbbing.

market. Two other COX-2 inhibitors—valdecoxib (Bextra) and rofecoxib (Vioxx)—were removed from the market. Since then, all NSAIDs, including over-the-counter products, warn of heart-related risks and gastrointestinal bleeding. The risks are highest for people who have coronary artery disease or a history of stomach ulcers and for people who have had cardiovascular bypass surgery or a stroke or ministroke.

My doctor prescribed Vicodin for my severe back pain. Will I become addicted?

It's unlikely. Vicodin (hydrocodone plus acetaminophen) belongs to a class of pain-relieving drugs called opioids that

work by interfering with the way your brain processes pain signals. While opioids are very powerful drugs, when they are used properly, the risk of addiction is low. In one study of people who took these drugs for several weeks or even months to relieve chronic pain, just 3.2 percent became addicted, meaning that they suffered physical symptoms when they tried to stop taking the drug. And most of these people already had a history of substance abuse.

That said, Vicodin should not be taken long-term given the risks of liver damage with acetaminophen. If you have chronic back pain, talk to your doctor about options such as other pain relievers, physical therapy, and exercise.

Is it okay to mix herbs and arthritis drugs?

Check with your doctor or pharmacist first. In a study of 238 arthritis patients, 1 in 10 reported taking supplements known to interact with some arthritis medications. Five of 120 patients raised their risk of liver toxicity by

DRUG-FREE FIX

Exercise

At least 10 minutes of aerobic exercise—biking, fast walking, running on the treadmill—can significantly improve chronic pain, likely by releasing natural pain relievers called endorphins.

taking echinacea, and 10 percent of patients taking NSAIDs increased their risk of bleeding problems by taking ginkgo biloba, garlic, and devil's claw.

Why did my doctor prescribe an antiseizure medication for my nerve pain?

Two antiseizure medications, pregabalin (Lyrica) and gabapentin (Neurontin), have been approved for the treatment of chronic neuropathic pain. This type of burning, agonizing pain results from injury or damage to the nerves, often from diabetes or the viral disease shingles. Other prescription pain relievers such as morphine and oxycodone don't always work for neuropathic pain, but anticonvulsants seem to work quite well. Side effects can include headache, confusion, skin rash, nausea, vomiting, abdominal pain, weight gain or loss, and swollen feet. Anticonvulsants can also increase the risk of suicide, so tell your doctor immediately if you have any thoughts of hurting yourself.

☐ PARKINSON'S DISEASE DRUGS

Help! My husband's been taking the Parkinson's drug Apokyn for the past 3 months and has started to gamble compulsively. He's lost $10,000! What's going on?

Unfortunately, your husband is in a small minority of people in whom these drugs, known as dopamine agonists, cause pathological behavior such as excessive gambling, shopping, or even sex. In one study of nearly 300 people taking the drugs, 6 percent reported such behavior, primarily gambling. (In the general population, only about 1 percent of people are pathological gamblers.) The Parkinson gamblers typically played the slots and had lost an average of $100,000 each; many were close to divorce as a result.

Rather than blaming your husband, blame the medicine. Dopamine agonists, which include apomorphine (Apokyn), bromocriptine mesylate (Parlodel), pramipexole (Mirapex), and ropinirole hydrochloride (Requip), mimic the action of dopamine. Dopamine acts in areas of the brain related to pleasure and reward and contributes to addiction. Tell your doctor about your husband's gambling and ask that he be switched to a different medication. Even switching to a different dopamine agonist might work.

☐ PROSTATE ENLARGEMENT MEDICINES

Is it safe for a 79-year-old man to take a drug like Flomax for an enlarged prostate?

That depends on whether he has any other medical problems. Drugs like terazosin (Hytrin), doxazosin (Cardura), alfuzosin (Uroxatral), tamsulosin (Flomax), and prazosin (Minipress) work by relaxing smooth muscles in the prostate gland. But in doing so they also lower blood pressure. In fact, several of them were originally developed and marketed as blood pressure drugs.

The low blood pressure can lead to dizziness or even fainting when you stand up from a sitting or lying position. A review of six

DRUG-FREE FIX

Vitamin D

Does your pain persist despite high doses of narcotics? Ask your doctor to check your blood level of vitamin D. A recent study found that people with chronic pain who had low vitamin D levels needed nearly twice as much medication to control their pain. Other research suggests that low levels of vitamin D might contribute to unexplained muscle and bone pain.

studies involving these drugs found that this side effect was most common in men taking Hytrin, even those with untreated high blood pressure. Uroxatral showed similar effects, particularly in men older than age 75, those with heart problems, and those being treated with blood pressure medications. Flomax has the lowest risk of dizziness and fainting. The good news is that the dizziness with Hytrin and its cousins often disappear after a few days. In the meantime, to reduce the risk of falling, take Hytrin at night after getting into bed.

I take Flomax for my prostate and am having cataract surgery. Why did my doctor tell me to stop taking the medicine for 2 weeks before the surgery?

One published study evaluated more than 96,000 men who had cataract surgery and found that men who had taken tamsulosin (Flomax) within 14 days before their surgery had a 2.3 times higher risk of complications than men who didn't take the drug. Flomax is designed to relax the smooth muscle found in the prostate gland, so it stops clenching the top of the bladder, triggering the urge to pee while interfering with urination. However, the same chemical responsible for smooth muscle

DRUG-FREE FIX

Fish Oil for Rheumatoid Arthritis

If you have rheumatoid arthritis, take a fish-oil supplement containing at least 2.2 grams of eicosapentaenoic acid (EPA) a day. Numerous studies have found that the anti-inflammatory effects of fish oil can reduce the pain and morning stiffness of rheumatoid arthritis and cut the amount of nonsteroidal anti-inflammatory drugs (NSAIDs) required by more than a third.

contraction in the prostate also enables your pupils to contract. If it can't contract, it remains abnormally large, resulting in floppy iris syndrome. During surgery, floppy iris syndrome requires special instruments to hold back the iris, which increases the risk of damage. It can also cause other problems that increase the risk of surgery-related damage. The problems seems limited to Flomax; researchers didn't see any connection between floppy iris syndrome and other drugs for prostate enlargement.

☐ RHEUMATOID ARTHRITIS DRUGS

I've been taking prednisone for the past few weeks and it's really helped. But now my doctor wants to put me on Rheumatrex. Isn't that a cancer drug?

Corticosteroids such as prednisone help reduce inflammation

and pain and prevent joint damage. They are most often used when you have a flare-up of pain. And yes, they are terrific at relieving your symptoms. But steroids have significant side effects when used long-term, including an increased risk of diabetes, osteoporosis, weight gain, and cataracts. That's why your doctor doesn't want to keep you on the prednisone for too long.

Methotrexate (Trexall) is a disease-modifying antirheumatic drug (DMARD) often used for rheumatoid arthritis. Among other actions, it inhibits overactivity of the immune system, the causes of the disease, helping to suppress inflammation and protecting joints. Yes, it is also used to treat some cancers, but it has been used as a first-line treatment for rheumatoid arthritis for decades. If you have problems with side effects (primarily nausea or vomiting), ask your doctor about splitting the dose and taking it twice a week instead of once a week. You shouldn't drink alcohol while taking this medication because it can affect your liver.

Next week, I get my first treatment with Remicade. How long will it take before it works, and what side effects should I know about?

You should start feeling better in anywhere from a few days to a couple of weeks. Infliximab (Remicade) belongs to the newest generation of drugs for rheumatoid arthritis. The other medicines in this class are adalimumab (Humira) and etanercept (Enbrel). They work by putting the brakes on a chemical called tumor necrosis factor (TNF) that, in turn, stimulates the inflammation that is the root cause of the pain and disability of rheumatoid arthritis. The drugs not only relieve the pain, swelling, and stiffness of the disease but also slow the underlying disease to reduce or even halt additional damage. The greatest risk is that because the drugs suppress part of the immune system, they make you more susceptible to tuberculosis and other serious, potentially fatal infections. That's why your doctor will monitor you closely while you're on this medication. Call your doctor right away if you have any signs of an infection, such as a fever, cough, flulike symptoms, or skin that's red and painful while on the drug.

☐ SLEEP APNEA MEDICINES

I have sleep apnea. Even though I use a continuous positive airway pressure machine, I'm still very sleepy the next day. My doctor prescribed Provigil. Is it safe?

Modafinil (Provigil) is a stimulant approved for the treatment of excessive daytime sleepiness caused by obstructive sleep apnea, narcolepsy, or shift-work disorder. Like stimulants used to treat ADHD, it not only helps you feel more alert but also improves concentration. The most serious side effect is a rash bad enough to send you to the hospital. There have also been some reports of psychiatric symptoms such as mania, delusions, hallucinations, and thoughts of suicide. So, like any other drug, Provigil has risks and benefits. It should not be taken simply to perk you up after a rough week at the office, only for tiredness that is so severe that it interferes with your ability to

function. Make sure you discuss the pros and cons of this medication with your doctor.

☐ THYROID MEDICINES

I take thyroid replacement pills for low thyroid. Some over-the-counter medicines like cold medicines say not to take them if you have thyroid disease. Does that mean me?

Probably not. While you should always check with your doctor, it's generally understood that this warning is more for people with hyperthyroidism (overactive thyroid) than hypothyroidism (underactive thyroid). Because some cold medicines contain stimulants, they could overstimulate people with overactive thyroid or strain their hearts. That said, some people with low thyroid hormone levels do find that they become sensitive to ingredients in cold and sinus medicines like pseudoephedrine. Some doctors recommend trying a partial dose to see if you have a reaction before taking the full dose.

Does it really matter when I take my thyroid pill?

Yes. Ideally you should take it first thing in the morning before you eat anything. That said, if you normally take your thyroid medicine with food and your thyroid levels are good, don't change anything. Also, it's important to take your multivitamin (especially if it contains iron) and calcium pill at least 2 hours after taking your thyroid pill; otherwise they could interfere with your body's ability to metabolize the thyroid medication.

☐ **ULCER MEDICINES**

Why did my doctor give me more than one prescription for my ulcer?

Most ulcers are caused by the bacteria *Helicobacter pylori*. While it makes sense to think that an antibiotic would be all you need to wipe out the culprit, it's not so simple. For years, the therapy of choice was a three-drug regimen involving two antibiotics— amoxicillin and clarithromycin —and a proton-pump inhibitor such as lansoprazole (Prevacid), omeprazole (Prilosec), or pantoprazole (Protonix) to halt acid production while the ulcer healed. Now, though, *H. pylori* is becoming resistant to clarithromycin, so some doctors are using a new four-drug therapy. A small study comparing the three-drug regimen with a four-drug combo of Prevacid, the antibiotics metronidazole and tetracycline, and the ulcer-fighting mineral bismuth subcitrate found that both approaches worked equally well, though people taking the four-drug combo were more likely to have nausea, vomiting, diarrhea, and black stools than those in the three-drug group. An advantage to the four-drug regimen? It's cheaper because most of the drugs are generic.

FAQ Frequently Asked Questions

Vitamins, Herbs, and Other Supplements

Are expensive supplements better? How do I know which brand to buy?

A high price tag isn't necessarily a sign of high quality. Some supplement sellers charge more only to convince consumers that their products are superior or contain high-quality ingredients. But that may not be true. "Very high-priced supplements can be junk," says Tod Cooperman, MD, president of ConsumerLab.com, which tests the quality of dietary supplements.

Meanwhile, low price isn't necessarily a sign of poor quality. Many large chains can charge less for supplements because they buy in high volume. However, be leery of low-priced products marketed by companies you have never heard of. Even the quality of

dietary supplements sold by reputable companies can vary, since the companies may purchase ingredients from all over the world, making it difficult to maintain consistency. The best general advice is to shop for well-established brands. For a modest subscription fee, you can check whether specific brands passed the quality test at www.consumerlab.com.

You might also look for products bearing the seal of an independent product tester such as ConsumerLab.com, United States Pharmacopeia (USP), and NSF International. Their seals of approval indicate that a product is likely to contain the amount of active ingredient listed on the label and be free of contaminants. The seal of approval from one of these authorities is not proof that an herbal remedy or nutrient actually cures or prevents any condition.

I sometimes see "standardized extract" on the labels of herb bottles. What does it mean?

Supplement manufacturers use this phrase to indicate that a product contains a specific concentration of key compounds from a medicinal plant—and only those compounds, which are "extracted" from whole dried herbs. Many standardized extracts contain the same level of these compounds as products that have been tested in clinical trials, though manufacturers are free to decide how much a "standardized" dose should contain. By contrast, if you buy whole-herb supplements, the amounts of the key ingredient may vary greatly from brand to brand and even batch to batch due to differences in growing conditions. In addition, whole herbs may contain traces of lead and other heavy metals, which are typically removed from standardized extracts.

Can I take all of my supplements at the same time, or will some block absorption of others?

In general, it's okay to take all of your supplements at once, with some exceptions. If you take a large dose of any vitamin or mineral, it's probably wise to do it a few hours after taking your other supplements. Calcium supplements are a good example. Taking a multivitamin and a calcium supplement at the same time is a mistake; the large dose of calcium (which can be up to 600 milligrams per dose) may block your body from absorbing other minerals, such as iron, chromium, and manganese, in the multivitamin. Large doses of vitamin C

could block your body's ability to absorb vitamin B_{12}.

Two more good rules to follow:

- *Take your multi and other vitamin supplements at mealtime.* You need some fat in the digestive tract to properly absorb fat-soluble vitamins A, D, E, and K.

- *Take medications and multivitamins a few hours apart.* Some vitamins and minerals can block drugs from being absorbed, making them less effective. For instance, calcium can interfere with thyroid medications. Some drugs can have a similar effect on vitamins and minerals.

I'm a vegetarian. What supplements do I need? Are there some I should avoid?

If you eat dairy foods and/or eggs and plan your diet well, you probably don't need vitamin supplements. But vegans, who eat no form of animal food, may be deficient in certain nutrients,

particularly vitamin B_{12}. Eating foods fortified with this vitamin (such as soy milk and breakfast cereal) can fill the void. Otherwise, getting vitamin B_{12} from a supplement is a must. A typical multivitamin will do the job; it will also give you at least a portion, and possibly all, of the daily requirement for other nutrients that may be low in a vegan diet, including calcium, vitamin D, iodine, iron, selenium, and zinc.

Certain supplements are off-limits if you follow a strictly vegetarian lifestyle. If you don't eat seafood, then obviously fish-oil capsules are not an option (though you can purchase supplements made from algae, plants that are a rich source of omega-3 fatty acids). And if you're a vegan and you take vitamin D, look for supplements containing vitamin D_2, or ergocalciferol. Vitamin D_3, the most common form by far, is made from lanolin, which is derived from sheep's wool. It's probably wise to assume that any supplement sold as gel caps that are not labeled "vegetarian" contains gelatin, which is made from animal protein.

Should I just take the dose in the directions?

Not necessarily. Compare brands and you may find that the recommended dose for the same vitamin, mineral, or other supplement can vary by as much as 10-fold. The dose you

AVOID THIS MISTAKE

Taking Calcium on an Empty Stomach

The calcium in most supplements is bound to a form of salt called carbonate. Your stomach needs plenty of hydrochloric acid to break down calcium carbonate, so always take your supplement with a meal or snack. Food will cause your stomach to produce the acid.

need will depend on the condition you're trying to prevent or treat, your gender, your age, and other factors. Talk to your doctor or get a recommendation from a trustworthy source. The complementary medicine section of the University of Maryland Medical Center's web site, www.umm.edu/altmed, offers comprehensive information on herbs and supplements, including dosing advice.

Should I take a daily multivitamin?

Surprisingly, it turns out there's not much evidence that people who faithfully toss back a multivitamin every morning are any healthier than those who don't. Some studies have even hinted that taking a multivitamin may actually cause harm. For instance, a study of more than 300,000 men by the National Cancer Institute found that multivitamin users doubled their risk for prostate cancer. Other research linked the use of a daily multi to a modest increase in the risk for breast and colon cancers.

One concern voiced by skeptics is that taking a multivitamin may expose you to too much folic acid. This B vitamin is essential for pregnant women, since it prevents spina bifida and related birth defects. Some studies indicate that folic acid may lower the risk for heart

attacks and strokes, too. But getting too much has drawbacks. It can mask signs of anemia in older people. And some scientists suspect that large amounts may feed cancerous tumors or growths that could become cancer.

The Center for Science in the Public Interest, a health watchdog group, recommends taking a multivitamin, but only every other day to limit your exposure to folic acid (unless you're pregnant, in which case daily is still the way to go). The Harvard School of Public Health, meanwhile, argues that taking a daily multi is still the best plan, but if you do, it's best to avoid foods—particularly breakfast cereals—fortified with folic acid.

Should I take a multivitamin that's specially formulated for my age or gender, or for a specific medical concern?

Generally speaking, don't bother, especially if it's more expensive than a standard multivitamin. There are countless multis on the market aimed at men, women, and other niche groups. For example, a multivitamin for women over 50 may contain additional ingredients for relieving hot flashes (such as black cohosh) or strengthening bones (such as soy). A multivitamin offering "immune support" might have extra vita-

 AVOID THIS MISTAKE

Storing Supplements in the Medicine Chest

High humidity in the bathroom could damage supplements; store them in a cool, dry place instead. Other good storage habits:
• Don't keep your daily supplements in the refrigerator unless the label says you should. Removing them every day will allow condensation to build up inside the container.
• If you buy supplements in bulk, keep 3 months' worth available for daily use and store the rest in the refrigerator. When you're ready to use them, remove them from the fridge and allow the container to reach room temperature before opening.
• Keep supplements in their original bottles with the caps screwed on tightly to preserve potency.

min C, plus echinacea and zinc. Often, however, these formulations contain skimpy amounts of "bonus" ingredients—too little to have any therapeutic effect (assuming the ingredients have any health benefits at any dosage).

There are some exceptions to the rule. For instance, postmenopausal women should look for a supplement without iron, whereas women who have been advised to take iron may want to get it in a multi. Beware, however, that pills marketed to women who need extra iron (such as women of childbearing age) may contain herbs and other ingredients that you don't want or need.

Will any supplements increase my energy?

If you eat a healthy diet, megadoses of vitamins and minerals won't rev up your stamina or strength. And the evidence that other herbs and supplements will give you a lift is spotty, at best. What might help:

- *Iron supplements.* These are standard therapy for people suffering from anemia, which causes fatigue. A doctor may prescribe vitamin C in addition, which makes it easier for the body to absorb iron. But don't take iron on your own or without having your blood iron levels tested first to confirm that you're low.

- *Vitamin B_{12}.* The ability to absorb vitamin B_{12} from the diet begins to diminish at midlife, which is why people over 50 are advised to eat foods fortified with vitamin B_{12} or take supplements. (Ask your doctor how much you need; a dose of 25 to 100 micrograms is usually recommended. You'll find the lower amount in many multivitamins.) Lack of other B vitamins, including biotin (vitamin B_7) and pantothenic acid (vitamin B_5) can cause fatigue, too, but that's less common. To be on the safe side, though, you may want to take a vitamin B complex supplement, which contains a daily dose of these important nutrients. B_{12} supplements may be prescribed for treating fatigue related to pernicious anemia, though severe cases require injections.

Beware of these alleged energy-boosters:

- *Ginseng.* This herb's reputation as a performance-booster came from poor-quality studies; there's little solid proof that it makes you work any harder or faster.

- *Guarana.* It sounds exotic, but this herb is nothing more than a natural source of caffeine.

- *Taurine.* This amino acid allegedly puts the zip in popular energy drinks, though the evidence is spotty—and the energized feeling the drinks

offer probably comes from caffeine and sugar.

Are joint-relief formulas effective?

Some may be at least marginally effective. The cause of your joint pain should dictate which you try.

- *Osteoarthritis.* For the most common type of arthritis, glucosamine and chondroitin—alone or in combination—appear to be the supplements that offer the most reliable relief, though not all studies have been positive, and the effects may be modest. Some studies suggest that the supplement SAM-e relieves arthritis-related inflammation as well as ibuprofen and other pain relievers. Some arthritis sufferers turn to ginger, devil's claw, and methylsulfonylmethane (MSM), too, but the science behind these supplements isn't as solid.

- *Rheumatoid arthritis.* This condition results when the immune system mistakenly attacks the joints. Some studies suggest that fish oil and evening primrose oil may ease the pain, but others found no benefit. A 2009 review determined that MSM and a related compound, dimethyl sulfoxide (DMSO), don't help. Other products, including bromelain and selenium, seem promising, but more research is necessary.

What is the best supplement for boosting my immune system?

Eating a well-balanced diet is the best way to strengthen your immune system. That's especially true if you consume plenty of foods rich in vitamin A (which takes the form of beta-carotene and other related compounds in fruits and vege-tables) and vitamin D (salmon is a good source). That said, some studies suggest that a few dietary supplements may help shore up your body's defense against germs.

- *Andrographis.* The herb, sometimes called Indian echi-nacea, may prevent colds and alleviate symptoms by boosting the immune system, according to a handful of studies. Prelimi-nary research also suggests that pairing andrographis with Siberian ginseng may make flu symptoms less nasty.

- *Astragalus.* This herb's repu-tation as an immune-booster comes primarily from its use in traditional Chinese medicine. Studies have shown that astra-galus supplements may rev up immune cells more than echi-nacea pills. In China, some cancer patients receive astrag-alus preparations to strengthen the immune system and increase the effects of chemo-therapy.

- *Echinacea.* Echinacea is most widely used for prevent-ing and treating colds. One 2007 review of studies found that echinacea supplements cut the risk of developing a cold by 58 percent, though other research is less positive.

- *Zinc.* Even mild zinc defi-ciency can turn down immune system activity, and some evidence suggests that sup-plements can help reduce infections. In one study, people who took 45 milligrams of zinc daily cut their risk for developing colds, the flu, cold sores, eye infections, and other infections by 80 percent. But talk to your doctor before taking more than 40 milligrams of zinc per day. High doses can have a variety of side effects including, ironically, lowered immunity.

If antioxidants are so important in fighting dis-eases like cancer, shouldn't I take an antioxidant formula?

No. While eating foods rich in antioxidants, which neutralize damaging molecules known as free radicals, is one of the most important things you can do for your health, popping antioxi-dant pills just doesn't offer the same benefits—and could even backfire. In a 2007 study published in the *Journal of the American Medical Association*, Danish scientists posed a simple question: Do people who take antioxidant supple-ments live longer than the rest of us? No, they concluded after analyzing 68 clinical trials involving 232,606 participants. In fact, death rates were slightly higher among people who took high doses of beta-carotene, vitamin A, and vitamin E supplements. The evidence was mixed for vitamin C and the mineral selenium. The take-home mes-sage? Get your antioxidants at the dinner table, not from the supplement aisle.

Do I really need to check with my doctor before taking a supplement?

If you're healthy and you decide to start taking a stan-dard multivitamin, there's no reason to contact your physi-cian, though you should mention your new habit at your next visit. If you choose to take an individual vitamin or mineral supplement, don't exceed the recommended daily intake for your gender and age group (check a reliable source such as the web site of the Office of Dietary Supplements at www. ods.od.nih.gov) without con-sulting your doctor. In all other cases, it's wise to discuss your supplement use with a physi-cian. Your doctor can help you decide whether you really need a given supplement and what dose is appropriate. He can also explain potential side effects and tell you whether the supplement will interact with drugs you may be taking.

Don't some supplements just pass through your body without breaking down?

Some poorly formulated supplements may fail to dissolve in the digestive tract, rendering the pills useless. That's more likely to occur with tablets and caplets, less likely with capsules and chewable pills. To avoid wasting money on dud pills, look for supplements that bear a seal of approval from ConsumerLab.com or United States Pharmacopeia (USP). Either seal means the supplement passed a disintegration test.

To test a supplement on your own, ConsumerLab.com recommends heating a cup of vinegar to 98.6°F (use a food thermometer and don't rest it on the hot bottom of the pan). Add the pill and stir frequently for 30 to 45 minutes. If the pill doesn't dissolve, it won't dissolve in your body either. Note: This test does not work with enteric-coated tablets.

Do supplements lose their potency over time?

Yes, though you may be better off relying on your senses than the package label. In the United States and some other countries, manufacturers are not required to stamp an expiration date on the label of a dietary supplement. Many do so anyway, and the expiration date represents the last day the manufacturer guarantees a product's potency. However, experts say that properly stored vitamins and other supplements can maintain their potency for another year or more past the expiration date. As a general rule, toss out any vitamin or herbal product that has changed color, taste, or smell—it's probably no good (though expired supplements are unlikely to cause any harm).

Do acai berry pills really help you trim pounds? Are any other weight-loss herbs effective?

There may be good reasons to eat acai berries or drink their juice, but despite all the hype, there have been no published studies on acai (pronounced ah-sigh-EE) supplements as a diet aid, so we have no idea whether or not they work. The grape-size acai berry comes from palm trees that grow in South America. Several years ago, companies began selling acai pills on the internet, claiming their products would help you "flush pounds," "detoxify" your body, and more. Acai does contain vitamin C and other antioxidants, but so do oranges and plenty of other fruits.

Acai is hardly unique; most herbs and supplements touted as weight-loss aids have little in the way of solid evidence behind them. There's one intriguing exception, however. Results from nearly a dozen studies suggest that green tea extract may modestly speed up weight loss. Scientists believe that green tea's combination of caffeine and an antioxidant called EGCG helps the body burn extra calories and fat.

Are there any supplements that help prevent cancer?

There are none with a proven track record. Researchers have looked at a variety of supplements, including beta-carotene, vitamin E, the mineral selenium, and lycopene, a compound found in cooked tomatoes. Population studies showed that people who consumed large amounts of these nutrients had low rates of several major cancers. But studies have failed to show that supplements cut cancer risk. In fact, one study found that smokers who took beta-carotene supplements increased their risk for lung cancer by 18 percent.

At present, green tea extract may be the most promising anticancer supplement, though the evidence is inconsistent and far from conclusive.

COMMON SUPPLEMENTS

What the Science Says

When something ails you, be it depression or the common cold, supplements may—or may not—help. Wandering the supplement aisles can fill you with both hope and doubt. Before you shop, check out what the science says about the vitamins, herbs, and other supplements commonly used to treat your ailment.

ALLERGIES

Popular Supplement: **Butterbur**	**Is It Worth Trying?** In some studies, this herb has proven as effective as antihistamines for treating hay fever. Avoid raw butterbur, which may cause liver damage.	**Common Dose:** 50 to 75 milligrams a day

ANGINA

Popular Supplement: **Carnitine**	**Is It Worth Trying?** Several studies have found that this vitamin-like supplement may help relieve chest pain and allow longer periods of pain-free exercise in angina patients when taken in addition to standard drug therapy. You may see this supplement labeled as L-carnitine.	**Common Dose:** 1.5 to 2 grams a day
Popular Supplement: **Coenzyme Q10**	**Is It Worth Trying?** A few studies suggest that supplements of this energy-producing compound may provide greater stamina in angina patients, many of whom have low levels of coenzyme Q10.	**Common Dose:** 30 to 300 milligrams a day, though some studies used higher doses

ANXIETY

Popular Supplement: **Kava**	**Is It Worth Trying?** A review of 11 studies found kava to be mildly effective and safe for use up to 6 months. Safety beyond 6 months is unknown; some countries have banned kava because of concerns about liver toxicity. May slow reflexes and impair judgment.	**Common Dose:** 150 to 300 milligrams (30 to 70 percent kavalactones) a day
Popular Supplement: **Valerian**	**Is It Worth Trying?** Some research suggests that valerian has a calming effect in stressful situations, though better studies are needed. May cause drowsiness, which is why it's also used as a sleep aid.	**Common Dose:** 200 milligrams, three or four times a day

ARTHRITIS

Popular Supplement: Fish oil	**Is It Worth Trying?** A 2007 review found that fish-oil supplements significantly reduce joint pain, tenderness, and stiffness in patients with rheumatoid arthritis (the kind caused by a problem in the immune system). However, fish oil probably won't keep the condition from getting worse.	**Common Dose:** 3 grams a day has been used in some studies for rheumatoid arthritis
Popular Supplement: Glucosamine and chondroitin	**Is It Worth Trying?** Often combined in one pill, but also sold as separate supplements. Some of the enthusiasm about glucosamine and chondroitin has waned in recent years, thanks to several large studies that found they offer no relief from pain and stiffness. However, earlier studies showed that they can ease pain and may even slow the progression of arthritis. Many doctors aren't ready to dismiss these supplements just yet and continue to recommend them. A word of caution: ConsumerLab.com's testing has found that the potency of many chondroitin supplements doesn't match the amount claimed on the label.	**Common Dose:** 500 milligrams, three times a day (glucosamine); 400 milligrams, three times a day (chondroitin)
Popular Supplement: SAM-e	**Is It Worth Trying?** May be as effective as ibuprofen and other nonsteroidal anti-inflammatory drugs (NSAIDs), though it's not clear that SAM-e stops damage to joints. SAM-e is safe, though it's is also very expensive.	**Common Dose:** 600 to 1,200 milligrams a day, divided into two or three doses

BACK PAIN

Popular Supplement: Devil's claw	**Is It Worth Trying?** Several well-designed studies found that this herb relieves back pain. Devil's claw is relatively safe, but avoid it if you have stomach ulcers or take blood-thinning drugs.	**Common Dose:** 600 to 1,200 milligrams, three times a day
Popular Supplement: White willow bark	**Is It Worth Trying?** Contains salicin, which is closely related to the pain-relieving chemical in aspirin. Don't combine it with aspirin or NSAIDs.	**Common Dose:** 400 to 800 milligrams (standardized to 15 percent salicin), twice a day

BONE LOSS

Popular Supplement: Calcium	**Is It Worth Trying?** Many, though not all, studies show that calcium supplements slow bone loss that occurs with aging and reduces the risk of fractures. Calcium appears to be most beneficial when taken with vitamin D supplements. It's possible to get adequate calcium from your diet, but doctors often recommend supplements as insurance.	**Common Dose:** 1,000 milligrams (age 50 and younger) and 1,200 milligrams (51 and older) a day; take no more than 500 milligrams at a time, with food, for best absorption
Popular Supplement: Isoflavones	**Is It Worth Trying?** Soy extract and other sources of these plant compounds (such as red clover) may bolster bone strength, but the benefit is probably modest at best. Some doctors worry that high doses of soy, which contains chemicals similar to the hormone estrogen, may stimulate the growth of cancerous or precancerous breast tumors.	**Common Dose:** 50 milligrams of soy isoflavones; up to 85 milligrams of red clover isoflavones
Popular Supplement: Vitamin D	**Is It Worth Trying?** The body requires vitamin D to absorb calcium, which is why these two supplements are often paired in the same pill. Sunlight triggers vitamin D production, so you may not need these supplements if you spend adequate time outdoors without sunblock. Milk and some other foods are fortified with vitamin D.	**Common Dose:** 200 International Units, (age 50 and younger), 400 IU (51 to 70), and 600 IU (71 and older) a day; doctors may recommend higher doses
Popular Supplement: Vitamin K	**Is It Worth Trying?** The minerals that form bone need vitamin K in order to bind. Leafy green vegetables are a good source, but a growing number of women take vitamin K supplements. Studies show that many women who develop fragile bones have low levels of vitamin K, but so far, there's no solid evidence that taking these supplements helps.	**Common Dose:** 120 micrograms (men) and 90 micrograms (women)

COLDS

Popular Supplement: Echinacea	**Is It Worth Trying?** A 2007 review of 14 studies found that this herb reduces the risk of colds by 58 percent and shortens their duration by more than a day. Echinacea turns up immune activity, so don't take it if you have an immune system disorder such as multiple sclerosis or rheumatoid arthritis. Don't take echinacea longer than 8 weeks at a time; some experts worry that long-term use could cause liver damage.	**Common Dose:** 300 milligrams, three times a day

COLDS (continued)

Popular Supplement: Vitamin C	**Is It Worth Trying?** It's a popular choice, but vitamin C does not prevent colds, according to a review of 30 studies. High doses may slightly shorten the duration of a cold, but not enough to recommend vitamin C for that purpose.	**Common Dose:** 25 to 1,500 milligrams a day
Popular Supplement: Zinc	**Is It Worth Trying?** Zinc lozenges might shorten the duration and relieve the symptoms of a cold, according to some studies, though others have found no benefit. Don't use nasal sprays, gels, or swabs containing zinc, which could ruin your sense of smell—permanently. Don't take zinc supplements longer than a few days without your doctor's okay, and avoid high doses, which can lower immunity. Don't chew zinc lozenges; allow them to dissolve in your mouth.	**Common Dose:** 13.3 to 23 milligrams, every 2 hours during the day

CONGESTIVE HEART FAILURE

Popular Supplement: Coenzyme Q10	**Is It Worth Trying?** Taking coenzyme Q10 supplements in addition to prescription drugs may improve the heart's pumping ability and relieve some symptoms (such as leg swelling), but study results have been inconsistent.	**Common Dose:** Up to 300 milligrams a day (or higher in some cases)
Popular Supplement: Hawthorne	**Is It Worth Trying?** A 2009 review of 10 studies, involving 855 patients, found that hawthorn supplements (taken in addition to drug therapy) significantly relieved common symptoms, such as shortness of breath and fatigue.	**Common Dose:** 160 to 900 milligrams a day, divided into three doses

CONSTIPATION

Popular Supplement: Psyllium	**Is It Worth Trying?** Yes, though you should talk to your doctor if you have chronic constipation. Produced from seed husks, psyllium is high in fiber and absorbs water in the gut, which makes stools bulkier and easier to pass.	**Common Dose:** Take enough to bring your daily fiber intake up to 25 to 30 grams a day, divided into several doses
Popular Supplement: Senna	**Is It Worth Trying?** This plant contains a potent "stimulant" laxative that forces the bowel muscles to contract. Like all stimulant laxatives, it should be used sparingly, if at all, since your colon may become dependent on it. Long-term abuse can cause serious complications, including chronic diarrhea and loss of vital nutrients, and can even prove fatal.	**Common Dose:** 0.6 to 2 grams a day

DEPRESSION

Popular Supplement: St. John's wort	**Is It Worth Trying?** Most scientists agree that this popular herb can be an effective treatment for mild depression. Some studies suggest it works as well as Prozac and similar antidepressants. St. John's wort is generally safe, but may make you more vulnerable to sunburn. It also interacts with many widely prescribed medications, so check with your doctor before taking it.	**Common Dose:** 300 milligrams (standardized to 0.3% hypericin), three times a day
Popular Supplement: SAM-e	**Is It Worth Trying?** A number of studies suggest that this naturally occurring compound relieves depression as well as older antidepressants known as tricyclic antidepressants, but without unpleasant side effects. However, many of those studies used injected SAM-e.	**Common Dose:** 200 to 1,600 milligrams a day

DIABETES

Popular Supplement: Bitter melon	**Is It Worth Trying?** This Chinese herb activates enzymes that lower blood sugar by making your muscles use glucose more efficiently. However, there has been very little formal study of bitter melon's benefits for people with diabetes.	**Common Dose:** 200 milligrams, two or three times a day
Popular Supplement: Chromium	**Is It Worth Trying?** Your body needs this trace mineral to maintain healthy blood sugar levels. However, chromium deficiency is rare, and studies have failed to show consistently that these mineral supplements improve blood sugar control.	**Common Dose:** 200 micrograms, one to three times a day
Popular Supplement: Ginseng	**Is It Worth Trying?** A few studies have found that this herb lowers blood sugar in people with type 2 diabetes, but more research is needed. There are several types of ginseng; most of the promising studies used the American variety.	**Common Dose:** 100 to 200 milligrams of American ginseng, one to three times a day

ECZEMA

Popular Supplement: Evening primrose oil	**Is It Worth Trying?** Evening primrose oil may clear up the rash, itching, and other symptoms of eczema, according to some studies. However, you must take large doses for an extended time, and other research suggests it may not work.	**Common Dose:** 4 to 6 grams a day

ERECTILE DYSFUNCTION (ED)

Popular Supplement: Arginine	**Is It Worth Trying?** This amino acid boosts nitric oxide levels, which causes blood vessels to relax and expand. That promotes increased blood flow, which is necessary for producing an erection. Arginine is often added to combination products advertised as "natural Viagra" supplements. Yet the evidence that these supplements cure ED is modest at best.	**Common Dose:** 2 to 8 grams a day
Popular Supplement: Asian ginseng	**Is It Worth Trying?** A half-dozen studies have found that this herb is an effective treatment for ED. However, the studies were small and their quality, questionable.	**Common Dose:** 200 milligrams a day
Popular Supplement: Yohimbe	**Is It Worth Trying?** This tree bark extract contains a chemical, yohimbine, that is also available as a prescription drug for ED. There has been little research on yohimbe but studies show that yohimbine is only modestly effective. Yohimbine can cause high blood pressure and other side effects, so beware of this herb.	**Common Dose:** 15 to 30 milligrams a day

FATIGUE

Popular Supplement: Ginseng	**Is It Worth Trying?** Despite its popularity as an energy-booster, studies do not consistently show that ginseng will give you more pep or stamina. However, some research suggests that this herb may stave off mental fatigue.	**Common Dose:** Up to 200 milligrams a day
Popular Supplement: Guarana	**Is It Worth Trying?** This herb is often added to energy supplements and beverages. Guarana is a natural source of caffeine, so it may make you feel more alert for a short time, but no more so than a cup of coffee or tea.	**Common Dose:** 50 milligrams (of caffeine)
Popular Supplement: Vitamin B_{12}	**Is It Worth Trying?** About 15 percent of adults over 65 are deficient in vitamin B_{12}, which may cause anemia; supplements can relieve fatigue and other symptoms of anemia. If your vitamin B_{12} levels are fine, there is little evidence that these supplements will fight everyday fatigue.	**Common Dose:** 25 to 100 micrograms a day

HEADACHES

Popular Supplement: Butterbur	**Is It Worth Trying?** One study found that butterbur supplements reduced the frequency of migraines by 50 percent after 3 to 4 months, though more research is needed.	**Common Dose:** 75 milligrams twice a day has been used in some studies

HEADACHES (continued)

Popular Supplement: Feverfew	**Is It Worth Trying?** This herb reduced the incidence of migraines by 24 percent in some studies. However, in other studies, feverfew failed to prevent these severe headaches.	**Common Dose:** 100 to 300 milligrams, up to four times a day
Popular Supplement: White willow bark	**Is It Worth Trying?** This herbal extract contains salicin, which is similar to the pain-relieving chemical in aspirin. Doctors in Germany and other countries commonly recommend white willow bark for pain relief, including headaches.	**Common Dose:** 400 to 800 milligrams (standardized to 15 percent salicin), twice a day

HERPES

Popular Supplement: Lysine	**Is It Worth Trying?** Herpes sufferers who take high doses of this amino acid, found in many foods (such as chicken and potatoes), may have fewer, less-severe outbreaks, though not all studies have found it to be effective. Don't take lysine if you have heart disease, high cholesterol, or high triglycerides.	**Common Dose:** 1 to 3 grams a day

HIGH BLOOD PRESSURE

Popular Supplement: Coenzyme Q10	**Is It Worth Trying?** This antioxidant lowers blood pressure effectively, according to a growing body of research. In one study, half of the subjects given coenzyme Q10 supplements were able to quit taking one or more blood pressure drugs. Benefits may take several months to emerge.	**Common Dose:** 30 to 300 milligrams a day
Popular Supplement: Garlic	**Is It Worth Trying?** Several recent reviews have persuaded some scientists that these pills may be worth a try, though earlier research failed to show that garlic supplements improve blood pressure.	**Common Dose:** 600 to 900 milligrams a day

HIGH CHOLESTEROL

Popular Supplement: Garlic	**Is It Worth Trying?** A 2009 review of 13 studies involving more than 1,000 patients found no evidence that garlic supplements lower cholesterol.	**Common Dose:** 900 milligrams a day
Popular Supplement: Guggul	**Is It Worth Trying?** Although some research indicates that this tree resin lowers cholesterol, a study in the *Journal of the American Medical Association* found that high doses of guggul actually raised LDL ("bad") cholesterol.	**Common Dose:** 1,000 to 2,000 milligrams, up to three times a day

HIGH CHOLESTEROL (continued)

Popular Supplement: Red yeast rice	**Is It Worth Trying?** This supplement is a natural source of lovastatin, the same compound found in Mevacor, a drug prescribed to lower cholesterol. The FDA has warned consumers to avoid these supplements. The reason: A red yeast rice product that lists any amount of lovastatin as an ingredient on the label is an unapproved drug. Consequently, most products do not list their lovastatin content, making it impossible to determine how much a pill contains—and the amounts can vary wildly. Red yeast rice supplements can cause some of the same side effects as Mevacor and other statin drugs, such as muscle pain.	**Common Dose:** 600 milligrams, two to four times a day
Popular Supplement: Soy	**Is It Worth Trying?** Soy supplements can lower LDL cholesterol by up to 7 milligrams per deciliter, according to Japanese researchers. That's a modest but valuable reduction in blood fats.	**Common Dose:** 20 to 80 grams of soy protein a day

HOT FLASHES

Popular Supplement: Black cohosh	**Is It Worth Trying?** Maybe, but study results have been conflicting. Much of the research showing that it works has been poor quality; other trials find it to be no more effective than a sugar pill.	**Common Dose:** 40 to 80 milligrams a day
Popular Supplement: Red clover	**Is It Worth Trying?** Research has been inconsistent, but the largest study of red clover for treating hot flashes failed to show any benefit.	**Common Dose:** 40 to 160 milligrams a day
Popular Supplement: Soy	**Is It Worth Trying?** Three out of five studies found that soy supplements modestly reduce the number of hot flashes—by about one per day, for the typical user. Some experts believe high doses of soy extract could increase the risk for breast cancer.	**Common Dose:** 40 to 80 milligrams a day

INSOMNIA

Popular Supplement: Kava	**Is It Worth Trying?** This Polynesian herb contains muscle-relaxing chemicals, but it has not been well-studied as a sleep aid. There have been rare—but alarming—reports of liver failure linked to kava supplements.	**Common Dose:** 210 milligrams kavalactones 1 hour before bedtime

INSOMNIA (continued)

Popular Supplement: Melatonin	**Is It Worth Trying?** Most studies show that melatonin can ease sleeplessness caused by jet lag. The evidence is less solid that this hormone cures everyday insomnia, though it seems to induce shut-eye in some users.	**Common Dose:** 3 milligrams 1 hour before bedtime
Popular Supplement: Valerian	**Is It Worth Trying?** Valerian appears to act as a mild sedative. Its track record for treating insomnia is mixed. Although many people take valerian for occasional sleeplessness, one large study found that the herb is most effective when taken for a month or longer.	**Common Dose:** 250 to 600 milligrams

LEG PAIN AND VARICOSE VEINS

Popular Supplement: Gotu kola	**Is It Worth Trying?** In one study of 94 patients with poor circulation in the lower limbs, a majority who took supplements containing this herb reported feeling less heaviness, pain, and swelling in their legs.	**Common Dose:** 30 to 90 milligrams a day
Popular Supplement: Horse chestnut	**Is It Worth Trying?** Solid research shows that horse chestnut relieves pain and swelling in the legs and ankles caused by varicose veins.	**Common Dose:** 300 milligrams, twice a day
Popular Supplement: OPCs	**Is It Worth Trying?** Oligomeric proanthocyanidin (OPC) complexes are antioxidants found in many plants. Grapeseed extract is one top source, and it improved symptoms in 75 percent of patients with poor leg circulation in one study. Some research suggests that another good source of OPCs, pine bark extract (sold in a product called Pycnogenol), may also be effective. Pine bark lowers cholesterol, too.	**Common Dose:** 100 to 300 milligrams a day (grapeseed); 360 milligrams a day (pine bark)

LIVER PROBLEMS

Popular Supplement: Milk thistle	**Is It Worth Trying?** Milk thistle is sometimes called the drinker's friend, thanks to a belief that this herb defends the liver against toxins, notably alcohol. But the protection milk thistle offers against alcohol and other toxins is modest at best, and many studies show that it has no effect. A 2008 review found no evidence that milk thistle can prevent or treat hepatitis (liver inflammation) caused by infections such as hepatitis C.	**Common Dose:** 200 to 400 milligrams, one to three times a day

MEMORY PROBLEMS AND MENTAL FUZZINESS

Popular Supplement: **Asian ginseng**	**Is It Worth Trying?** A few studies suggest that ginseng (especially the Asian variety) may make you think faster or more clearly. However, some of the optimistic research was flawed, say skeptics, and other studies have failed to show that ginseng offers any boost to brainpower.	**Common Dose:** 200 milligrams a day
Popular Supplement: **Ginkgo biloba**	**Is It Worth Trying?** It probably won't improve your memory or make you feel sharper if you're otherwise healthy. And a large 2008 study found that ginkgo biloba does not prevent Alzheimer's disease or other forms of dementia. However, some evidence suggests that people who develop these diseases may benefit from this herb.	**Common Dose:** 120 to 240 milligrams a day
Popular Supplement: **Vitamin E**	**Is It Worth Trying?** This antioxidant protects cells from damage by oxidative stress, which some scientists believe may contribute to Alzheimer's disease. So far, however, studies have not consistently shown that taking vitamin E supplements prevents this devastating condition.	**Common Dose:** 800 IU and higher have been used in studies, though few experts recommend taking more than 400 IU

NAUSEA

Popular Supplement: **Ginger**	**Is It Worth Trying?** Ginger is effective for motion sickness, morning sickness, and nausea related to drugs or surgery. In one study of naval cadets, ginger reduced seasickness by 38 percent. To prevent seasickness, experts suggest taking a ginger supplement 30 minutes before setting sail, then another dose every 4 hours if you develop any symptoms.	**Common Dose:** 1 gram every 4 hours

PROSTATE ENLARGEMENT

Popular Supplement: **Beta-sitosterol**	**Is It Worth Trying?** Four small, short-term studies found that these plant extracts may help increase urine flow and relieve other symptoms of enlarged prostate. A plus: beta-sitosterol may also lower cholesterol.	**Common Dose:** 60 to 130 milligrams a day
Popular Supplement: **Pygeum**	**Is It Worth Trying?** A few small studies suggest that this supplement (which comes from the bark of the African plum tree) may offer modest relief from prostate enlargement, known as benign prostatic hyperplasia, or BPH.	**Common Dose:** 75 to 200 milligrams a day

PROSTATE ENLARGEMENT (continued)

Popular Supplement: Saw palmetto	**Is It Worth Trying?** Many older studies have shown saw palmetto to be as effective as commonly prescribed BPH drugs. However, in two major studies published since 2003, the herb was no better than a sugar pill.	**Common Dose:** 160 milligrams, twice a day

PSORIASIS

Popular Supplement: Capsaicin	**Is It Worth Trying?** Several small studies have found that skin creams containing capsaicin, the chemical that puts the heat in hot peppers, can relieve the pain and itching of psoriasis.	**Common Dose:** Follow label instructions
Popular Supplement: Fish oil	**Is It Worth Trying?** Fish-oil capsules may offer moderate relief of this painful skin condition.	**Common Dose:** 3 to 4 grams a day

ULCERS

Popular Supplement: Ginger	**Is It Worth Trying?** Herbalists have long recommended ginger as ulcer therapy. Recent research suggests that it blocks the ill effects of the bacteria that cause most ulcers, *Helicobacter pylori* (though you will still need to take antibiotics to kill this ulcer-causing bug).	**Common Dose:** 1 to 4 grams a day, divided into several doses
Popular Supplement: Licorice root	**Is It Worth Trying?** Supplements may speed the healing of ulcers as effectively as standard acid-blocking drugs, some studies say (though, again, antibiotics are necessary to eliminate *H. pylori*). Look for supplements labeled DGL, for "deglycyrrhizinated," which have been stripped of a compound that may raise blood pressure. Licorice has hormonelike effects and should not be taken by women who are pregnant or nursing, or who have had breast cancer. Licorice supplements can also reduce testosterone levels in men. Note that licorice candy is not a substitute for supplements.	**Common Dose:** 0.4 to 1.6 grams, three times a day

VISION PROBLEMS

Popular Supplement: Bilberry	**Is It Worth Trying?** Some people take these antioxidant-rich supplements to improve night vision. However, a 2004 analysis found no evidence that bilberry will help you see better in the dark.	**Common Dose:** 40 to 480 milligrams a day, divided into two or three doses
Popular Supplement: Lutein and zeaxanthin	**Is It Worth Trying?** These antioxidants help protect the retinas from damaging light. One large study found that women who consume the most lutein and zeaxanthin cut their risk for cataracts by 18 percent. Scientists are studying whether they prevent macular degeneration.	**Common Dose:** 10 milligrams a day (lutein); 2 milligrams a day (zeaxanthin)
Popular Supplement: Zinc	**Is It Worth Trying?** A National Eye Institute (NEI) study found that zinc supplements (with or without beta-carotene, vitamin E, and vitamin C) slow the progression of macular degeneration in high-risk patients by about 25 percent; it may keep vision sharp, too. However, this study used high doses of zinc, which can cause stomach upset and lowered immunity.	**Common Dose:** The NEI study used 40 to 80 milligrams a day, but researchers are now studying whether 25 milligrams is beneficial

Vitamins, Herbs, and Other Supplements

☐ BETA-CAROTENE

I've heard that beta-carotene protects against heart disease and cancer. Is there any reason to avoid beta-carotene supplements?

Yes. While cancer rates are lower in people who eat lots of foods rich in beta-carotene, such as green and orange vegetables, there's no indication that taking supplements reduces your risk of disease. What's more, a large study involving more than 29,000 male smokers found that beta-carotene supplements actually increased the risk for lung cancer by 18 percent. A later study reached a similar conclusion. So avoid beta-carotene if you smoke.

Should I take beta-carotene to protect my vision?

No. You'd be better off simply eating more spinach, carrots, and sweet potatoes. These are all good sources of beta-carotene, which the body uses to make vitamin A. You need vitamin A for healthy retinas; it's particularly important for ensuring that your eyes adapt to darkness. People whose diets are rich in beta-carotene and similar compounds, known

collectively as carotenoids, tend to have a low risk for vision loss, cataracts, and macular degeneration. But there's little evidence that these supplements improve vision or prevent eye disease. (One large clinical trial showed that supplements containing beta-carotene, vitamins C and E, and zinc lowered the risk for macular degeneration. However, zinc appeared to confer the most protection.)

☐ CALCIUM

Will calcium supplements really protect my bones?

Yes, but keep in mind that building stronger bones takes more than calcium, whether you get it from pills or food. Bones start to become thinner and more fragile at midlife. Most studies show that people who consume little calcium are more likely to suffer bone fractures as they age. Increasing calcium intake won't stop bone loss, but it can slow the process.

Adults 50 and younger should consume 1,000 milligrams of calcium daily, while people over 50 need 1,200 milligrams. Dairy foods and leafy greens are good sources, but studies show that supplements protect bones, too. An analysis of 15 studies found that women over 45 who took supplements containing at least 400 milligrams of calcium daily cut their risk for fracturing a vertebra by 23 percent; protection against other bone breaks was more modest.

The message is clear: Calcium alone won't save your skeleton. Consuming adequate vitamin D is critical, too, since your bones can't use calcium without it. Meanwhile, exercise—especially activities that involve lots of footwork, such as walking, jogging, and dancing—strengthens bones, too.

Can calcium supplements give me constipation? Which ones won't?

Some people find that the most common form of calcium supplements, calcium carbonate, causes constipation. One solution is to purchase calcium citrate supplements. This form of calcium breaks down more readily during digestion, so it doesn't cause gastrointestinal discomfort. However, calcium citrate tends to be more expensive. As an alternative, you may be able to stick with calcium carbonate and avoid constipation if you divide your daily dose into two or three smaller doses. For example, if your regimen calls for 1,000 milligrams a day, take 500 milligrams in the morning and another 500 milligrams in the evening. Always take calcium with food to ensure that your stomach generates enough acid to break down the tablets.

I'm a man. Do I need calcium supplements?

You might. Despite what many men believe, they require the same amount of calcium every day as women do: 1,000 milligrams for adults 50 and younger, 1,200 milligrams a day for adults over 50. The best sources are low-fat and nonfat milk, yogurt, and other dairy products, as well as kale, collard greens, beans and other legumes, and fortified foods and beverages (such as orange juice). If your diet doesn't include plenty of these foods, you're probably a good candidate for calcium supplements.

It's worth talking to your doctor, though, before upping your calcium intake. Some studies have found that men who consume lots of this mineral have an increased risk for prostate cancer, though others have failed to confirm the link (and the results of at least one study suggest that calcium may even *prevent* prostate cancer in some men). The best advice: Don't exceed the recommended intake of calcium for your age group. The worrisome studies found that men had the greatest risk if they consumed very high levels— 1,500 milligrams a day or more.

☐ COENZYME Q10

I take a statin drug to lower my cholesterol, and my doctor suggested I also take coenzyme Q10. Why?

To prevent muscle pain, fatigue, memory problems, and other side effects statins may cause, though coenzyme Q10 (CoQ10) may or may not get the job done. Simvastatin (Zocor), atorvastatin (Lipitor), and other statin drugs reduce levels of CoQ10, a vitamin-like substance that acts as an antioxidant and helps cells produce energy. Some doctors believe that depletion of CoQ10 causes many of the side effects often reported by statin-users, particularly muscle pain, though this theory is controversial. One study found that CoQ10 supplements help prevent muscle pain, but two other studies did not. Nonetheless, some physicians swear that their patients who take statins are less likely to suffer side effects if they add CoQ10 supplements to their regimens. Other strategies for coping with statin-related muscle pain include switching brands and taking a lower dose.

I'm always short of breath. Will CoQ10 supplements help?

They might, but talk to a doctor about your problem. Frequently feeling out of breath may simply be a sign that you need to get more exercise. But it's also a common symptom of a serious condition, including congestive heart failure, which weakens the heart, reducing its ability to pump blood throughout the body. Patients with heart failure tend to have low levels of CoQ10. Some studies (though not all) have found that CoQ10 supplements increase the heart's pumping capacity and prevent fatigue and other symptoms (such as swollen ankles) in people with heart failure. If you have congestive heart failure, your doctor will prescribe medications and lifestyle changes to help you cope with the condition. He or she may suggest that you take CoQ10 supplements, too. CoQ10 is believed to be reasonably safe, though it may lower blood pressure or blood sugar, so it's essential for your physician to know if you decide to take it.

☐ DHEA

I'm getting up there in years. Can DHEA help me look and feel younger?

Don't buy the hype. Neither the age-defying benefits nor the safety of these supplements has been proven. DHEA is a hormone produced by the adrenal glands that your body converts to testosterone and estrogen. DHEA production starts to drop off in your mid-twenties, so researchers wondered if synthetic supplements could restore youthful vigor in people middle-age and beyond. In the late 1990s, one study suggested that the supplements helped older men build muscle and trim fat, while another found that the pills improved libido in older women diagnosed with low DHEA. Since then, however, a number of studies have failed to show that DHEA produces these rejuvenating changes.

Some doctors fear that because of DHEA's potential to boost estrogen and testosterone levels, the supplements may increase the risk for breast cancer, prostate cancer, and other cancers. Also, in some studies, people who took DHEA supplements developed unwelcome side effects, such as a drop in HDL ("good") cholesterol, a rise in blood pressure, and growth of facial hair in women. DHEA supplements have a role in medicine (they may relieve symptoms of lupus, for example). But dodging Father Time isn't one of them.

☐ ECHINACEA

Should I take echinacea all the time or just during cold season?

Don't take echinacea every day, year-round. It's not known for certain, but there's reason to worry that taking this herb for longer than 2 months at a time may cause serious side effects, such as liver damage. Instead, use it in specific situations.

● *Before cold season.* To use echinacea to prevent the sniffles, start taking it a week or two before cold season starts. That's a tricky date to pin down, depending on where you live, though in many parts of the world, that means late summer or early fall. If you take echinacea for the entire cold season, take at least a 1 week break every 2 months.

● *At the first signs of a cold.* Start taking it right away and you might feel better sooner.

● *Before you fly.* You might consider starting it a week before you'll be exposed to others who might have colds, such as traveling by air, says University of Connecticut professor of pharmacy Craig I. Coleman, PharmD.

The usual dose is 900 milligrams per day of echinacea extract or 2,700 milligrams of dried herb powder.

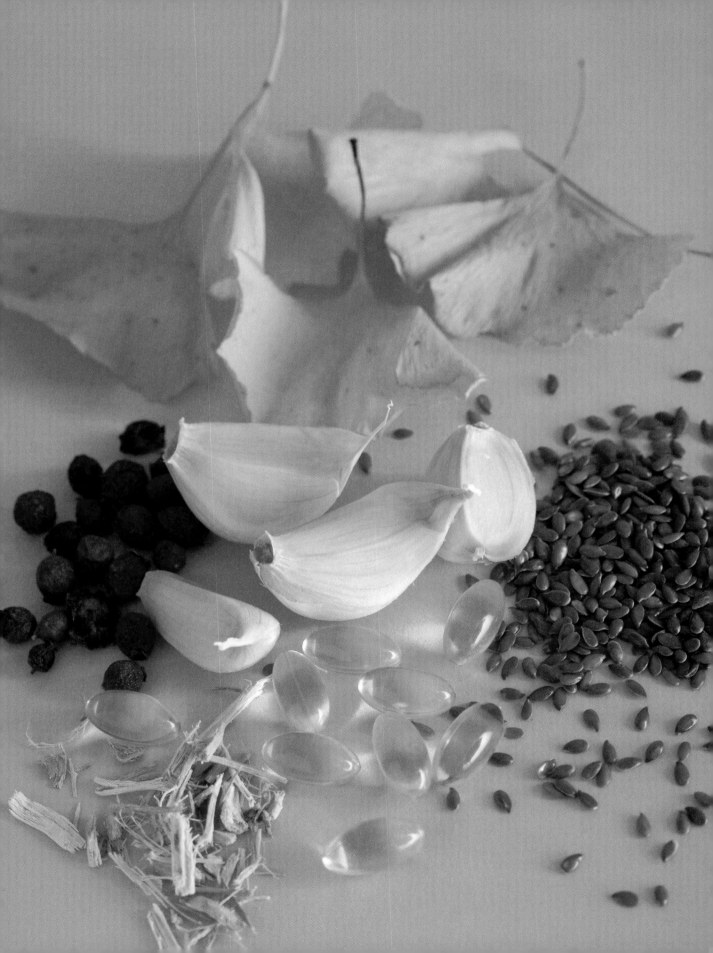

☐ EVENING PRIMROSE OIL

Does evening primrose oil relieve PMS?

The research isn't clear on this; some studies show it helps, others don't. The oil contains certain essential fatty acids that your body uses to form hormonelike substances called prostaglandins. Some scientists theorize that low levels of prostaglandins cause the symptoms of premenstrual syndrome (PMS), such as fatigue, mood swings, bloating, and breast tenderness. The best advice is to try the oil and see if it works for you. Evening primrose is considered quite safe, so you can take it daily. Some herbalists recommend 250 to 500 milligrams a day, though up to 3 grams daily (divided into several smaller doses) has been used in some studies of women with breast pain related to PMS.

☐ FISH OIL

I hate fish. Should I take fish-oil capsules?

Yes, if your doctor thinks they're right for you. Eating seafood two or three times a week—especially oily fish such as salmon and sardines—cuts the risk for heart disease by up to 36 percent, according to more than 30 studies. Fish-lovers also suffer fewer strokes, and mounting evidence suggests

that fish oil fights depression and boosts brainpower.

But none of that matters if you don't eat fish very often. Fish-oil supplements can fill the void. And you don't need as much as you might think. While there is no official recommended intake for fish oil in the United States, authorities in many countries advise healthy people to consume 300 to 500 milligrams of DHA and EPA—the fatty acids in fish oil—every day. Much larger amounts of DHA and EPA, up to 5,000 milligrams a day, are prescribed for treating specific conditions, such as lowering triglycerides. Important: The dosage listed on the front label is the total amount of fish oil per serving, *not* the amount of DHA and EPA. Fish oil contains other fatty acids, so buy products that list the amount of DHA and EPA on the ingredient list. (Some fish-oil supplements contain as little as 30 percent DHA and EPA; more expensive brands contain up to 90 percent.)

Fish-oil supplements are generally safe, though they may cause mild gastrointestinal

problems. People who use warfarin, a blood-thinning medication, shouldn't take fish-oil supplements, which may increase the drug's effects.

Is there mercury in fish-oil supplements?

Most fish-oil supplements are either mercury-free or contain barely detectable amounts—not enough to worry about. Virtually all fish contain at least a trace of mercury, a toxic heavy metal from pollution and natural sources (such as volcanoes) that contaminates fresh and saltwater. Consuming too much mercury has been linked to brain damage in infants and, more recently, heart disease.

Most fish-oil supplements are made from short-lived species, which accumulate very little mercury compared to longer-lived predators, such as shark and swordfish. Furthermore, many manufacturers purify fish oil, which removes mercury, as well as PCBs, dioxins, and other contaminants. When

Harvard scientists sampled five over-the-counter fish-oil supplements they found, at most, "negligible" amounts of mercury. A larger sampling by ConsumerLab.com failed to find any supplements that contained detectable levels of mercury.

What can I do about fishy burps?

Taking a few steps may help eliminate this annoyance.

• *Try enteric-coated capsules.* These break down in the intestines, not in your stomach, so they are much less likely to cause burping and an unpleasant aftertaste. Beware, though, that ConsumerLab.com has found that some enteric-coated pills don't perform well in the digestive tract; a few brands release oil while still in the stomach, which can give you fishy breath. (Some others release oil too late, so it's not well-absorbed.)

• *Store fish-oil supplements in the freezer.* The pill will break down more slowly, which may help minimize fishy burps.

• *Take fish-oil supplements with a meal.* Other food ingredients may be able to neutralize the strong taste of fish oil.

• *Buy highly concentrated fish oil.* If you don't mind paying more, purchase fish-oil capsules that contain large amounts of DHA and EPA. They tend to be smaller than other capsules, since nonbeneficial fatty acids are removed.

That means less fishy-smelling oil in your system.

☐ GARLIC

Do garlic supplements prevent cancer or anything else?

Taking garlic supplements may help fight some types of cancer, though the evidence is preliminary. We know that people who eat lots of garlic have a lower risk for colon cancer, for instance, so some researchers are trying to find out if garlic supplements help fight this disease. Japanese scientists gave highly concentrated garlic pills to one group of patients who had precancerous tumors (called adenomas) removed from their colons, meaning that they had a high risk for colon cancer. A similar group of patients received placebo pills. After a year, patients in the placebo group had developed additional adenomas; those

taking garlic supplements had not. Most experts agree, however, that far more research is needed to determine whether it's worth taking garlic supplements to lower the risk for colon cancer or any other form of the disease. It's worth noting that a 2009 scientific review found no evidence that garlic prevents stomach, breast, lung, or endometrial cancer.

Garlic has been used to treat many other conditions dating back to ancient times. Two conditions it's more commonly used for today are:

• *Colds.* In one study with 146 volunteers, people taking garlic supplements had roughly one-third as many colds as others who took sugar pills. However, this is the only decent study of garlic for preventing colds, so more are needed.

• *Heart disease.* Garlic supplements may modestly lower cholesterol and blood pressure, though not all studies show this to be true.

FACT OR FICTION

Flax Seed–Oil Supplements Are As Good As Fish-Oil Supplements

Fiction. Fish oil is good for you because of its omega-3 fatty acids, specifically, types called DHA and EPA, which protect the heart and brain by fighting inflammation, preventing blood clots, nourishing cell membranes, and more. Flax seed contains omega-3's, too, but a different kind, called ALA. The body converts ALA to DHA and EPA, but not very efficiently. Get your omega-3's from seafood or fish-oil supplements.

My garlic pills give me bad breath. What should I do?

Buy enteric-coated garlic supplements. These survive exposure to your stomach acid and don't dissolve until they reach the intestines, making them far less likely to produce garlic breath or body odor. Enteric-coated pills are probably more effective, too. That's because stomach acid neutralizes the healing compounds in garlic. Beware, though: Some enteric-coated supplements may as well be sealed in kryptonite, since they pass through the digestive tract without dissolving. Look for the USP or ConsumerLab.com seal for high-quality supplements that break down properly.

☐ **GINKGO BILOBA**

Will ginkgo boost my memory?

If you're overworked and over-scheduled but otherwise healthy, probably not. Millions of people take ginkgo biloba supplements, which are derived from one of the oldest species of tree in the world, in the belief that this herb will help them remember appointments, quit forgetting names, and—yes—find their darned keys. Ginkgo biloba is an antioxidant, so it protects cells from damage by free radicals. It also increases blood flow by dilating blood vessels, which would seem to benefit the

brain, an organ that needs a plentiful, uninterrupted supply of blood to stay healthy and function efficiently. The herb also makes the blood less likely to form artery-plugging clots.

But most studies offer little reason to think it will help your memory. In one trial, healthy people age 60 and older took ginkgo biloba for 6 weeks, then underwent a battery of psychological tests designed to measure their memory, attention span, and other cognitive skills. They scored no better than similar men and women who didn't use the herb.

Ginkgo biloba supplements probably won't lessen your risk for developing conditions that rob memory and other intellectual capacities, including Alzheimer's disease or other forms of dementia. However, if a loved one has been diagnosed with dementia, take note that some research suggests that the herb could help to lessen the devastating symptoms. Ginkgo biloba preparations are widely used to treat dementia in Europe, and several studies have found that it appears to slow down the loss of memory and other mental functions in dementia patients.

My legs ache when I walk and a friend said that ginkgo might help. Could it?

Ginkgo biloba may help if your pain is caused by intermittent

claudication, a condition caused by poor blood flow in the legs. Just as the arteries in your heart can become clogged with cholesterol, fat, and other gunk, so can the blood vessels in your legs. As blood flow in your legs is reduced, you'll likely find it difficult to walk long distances without pain. Eventually, your legs may ache even at rest.

Ginkgo biloba's potential for improving circulation has made it a popular choice for people suffering from intermittent claudication and other circulation problems. But if it actually helps—doctors don't agree—the benefit is probably modest. By one estimate, the supplements will increase your ability to walk for an extended distance, but only by about an extra 70 yards, or about two-thirds of a football field. If you decide to try the herb, a daily dose of 120 to 240 milligrams of extract is typical.

Will ginkgo stop the ringing in my ears?

Unfortunately, no. A few old, poorly designed studies suggested that ginkgo biloba might help restore the peace for tinnitus sufferers, who hear ringing, hissing, or buzzing sounds. But more recent research using higher standards of proof show that it won't.

☐ GINSENG

I think stress is making me sick. Can ginseng help me cope better?

Don't bet on it. Herbalists claim that ginseng is an adaptogen, a substance that helps the body adapt to stress and change. However, there is little scientific evidence that ginseng will help you get through a chaotic day and keep you on your feet. Most of the research suggesting that ginseng might be a stress-buster comes from animal studies. Some, though not all, of these studies show that mice fed ginseng have greater endurance and react better to stressful situations (like being plunged into icy water). However, these same benefits don't seem to transfer to humans, according to a 2009 review. In fact, one study even found that Siberian ginseng actually *increased* levels of the stress hormone cortisol. There are better ways—everything from exercise to meditation—to ease emotional stress.

☐ GLUCOSAMINE

Is glucosamine effective for joint pain if I take it alone? Or should I take it combined with chondroitin?

First of all, there's no guarantee that glucosamine or chondroitin—taken alone or separately— will relieve your joint pain. Glucosamine and chondroitin are naturally occurring substances found in cartilage, which is the flexible tissue that protects the ends of joints. These compounds are marketed for the relief of joint pain and stiffness from osteoarthritis, but study results have been mixed—some found them to be effective, while others showed that they're no better than sugar pills.

If you decide to try a supplement for joint pain, there is no evidence that pairing glucosamine and chondroitin produces better results than taking one or the other. Which type of glucosamine you choose may matter, however. Some scientists believe that glucosamine sulfate produces better results than another common form, glucosamine hydrochloride, though other experts say both are acceptable. It may be several weeks or longer before you feel any benefit from glucosamine and/or chondroitin, but if you don't notice any improvement in pain and stiffness after 2 months, these supplements probably aren't going to help.

☐ GRAPESEED EXTRACT

Will grapeseed extract give me the benefits of wine without the alcohol?

Not exactly. As many studies have shown, having a glass of wine or two every day may lower your risk for heart disease and other conditions. Mounting research now suggests that many of wine's health benefits come from an antioxidant called resveratrol, which some scientists believe could fight heart disease, cancer, obesity, and aging itself. Resveratrol is found mostly in grape skins (that's why red wine contains much more resveratrol than white varieties; winemakers remove grape skins when making white wine).

That doesn't mean grape seeds aren't useful, though. They are a great source of vitamin E, as well as potent antioxidants called oligomeric proanthocyanidins (OPCs). Although there hasn't been a great deal of research on grapeseed extract, some investigations suggest that it may be useful for treating some conditions, such as varicose veins.

☐ HAIR & SKIN FORMULAS

Do supplements for healthy skin work?

There is no question that your body needs vitamins, minerals, and other nutrients to maintain healthy skin. Beta-carotene, vitamins C and E, and other antioxidant compounds fight the damaging effects of destructive free radicals generated by overexposure to the

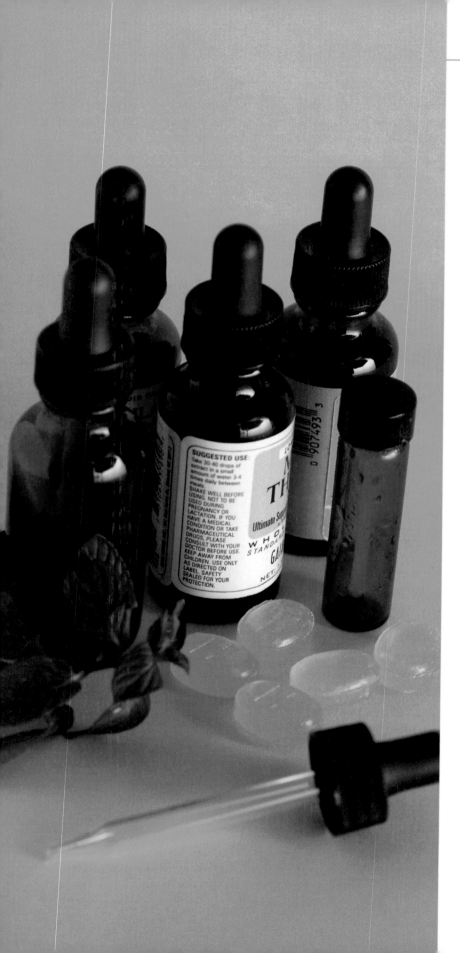

sun, smoking, and other influences that age the skin. There is some evidence that high doses of antioxidants may give skin a more youthful appearance. German researchers gave two groups of subjects supplements containing various combinations of beta-carotene and two other carotenoids (lutein and lycopene), vitamin E, and selenium. After 12 weeks, the skin of people in these groups was less rough and dry than other study subjects who took placebo pills.

Yet there has been at least one study suggesting that it may not be safe to use these supplements long-term. A 7.5-year French study found that women taking antioxidant supplements were 68 percent more likely to develop skin cancer. (The researchers speculated that it may have been too late to block the DNA damage done by sun exposure, which occurs over many years, and that high doses of antioxidants may actually have protected tumors from the body's natural cancer-fighting defenses.) Most dermatologists say that a healthy diet provides all the antioxidant protection most people need to keep their skin healthy-looking, though adding a multivitamin to the mix may be a good idea.

Less is known about the benefits of green tea, grapeseed extract, pine bark extract, and other supplements that are often included in skin products.

I'm losing my hair. Which supplements will help?

Probably none. Herbalists recommend saw palmetto, licorice, and a variety of other plant extracts for male-pattern baldness, the most common cause of hair loss. But none has been properly tested. One study found that among men or women who developed bald spots due to a condition called alopecia areata, a combination of essential oils (thyme, rosemary, lavender, and cedarwood) massaged into the scalp helped fill in patches.

☐ IRON

Will iron supplements give me more energy?

Only if you are suffering from iron deficiency, the leading cause of anemia. (Fatigue and weakness are common symptoms of anemia.) You need iron to form hemoglobin, the protein in red blood cells that ferries oxygen to muscles and other tissues. Iron is also necessary to burn oxygen and produce energy. Researchers have given iron supplements to athletes to see if high doses make them faster or stronger. Answer: It only boosted energy and strength in athletes who were found to be iron deficient.

It's possible to have low levels of iron but not be anemic; however, it's not clear that iron supplements will give you more pep if that's the case. If you're healthy, a balanced diet provides all the iron you can use, since this mineral is plentiful in meat, fish, poultry, whole grains, leafy greens, and dried fruits.

Are iron supplements safe?

Iron overload can cause a serious condition called hemochromatosis, which may lead to liver damage, diabetes, and other complications. So take iron supplements only if a doctor says your body has too little of this mineral. (Iron deficiency is rare among non-vegetarian men and women who have reached menopause.) Some people who take iron supplements develop gastrointestinal problems, such as diarrhea and constipation. Of greater concern, preliminary research suggests that long-term use of iron supplements may increase the risk for heart disease, cancer, and Alzheimer's disease. Iron supplements are a leading cause of poisoning in children under age 6, so store them in a safe place.

☐ KAVA

I'd like to take kava to help me relax and fall asleep, but is it safe?

There are several reasons to be careful with kava. Pacific Islanders have long used the roots of this plant to make a beverage that's sipped during special ceremonies or simply to relax and unwind. At one time, the biggest concern about kava was that consuming too much can cause intoxication. Motorists have been arrested for driving under the influence of kava, but typically after consuming many cups of kava tea or some other potable containing the herb.

However, in recent years, another significant concern about kava has emerged: liver damage. Although the risk may be small, there have been enough reports of cirrhosis, hepatitis, and liver failure in kava-users to prompt health authorities in some countries to ban the sale of the herb. Others, including the U.S. Food and Drug Administration, caution consumers to speak with a physician before using kava, report any signs of liver problems (such as yellowing skin or brown urine), and avoid this herb altogether if you have any form of liver disease.

☐ MAGNESIUM

I have diabetes and I'm struggling to lower my blood sugar. Can magnesium supplements help?

They might, though simply eating more fruit, vegetables,

whole grains, and other magnesium-rich foods might be just as effective.

Your body needs magnesium to process carbohydrates in food and keep blood sugar from rising. Studies show that people who don't get much magnesium from their diets increase their risk for type 2 diabetes by more than 30 percent. A number of studies have examined whether magnesium supplements (usually in the range of 300 to 400 milligrams a day) can improve blood sugar control. The research suggests that they may help maintain lower blood sugar immediately following a meal, but that they have only a slight impact on overall blood sugar control. People who take magnesium supplements achieve only a modest drop in their A1C level, the blood measurement your doctor cares about most.

WHAT YOU DON'T KNOW

Magnesium Could Save Your Hearing

If you blast music on your headphones, work in a factory, or expose yourself to other sources of loud noise, the best advice is to turn down the volume or wear a good set of earmuffs. But getting a little extra magnesium could help protect your ears. Scientists believe that this mineral may block noise-induced damage to hair cells, which are responsible for receiving sound signals. One study found that taking 167 milligrams of magnesium per day protected army recruits exposed to the sound of gunshots and other loud noises from permanent hearing loss. A typical magnesium supplement provides 250 milligrams. Ask your doctor before taking one.

☐ MELATONIN

Will popping a few melatonin pills before a flight prevent jet lag?

Taking melatonin will probably make you less likely to experience insomnia, fatigue, headache, and other symptoms of jet lag. Melatonin is a naturally occurring hormone that helps to regulate your sleep patterns. Your pineal gland makes large amounts as darkness falls; during the day, light blocks melatonin production. Some experts say you should begin taking melatonin (5 milligrams is the usual dose) about an hour before bedtime a few days prior to traveling, while others recommend starting when you arrive at your destination. In one large study, Swiss researchers found that travelers who took 5 milligrams at bedtime for the first 4 days after a flight said they slept better, drifted off faster, and felt less groggy during the day. Research shows that melatonin is more effective when you travel eastward, since you will see less daylight and nightfall arrives earlier. It appears to have the most benefit for air travelers who cross at least five time zones.

Will melatonin help me get a good night's sleep?

It could, though the results of studies have been mixed. Some experts believe that these supplements will only help you sleep better if you have naturally low levels of melatonin. Another open question is how to use melatonin in order to get the most benefit and avoid feeling drowsy the next day. Most experts advise taking a melatonin supplement an hour or so before turning in. (The usual dose for insomnia is 3 to 6 milligrams.) However, one study found that taking melatonin 5.5 hours before bedtime on a Sunday night helped people reestablish a normal sleep routine after staying up later than usual on the weekend.

☐ PROBIOTICS AND PREBIOTICS

What are probiotics?

Probiotics are beneficial bacteria and other live microbes (including some forms of yeast) that are sold as dietary supplements. They are also used to make certain foods, such as yogurt and other fermented dairy products. Your body is already teeming with naturally occurring probiotics, which live in the gut and, in women, the vagina. The many different strains of healthy bacteria that dwell in humans help maintain control of germs that find their way into your system every day.

Taking probiotic supplements ensures a thriving population of beneficial bacteria in the gut. This may leave less food and other resources to go around, so bad bacteria can't grow. Also, some scientists believe that good bacteria make the digestive tract acidic, which kills off germs. Whatever the case, your body needs good bacteria, and probiotic supplements provide reinforcements. Some studies show that probiotics may help prevent and treat some digestive problems, particularly diarrhea caused by infections or that occurs as a side effect of taking antibiotics (which can wipe out healthy bacteria). Probiotics also strengthen your defense against infections by making white blood cells, the immune system's foot soldiers, more aggressive against germs.

What are prebiotics?

Think of prebiotics as fuel that your body uses to make more probiotics. Prebiotics are food

ingredients that your body can't digest but that trigger production of healthy bacteria. The names of common prebiotics probably won't ring many bells; a few include fructo-oligosaccharides, inulin, and galacto-oligosaccharides. You consume a few grams of prebiotics every day, since they occur in plant foods. Garlic, bananas, and wheat are good sources.

Some experts recommend taking a probiotic *and* a prebiotic supplement to get the full range of benefits these digestive aids offer. However, if you're bothered by diarrhea, a probiotic is more likely to help, while prebiotics seem to be more useful in relieving constipation.

How do I choose the right probiotic? Does it need to be refrigerated?

Probiotics are a diverse bunch of bacteria, and each strain appears to have particular skills. You may be familiar with *Lactobacillus acidophilus*, often added to yogurt, which is a kind of all-purpose probiotic that's recommended for various conditions. However, there is at least preliminary research showing that these lesser-known strains and species may help with these specific conditions:

- *Diarrhea caused by antibiotics: Saccharomyces boulardii*

- *Diarrhea caused by infection: Lactobacillus rhamnosus* and *L. casei*

- *Irritable bowel syndrome: Bifidobacteria* or *Lactobacilli* species, alone or in combination

- *Ulcerative colitis:* A mix of *Bifidobacteria, Lactobacilli,* and *Streptococcus* species (sold as VSL#3)

- *Vaginal infections: Lactobacillus rhamnosus GR-1* and *Lactobacillus reuteri RC-14*

Package labels don't always say which strains of probiotics a supplement contains. Avoid such a product or call the company and ask which strains it contains. Always follow storage instructions closely. Since probiotics are live strains of bacteria, some experts believe that these supplements should always be refrigerated, whether or not the instructions tell you to do so, in order to keep them viable.

Will taking probiotics before a trip help prevent traveler's diarrhea?

Yes. In some parts of the world, as many as 50 percent of visitors develop traveler's diarrhea. While it's still wise to follow that old advice—"don't drink the water"—and take other commonsense measures in some countries, studies show that arming your stomach with probiotics can crowd out infectious bacteria you may consume in contaminated food or beverages. Look for supplements containing *Saccharomyces boulardii, Lactobacillus acidophilus,* and *Bifidobacterium bifidum,* which seem to be the most effective choices. Some experts recommend starting a course of probiotics 1 week before you hit the road and continuing for 1 week after returning. Most products are labeled in terms of the number of viable bacteria and other organisms. In general, look for products that provide one billion or more organisms per day.

☐ PSYLLIUM

Can I lower my cholesterol with fiber supplements?

If your cholesterol is too high, taking fiber supplements can help a little. While statin drugs such as simvastatin (Zocor) and atorvastatin (Lipitor) slash cholesterol levels by up to 50 percent or more, studies show that taking fiber supplements every day (5 grams of psyllium is a typical dose) bring levels down by about 5 percent. However, every 1 percent drop in LDL cholesterol lowers the risk for heart attack by 2 percent, so adding fiber supplements to your regimen could be worthwhile.

☐ ST. JOHN'S WORT

I need an antidepressant, but I'm concerned about side effects. Is St. John's wort a good alternative?

It might be, depending on the severity of your condition.

Most experts agree that St. John's wort is probably not a good choice for people with serious depression. But many doctors in Europe prescribe it for mild depression, and there's good reason to believe its effective, according to a 2008 review of studies. Researchers looked at 29 studies involving 5,489 patients and found that St. John's wort is just as effective as fluoxetine (Prozac) and other drugs prescribed for depression—and that people who take St. John's wort are 50 to 75 percent less likely to experience side effects linked to antidepressants, which can range from headaches and nausea to loss of libido.

While this herb causes few side effects, it does interact with many common medications, including antidepressants such as Prozac. Talk to your doctor if you're interested in trying it.

☐ SAW PALMETTO

Will saw palmetto relieve symptoms of an enlarged prostate?

You might give it a try, but keep your expectations in check. Many doctors recommend this herb (made from the dried berries of a small tree that grows in the southeastern United States) based on a number of small studies showing that it may provide modest relief from symptoms that include poor

urine flow and feeling as though you can't empty the bladder. But several recent studies found that saw palmetto supplements don't help. Nonetheless, some doctors still feel the weight of evidence is on saw palmetto's side. Since it is reasonably safe, you may want to give it a try (but tell your doctor about any side effects you may notice).

☐ SELENIUM

Does selenium prevent prostate cancer?

No, according to a large study sponsored by the National Cancer Institute. After 5 years, the men who took selenium supplements had the same odds of developing prostate cancer as a similar group of men who took placebo pills. Study officials decided to end the study early since there were some signs that selenium might increase the risk for diabetes. As far as we know, no other dietary supplement prevents prostate cancer.

☐ VITAMIN C

Are vitamin C powders better than tablets?

No; your body can't tell the difference. Companies that sell vitamin C powder often claim that it's "biologically active," suggesting that it's more

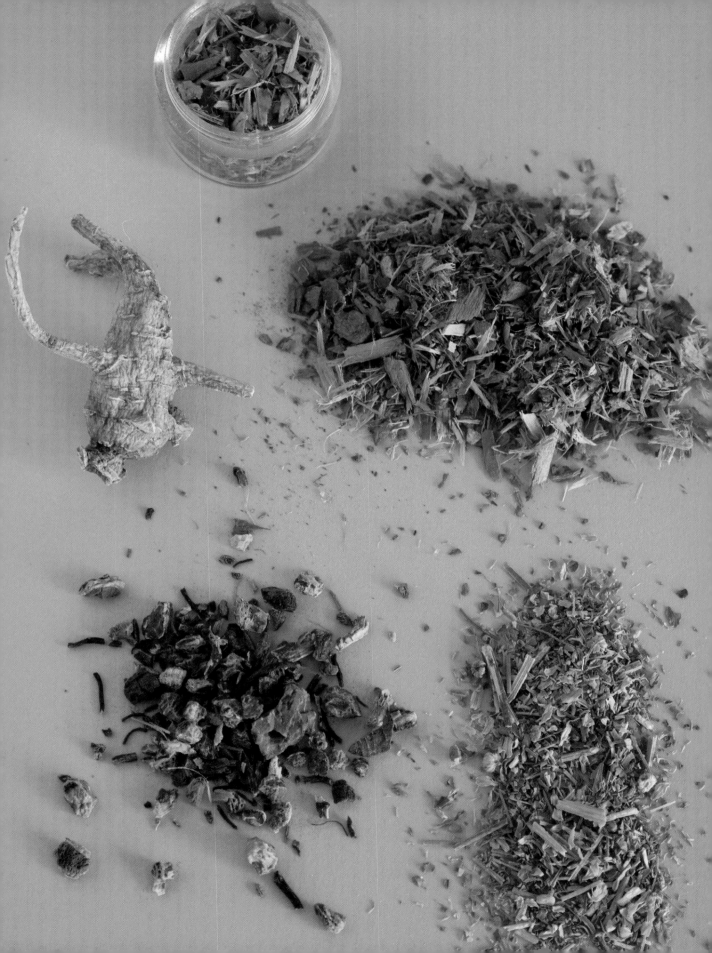

potent and gets to work faster than vitamin C tablets. But your body absorbs all forms of vitamin C in the same way. So go with whatever supplement suits you best. If you don't like swallowing pills, you can stir vitamin C powder into a glass of water or smoothie. If you choose pills, beware that some vitamin C tablets don't dissolve properly. Use the home test on page 161 to find out if your brand breaks down adequately.

☐ **VITAMIN D**

Vitamin D seems like the new miracle vitamin. Does it live up to all the hype?

Doctors and researchers are increasingly excited about the powers of this vitamin, with plenty of good reason. But keep in mind that supplements

go in and out of fashion faster than skirt lengths and necktie widths. (Remember when vitamin E was all the rage? See Vitamin E on the opposite page.) These days, vitamin D has taken center stage. You may already know that it helps your body absorb calcium, which is why these two nutrients are often teamed up in "bone health" supplements. But here are some of the findings that are creating buzz around this vitamin.

● *Autoimmune diseases.* Over the last 2 decades, scientists have discovered that vitamin D is necessary for a healthy immune system. Getting adequate amounts may help prevent autoimmune diseases such as type 1 diabetes, rheumatoid arthritis, and multiple sclerosis. One study of U.S. soldiers found those with the highest levels of vitamin D cut their risk for multiple sclerosis by 62 percent.

● *Cancer.* Lab studies show that vitamin D can block the growth of cancer cells. Some forms of cancer tend to be less common in sunny parts of the world, again hinting that high vitamin D levels may be protective. Population studies show that people who consume plenty of vitamin D tend to have a low risk for cancer, though it's not clear yet that taking supplements will help.

● *Heart disease and strokes.* Preliminary research shows that people with low levels of vitamin D are more likely to suffer heart attacks, heart failure, and strokes. One reason may be that vitamin D helps regulate blood pressure by turning down the activity of certain enzymes produced in the kidneys. Vitamin D deficiency has also been linked to chronic inflammation, another risk factor for heart disease. However, it's premature to recommend vitamin D supplements for preventing heart attacks and strokes.

● *Osteoporosis.* Vitamin D helps with calcium absorption, but now it seems that D helps fight osteoporosis on its own, too. The brittle bone disease is more common in Northern countries, where people spend less time in the sun (which generates vitamin D production in the body). Studies show that getting at least 800 IU of vitamin D per day (from food or supplements) in addition to 1,000 to 1,200 milligrams of calcium appears to cut the risk of bone fractures.

WHAT YOU DON'T KNOW

Smokers and Secondhand Smokers May Need Extra Vitamin C

Smokers need extra vitamin C, since lighting up depletes the body of this important antioxidant. But just living or working with a smoker may increase your need for it, too. One study found that 12 percent of nonsmokers who were regularly exposed to secondhand smoke had low blood levels of C. The recommended daily intake for smokers is 35 milligrams higher than for nonsmokers. There are no formal recommendations for people who breathe lots of secondhand smoke, but this may be reason enough to take a multivitamin, which typically provides 60 to 90 milligrams of C.

So should I take a vitamin D supplement?

That's up to you and your doctor, but certain groups of people are at high risk for vitamin D deficiency, making them potential candidates for supplements. For instance, the American Academy of Pediatrics recommends that infants who are exclusively or partially breastfed receive a supplement containing 400 IUs of vitamin D per day, since breast milk is low in vitamin D. Other groups are at risk for vitamin D deficiency, too, according to the National Institutes of Health's Office of Dietary Supplements. Ask your doctor if you should take a vitamin D supplement, and how much you need, if you fall into any of these groups:

- *You're age 50 or older.* As you age, your body becomes less efficient at creating vitamin D from sunshine.

- *You get little sun exposure.* That includes people who live in Northern latitudes, women who wear long robes and head coverings, and anyone who spends most of their days indoors.

- *You have dark skin.* The pigment melanin interferes with the skin's ability to make vitamin D when exposed to sunlight.

- *You have a condition that interferes with fat absorption.* Vitamin D requires fat in the gut in order to be absorbed. People

Vitamin D_3 is More Effective than Vitamin D_2

Fact. Vitamin D_3 is the kind your body produces when you stand in the sun; it's also the primary form found in foods such as cheese and eggs. Vitamin D_3 supplements are derived from lanolin. Some studies have shown that vitamin D_3 supplements increase blood levels of this important nutrient much more efficiently than vitamin D_2 pills, derived from yeast. But supplements containing either variety will get the job done, most doctors agree. A 2007 trial involving 68 adults found that 1,000 milligrams daily of vitamin D_2 or D_3 were equally effective at raising blood levels of the vitamin.

with certain forms of liver disease, as well as conditions such as cystic fibrosis and Crohn's disease, may not absorb fat properly, making a vitamin D supplement necessary.

- *You're obese.* People who have a body mass index of 30 or higher tend to have low blood levels of vitamin D. Gastric bypass surgery may worsen this problem, since the gastrointestinal tract is routed around the upper small intestine, where vitamin D is absorbed.

☐ **VITAMIN E**

I've heard a lot of conflicting information about vitamin E. Is it still worth taking?

Probably not. The evidence that vitamin E supplements will keep you from getting sick is weak, at best, and there are some clues that it could actually harm you. Interest in vitamin E arose thanks to large population studies showing that people who consume lots of this antioxidant nutrient, found in nuts and vegetable oil, have a low risk for certain diseases. However, vitamin E supplements have flunked when tested in formal clinical trials.

- *Alzheimer's disease.* Scientists theorized that vitamin E might block oxidative damage to cells in the brain and prevent Alzheimer's disease and other forms of dementia. A 3-year study, however, found that taking large daily doses of vitamin E did not prevent dementia.

- *Cancer.* A 10-year study of 39,000 women found that those who took vitamin E supplements gained no protection against developing or dying of cancer. A 7-year Canadian study reached the same conclusion.

• *Diabetes.* Some evidence suggests that vitamin E supplements may help manage blood sugar, though there's no proof that these pills will prevent diabetes complications such as blindness or kidney disease.

• *Heart disease.* In a number of studies, doctors gave vitamin E pills to one group of subjects and compared them with others who took placebos. The majority of these studies found that vitamin E supplements don't prevent heart attacks. Even worse, a 2005 study discovered that vitamin E users had a slightly elevated risk for heart failure. Some experts say vitamin E may still be a heart-saver, however—if you choose the right type. They point out that many of the negative studies used synthetic vitamin E, which has half the potency of natural E, the kind found in foods (look for "d-alpha" on labels).

A Bad Mix: Supplements and Medications That May Interact

A calcium or vitamin C tablet might seem harmless enough, but these and other supplements can block or exaggerate the effects of drugs you take. This chart lists common interactions between supplements and medications; there are many others. It's smart to check with your doctor before taking any supplement.

SUPPLEMENT	COULD INTERACT WITH	INTERACTION
Calcium citrate	Antacids that contain aluminum	May increase blood levels of aluminum and cause kidney damage
Chromium	Insulin and oral diabetes drugs	May cause low blood sugar
Echinacea	Drugs that suppress the immune system, such as cyclosporine and prednisone	May offset the action of these drugs by increasing immune system activity
Evening primrose oil	Tranquilizers such as chlorpromazine	Increases risk of epileptic seizures
Fish oil	Blood thinners such as aspirin and warfarin	May increase risk of bleeding (though this risk is theoretical and not well-documented)
Folic acid	Tetracycline antibiotics	May make tetracycline less effective; take folic acid and tetracycline several hours apart
Garlic	Blood thinners such as aspirin and warfarin, diabetes drugs such as sulfonylureas, HIV drugs such as saquinavir	May cause bleeding, lower blood sugar, and make some drugs less effective
Ginkgo	Blood-thinning drugs, including aspirin and warfarin	May increase the risk of bleeding
Ginseng	Insulin and oral diabetes drugs such as sulfonylureas and blood thinners such as warfarin	May cause low blood sugar when taken with diabetes drugs and block the effects of warfarin

☐ ZINC

Is it true that using zinc for colds could ruin my sense of smell?

Yes, if you use it in nasal spray form. This mineral is critical for a healthy immune system. Some studies have found that zinc supplements can ward off colds. However, the FDA received 130 reports of anosmia, or loss of the sense of smell, from people who used nasal sprays containing zinc, so the agency cautioned consumers to avoid these products. If you decide to try zinc, stick with lozenges or tablets. Many foods contain zinc, too, including oysters, breakfast cereal, pork, and beans.

SUPPLEMENT	COULD INTERACT WITH	INTERACTION
Iron	Antibiotics including tetracyclines and quinolones, blood pressure drugs called ACE inhibitors including captopril and others, thyroid drugs such as levothyroxine, and drugs for Parkinson's disease such as levodopa	May interfere with absorption of these drugs and make them less potent
Kava	Antianxiety drugs such as clonazepam, antiseizure drugs such as pentobarbital, alcohol, and any other sedative	May cause drowsiness and other side effects
Licorice	Antibiotics such as nitrofurantoin, birth control pills, blood thinners such as warfarin, diuretics such as hydrochlorothiazide or furosemide, heart failure drugs such as digoxin, hormone replacement therapy	May cause bleeding, loss of potassium, and other side effects; could interfere with hormonal drugs, including birth control pills
Magnesium	Antibiotics including tetracyclines and quinolones	May interfere with absorption of these drugs, so take them several hours apart
Psyllium	Antidepressants, blood thinners, lithium, and several other drugs	May reduce amount of drug absorbed, though this can be avoided by taking psyllium several hours after other medication
St. John's wort	Antidepressants (Prozac), allergy drugs, antibiotics, birth control pills, blood thinners (warfarin), heart failure drugs (digoxin), chemotherapy drugs, and other medications	May increase or decrease the potency of drugs; taken with antidepressants, can cause serotonin syndrome (muscle rigidity, confusion, fever)
Vitamin A	Blood thinners such as aspirin and warfarin, retinoic acid (for acne, other skin conditions)	May cause bleeding, headaches, vomiting, and other symptoms of vitamin A toxicity
Vitamin C	Acetaminophen and antacids containing aluminum	High doses may exaggerate side effects such as liver problems and constipation
Vitamin E	Blood thinners such as warfarin, heart failure drugs such as digoxin	May cause bleeding; digoxin dose may need to be reduced

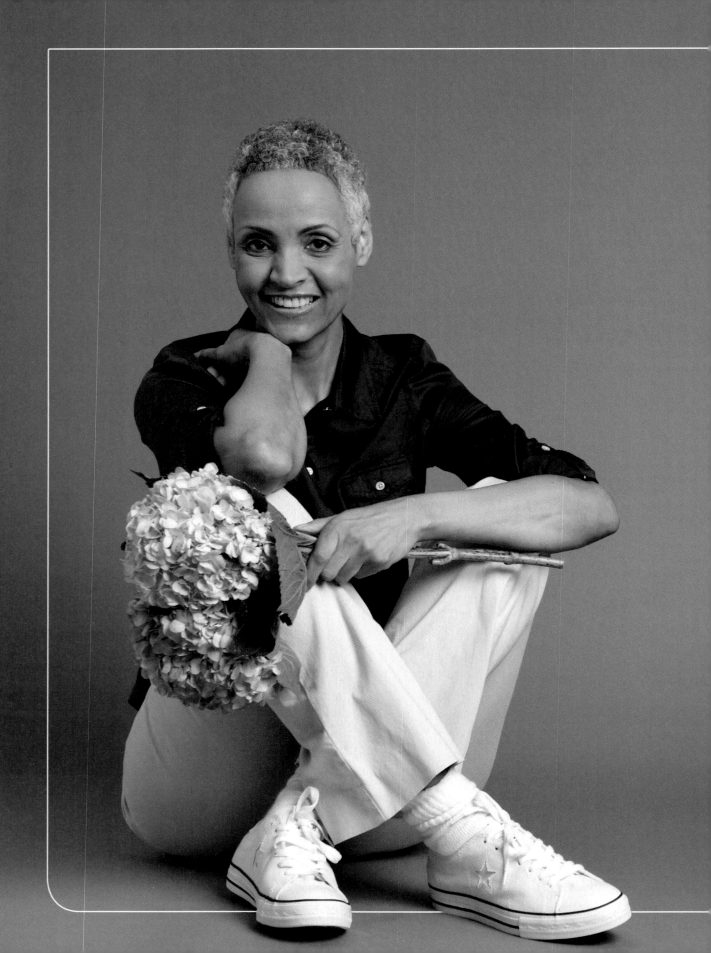

PART THREE

Common Health Conditions

Whether you have a cold or cancer, back pain or bronchitis, chances are you have questions to go with it. What's wrong—and what will make it go away? How can I get better faster? When is it time for surgery? Here, the answers, advice, and information you deserve.

FAQ Frequently Asked Questions

Common Health Conditions

Can stress really make you sick?

Absolutely. Feeling on edge or anxious now and then is perfectly normal and nothing to worry about. In fact, your body's natural stress response makes you more alert and able to react in a crisis. But chronic stress from financial concerns, marital problems, or any of life's woes can be disastrous for your overall health, and not just because people tend to cope with stress by smoking, drinking, overeating, and resorting to other unhealthy habits. It exposes your body to a daily blast of stress hormones, which, over time, can raise blood pressure, increase inflammation in the arteries, and cause other cardiovascular chaos. A recent study of more than 10,000 civil service employees in London found that those who reported feeling the most chronic emotional strain on the job were 68 percent more likely to suffer a heart attack.

Stress has been linked to a long list of additional health threats, including insomnia, diabetes, headaches, gastrointestinal problems, asthma, arthritis flare-ups, depression, and many others. Finding a way to cope with stress—whether it's deep breathing, yoga, prayer, exercise, or simply talking with a close confidante—could be a lifesaver.

My doctor tells me things on a need-to-know basis, and I often have questions I never get to ask. How can I get more information out of him?

The communication gap with your doctor isn't just frustrating—it may bad for your health. Many studies show that patients fare better when they have a free exchange of information with their physicians. To get more out of your office visits:

● *Be honest with your doctor.* Tell him that you feel in the dark about your own health and want more information. Be specific about your concerns.

● *Mention right away that you have questions.* Time-pressed doctors sometimes become annoyed when patients start asking questions at the end of an exam or office visit.

● *Bring a written list of questions.* Keep it short, and check off each question as your doctor answers it.

● *Don't worry about sounding stupid.* Surveys show that even doctors worry about asking dumb questions when they are patients. But there are no dumb questions in an examination room.

If you're dealing with a chronic condition, your doctor may have to spend most of your allotted appointment time discussing test results and changes in treatment. If there's no time for all your questions, ask if you can schedule a follow-up appointment to talk about your health more generally.

If you still feel that your doctor is always rushing you out the door, it's time to find another doctor.

I can never remember everything my doctor says during appointments, and he talks too fast for me to write it all down. What should I do?

Learn to ask this simple question: "Could you repeat that?" Better yet, ask your doctor to discuss your case in plain English and explain any medical jargon he uses. It is your right as a patient to leave an office visit with a full understanding of your diagnosis and treatment plan.

Other strategies that may help: Bring a friend or relative to your appointments to serve as a second set of ears; she may think of questions you forgot to ask, too. You might also consider bringing a small tape recorder to your office visits, which will free you from playing stenographer. Many cell phones have a voice-recorder function now, too.

What's the difference between a medical doctor, an osteopath, and a naturopath?

All three of these healers call themselves doctors, but there are important differences in how they are trained to treat patients.

- *Medical doctor.* After receiving a bachelor's degree, a candidate for a doctor of medicine degree (MD) attends a 4-year program, then performs a 1-year internship. Specialists, such as cardiologists and oncologists, require several additional years of training.

- *Osteopath.* A doctor of osteopathic medicine (DO) receives the same 4-year medical education as an MD and may also become a specialist. They also receive extra training in skeletal manipulation. When it comes to treating ailments, these doctors focus on the body as a whole rather than on one system or body part. They often use their hands to manipulate the musculoskeletal system in the belief that doing so will free the body to better heal itself.

- *Naturopath.* A doctor of naturopathic medicine (ND) attends a 4-year program that includes essential courses in medical sciences. However, they also learn about herbs, homeopathy, and other forms of holistic medicine. Some naturopaths receive additional training in specialties such as acupuncture or natural childbirth. To obtain a license to practice, a naturopath must pass a professional board exam.

I want to try acupuncture for my condition, but my doctor implies that I'm wasting my time. Am I?

Your doctor shouldn't be so quick to dismiss acupuncture, though whether it works may depend on what ails you. Practitioners of traditional Chinese

✋ AVOID THIS MISTAKE

Sticking with a Doctor You Don't Like

If you and your doctor just don't click, it's worth the time and effort to find another. Feeling uncomfortable or at odds with a doctor can lead you to question his judgment. Research confirms that patients who don't trust their doctors fare worse than other patients, possibly because they're less likely to follow care instructions. A 2000 study found that distrustful patients often failed to adhere to their doctors' advice—and were 30 percent less likely to get better.

medicine say that inserting acupuncture needles at precise points in the body treats diseases by restoring the healthy flow of energy, known as qi (pronounced CHEE), in the body. Modern medicine doesn't recognize the existence of qi, but solid research suggests that acupuncture does *something* beneficial. A panel of experts convened by the National Institutes of Health back in 1997 determined that it's effective for several conditions including:

- Nausea and vomiting following an operation or chemotherapy
- Nausea during pregnancy
- Pain from dental procedures

The panel also found that acupuncture might be helpful as an additional or alternative therapy for headaches, low back pain, asthma, menstrual cramps, addiction, and several other conditions.

I see a chiropractor for back pain, but lately she has been offering me general medical advice. Is she qualified to do that?

Few chiropractors have medical degrees, an important fact to keep in mind before you accept general medical advice from your practitioner. Like physicians, chiropractors attend

4-year schools that require them to study basic medical science and do hands-on work in a clinic. However, chiropractic is based on the concept that misalignments in the spinal cord, called subluxations, create disorder in the nervous system and affect general health. That's a controversial theory, and most medical doctors don't buy it.

Chiropractors are not allowed to perform surgery or prescribe drugs. Some practice acupuncture, herbal medicine, and other alternative therapies. While research suggests that chiropractic can provide short-term relief for low back pain, it's far less clear whether spinal manipulation is effective for any other condition.

The standard therapy for my condition isn't working. Is it safe to enter a clinical trial?

Enrolling in a clinical trial could mean that you receive a break-through therapy that cures your disease or relieves symptoms. Yet you must accept the hazards that come with being a human guinea pig.

- *You might not get the experimental therapy.* In most clinical trials, scientists give an experimental drug or treatment to one group of subjects, while a similar group receives a

placebo, or fake treatment. This type of study is necessary to determine whether a novel therapy truly works. But it also means you may be swallowing a sugar pill instead of medicine.

- *The therapy might not work.* Treatments that look promising in preliminary animal studies often prove useless in humans.
- *The therapy could make you sick.* Side effects may be mild, such as headaches or upset stomach. But many clinical trials have been stopped early because subjects who took an experimental treatment became seriously ill or died.

How do I find out how risky a certain procedure is?

Ask your doctor. He should be able to list any potential complications that may occur during or as a result of a medical procedure—and how likely they are to happen. Press for specifics, if possible. Ideally, instead of saying "knee replacement surgery is reasonably safe," your doctor should be able to tell you that a small number of patients who undergo the procedure develop serious complications such as nerve damage or blood clots in the leg veins or lungs. (The precise figure is 2 percent of patients, though such detailed information isn't available for all medical procedures.) Keep in mind that complication rates are only averages, and that many factors influence your risk. Ask whether your age, weight, and overall health make you more or less likely to experience problems.

How do I make sure my surgeon is the best one for my surgery?

If you need surgery, your primary care physician or health insurance plan will recommend a doctor to perform the procedure. That's a good start, but doing your homework will boost your chances of undergoing safe, successful surgery.

- *Ask around.* You may be surprised to find out how many people in your life have needed the same procedure or know someone who did. One study found that when women who needed breast cancer surgery asked friends and colleagues to recommend doctors with the best reputations, they were more likely to be treated by experienced doctors at high-quality cancer centers.

- *Find out if the surgeon is board certified.* Believe it or not, any doctor can perform surgery in many states, whether or not he has the proper training. Surgeons certified by the American Board of Medical Specialties must undergo years of training and pass rigorous exams; check the board's web site at

www.abms.org and look for the link "Is Your Doctor Certified?" or call (866) ASK-ABMS.

- *Look for a "high-volume" surgeon.* Like pitchers and pianists, surgeons get better with practice. Research shows that surgeons who perform the same surgeries over and over again are more likely to perform safe, successful procedures, whereas patient death rates from certain operations can be more than three times higher in the hands of an inexperienced surgeon, according to one study. What qualifies as "high volume?" There's no set definition, so go with the doctor who performs the most in your area.

- *Check the surgeon's record for complaints.* Contact your state licensing board or use DocInfo (https://s1.fsmb.org/docinfo), run by the Federation of State Medical Boards, to find out if the doctor has ever been disciplined (such as having a license suspended) for a professional or ethical lapse.

AVOID THIS MISTAKE

Choosing a Surgeon Who Doesn't Have Hospital Privileges

Don't have surgery in an office or stand-alone clinic unless the surgeon has admitting and operating privileges at a local hospital. If something goes wrong during the procedure, you could end up in an emergency room, where your doctor would not be able to provide your care. Also, lack of operating privileges may be a sign that your local hospital does not think the surgeon is competent.

I'm having a major medical procedure at a teaching hospital. Does that mean that my doctor will be a student— and is that safe?

There's little need for concern. In fact, patients treated at teaching hospitals often fare better than those who receive care at other medical centers, according to some research. Much of the care at teaching hospitals (also called university hospitals or academic medical centers) is provided by fellows, residents, and interns, all of whom are medical school graduates in various stages of their post-doctoral training. Current medical students see patients, too. However, all evaluation and treatment in a teaching hospital is supervised by board-certified attending physicians.

A 2000 study looked at the outcomes of nearly 17 million patients in the United States who were admitted to hospitals for 10 common conditions and 10 surgical procedures. Compared to all other types of hospitals, teaching hospitals had the lowest death rates.

How can I avoid having surgery that I don't really need?

You can start by getting a second opinion, which is standard procedure any time a doctor recommends surgery. Seek out another physician who specializes in treating your condition and find out whether he believes that going under the knife is the best solution for you. You can also do your own research. Check reliable sources and find out whether surgery is your only, or best, option. Some good web sites include the Mayo Clinic (www.mayoclinic.com), the Cleveland Clinic (www.clevelandclinic.org), and the National Library of Medicine (www.medlineplus.gov).

Ultimately, make sure you get satisfactory answers to all of the following questions before agreeing to have surgery.

- Why do I need surgery?
- What are the benefits?
- What are the alternatives to surgery?
- What are the risks of having the operation?

- What are the risks of not having the operation?

How can I tell if health information I find on the internet is accurate?

Ask some common sense questions before you trust information you find online.

- *Is the web site sloppy and amateurish?* The web sites of major hospitals, government health authorities, and other reliable sources of medical information tend to be well-designed and written. A slapdash-looking web site full of typos and poor grammar should raise a red flag.

- *Is it up to date?* A web site that doesn't appear to have been updated recently, or only mentions research that's more than 5 years old, may not provide you with state-of-the-art medical information.

- *Does the site ask for your credit card?* Does it offer to sell you something? A web site that tries to sell you dietary supplements or medical gizmos is probably best ignored.

- *Does it seem balanced?* Be skeptical of a web site that only describes one approach to coping with a medical concern.

- *Does it agree with what other web sites say?* Double-check any critical information you find with several other sources.

My doctor isn't treating my pain sufficiently. What should I do?

Ask for a referral to a pain specialist. For a variety of reasons, some physicians do a poor job of treating pain. Fear that patients may become addicted to pain-relief medication is one concern. Some doctors are simply not familiar with the scope of pain-relief therapies available. Thankfully, a growing number of doctors now specialize in treating pain, both acute (such as the pain following surgery or an injury) and chronic (such as ongoing back and joint

 AVOID THIS MISTAKE

Trying to Diagnose Yourself

No matter what web site you're using, remember that self-diagnosis is a bad idea. It's not as easy as it may seem and could lead you to incorrect conclusions. Feel free to research your symptoms, but let your doctor decide what's ailing you.

WHAT YOU DON'T KNOW

Your Brother's and Sister's Health Problems Count

As you compile your medical history, don't forget to include all of your close blood relatives who have had major health problems—not just your mother and father. Having a sibling with heart disease raises your own odds for cardiovascular trouble by 45 percent, whether or not you currently have any other risk factors such as high cholesterol. That makes it twice as risky as having a parent with heart problems.

pain). If your doctor doesn't know any pain specialists, check the American Academy of Pain Medicine web site (www.painmed.org/patient/index.html) to find one near you.

How can I determine my risk of disease?

You can start by checking the Disease Risk Index at www.diseaseriskindex.harvard.edu. Created by the Harvard School of Public Health, it estimates your risk for developing heart disease, stroke, diabetes, osteoporosis, and a dozen different forms of cancer. All you have to do is type in some basic information, such as your age, height, weight, and what sort of diet you eat.

If you have a family history of certain diseases, you can also undergo genetic testing for genes linked to an increased risk of colon and breast cancer, Alzheimer's disease, and rare disorders such as Huntington's disease. A genetic counselor at your local hospital can discuss the pros and cons of genetic testing.

I have a serious medical condition. Is it okay for me to plan an overseas trip?

Assuming that your condition is stable, it should be okay. Taking these steps before you hand over your passport will help ensure that you enjoy a safe, anxiety-free journey.

● *Check in with your doctor.* He can discuss what measures you should take before traveling, such as getting necessary vaccinations. You can check on the latter yourself at www.cdc.gov/travel.

● *Be sure you're covered.* Make sure your insurance pays the cost of health care provided abroad; get extra coverage, if necessary. Think about buying medical evacuation insurance, which will pay transportation costs, if needed.

● *Know where to turn for help.* Join the International Association for Medical Assistance to Travellers (www.iamat.org). Membership is free and provides (among other benefits) a directory of qualified English-speaking doctors in more than 90 countries and 350 cities. If you need further assistance in a medical crisis, contact the U.S. Embassy. (Check the State Department web site for a list of all U.S. embassies, consulates, and diplomatic missions at www.usembassy.gov.)

● *Learn some lingo.* When you look up how to hail a cab or order in a restaurant, make sure you also learn how to say "I need a doctor" and any other phrases you may need in an emergency. For instance, if you have diabetes, learn the phrase for "I need fruit juice or sugar" in case you develop hypoglycemia.

● *Pack smart.* Take extra medicine and supplies (such as inhalers or syringes). Bring copies of your prescriptions, and be sure the drugs are listed by generic name, since brand names vary by country. Obtain a letter from your doctor explaining your medical condition and the treatments you require. If necessary, notify officials at airport security checkpoints that you are carrying medical supplies.

Common Health Conditions

☐ **ACNE**

Do chocolate and greasy foods cause acne?

Most doctors have long dismissed this theory, chalking acne up to hormone shifts. But the answer may not be quite so simple. For instance, over the last half-century or so, scientists studying cultures as diverse as the Inuit of the Arctic Circle to the Kitavan Islanders near Papua New Guinea have noticed a trend: People who consume simple, traditional diets tend to have unblemished skin. Some researchers now believe that the typical high-calorie, sugar-laden Western diet drives up insulin levels, which may in turn lead to higher levels of androgens, the hormones linked to acne. This theory is controversial, and even if it's true, some skin may be more susceptible to the effects of junk food than others. But eating less sugar and grease certainly can't hurt.

I'm middle-aged and I still break out now and then. What can I use that will work for me?

Some simple steps may keep you in the clear; if not, your doctor can prescribe effective medications. Acne breakouts happen when skin oil, dead skin cells, and bacteria clog hair follicles. Keeping your skin clean and dry is a good start, but don't overdo it. Wash with mild soap and avoid vigorous scrubbing, which could worsen acne.

Over-the-counter medications can help with mild acne. Most contain either salicylic acid, which limits the shedding of skin cells and unclogs pores, or benzoyl peroxide, which kills bacteria.

For more resistant acne, see your doctor. He will most likely prescribe a skin lotion, cream, or gel containing retinoids, which are derived from vitamin A. Retinoids unclog pores and block the formation of whiteheads and blackheads. Products include adapalene (Differin), tazarotene (Avage, Tazorac) and tretinoin (retin-A, Renova). Note that these may dry or irritate skin. Doctors can also prescribe low-dose oral antibiotics and antimicrobial skin treatments that kill bacteria that feed the growth of acne.

If you're a woman and you need both acne help and birth control, consider an oral contraceptive that contains estrogen and progestin; these reduce production of skin oil and can help control acne in women. Talk with your doctor to make sure you're a good candidate.

What's the best treatment for acne scars?

Dermabrasion is generally considered the most effective way to remove or minimize acne scars. As the body tries to heal the inflammation-induced injury caused by acne it may leave behind pits, pock marks, and other disfiguring marks on the skin. During dermabrasion, a doctor uses a high-speed brush to remove the top layer of skin and smooth over scars. Dermabrasion can eliminate shallow scars and soften the appearance of deeper blemishes.

More serious acne scars may require surgery. In one common procedure called subcision, the surgeon makes cuts under the skin that "lift" scar tissue, making it level with the skin. Laser treatments are another option, as is skin grafting. These procedures are best done after the acne is cleared up; otherwise additional scarring could ruin the benefit of the scar-removal procedure.

☐ ADHD

I think my husband might have ADHD. What are the signs in adults? Are the treatments the same as for kids?

The basic symptoms of attention deficit hyperactivity disorder are similar in children and adults. People who have the condition are easily distracted, restless, and impulsive. However, ADHD *looks* different in adults. While a parent or teacher may first suspect ADHD in a child who can't sit still or pay attention in the classroom, the warning signs in adults may be less obvious. Does your husband:

● *Bounce from job to job?* People with ADHD often have a history of frequent firings due to poor performance. Or they quit steady jobs abruptly because they're bored.

● *Struggle to get things done?* Unpaid bills, home-improvement projects left half finished, missed appointments, and a general lack of organization are all red flags.

● *Have a spotty romantic track record?* If your spouse was a serial dater before you met, you may now know why.

● *Seem stressed out, frustrated, and guilt-ridden?* Constant failure can really grind down your psyche.

If you answered yes to most or all of these questions, consider asking your husband to be evaluated by a doctor or by a psychologist who specializes in treating ADHD. Don't be surprised if your husband resists at first, since many people remain skeptical about ADHD. Emphasize that effective treatment is available. Most adults with ADHD receive counseling on time management and other organizational skills, as well as

WHAT YOU DON'T KNOW

Stress Causes Acne

Does it seem like you break out only when a deadline looms or you're worried about a loved one? It may not be your imagination. Some research suggests that psychological stress worsens acne. In one study, dermatologists evaluated the skin of a group of college students before and after taking exams. Students who reported feeling the most stressed out during exams had the worst acne.

a prescription for amphetamine (Adderall) or similar medication. Research in children (and, to a lesser degree, adults) shows that these stimulant drugs help people with ADHD focus their attention.

What's the difference between ADD and ADHD?

Although some people use these abbreviations interchangeably, they don't mean exactly the same thing. Furthermore, the former has mostly fallen out of favor with doctors. ADD, which stands for attention deficit disorder, is the older of the two names for this condition. It was a clear improvement over some even older names, which included "minimal brain dysfunction." However, attention deficit disorder describes only one of the hallmark symptoms of the disorder, the inability to concentrate and focus on tasks. Scientists switched to the newer term in order to reflect restlessness and impulsivity, behaviors that may accompany inattentiveness—though not necessarily. (The American Psychiatric Association distinguishes between ADHD patients who are primarily inattentive, primarily hyperactive or impulsive, and a third group who are a mix of both.)

My child has ADHD, but I don't want him to take drugs. Will behavioral modification help?

Teaching a child with ADHD to follow a daily routine, use organizers, and adhere to other behavioral modification strategies might help tone down his erratic, unpredictable behavior. But research shows that the benefits are likely to be modest. Meanwhile, many studies have found that commonly prescribed medications—particularly stimulants such as amphetamine (Adderall) and methylphenidate (Ritalin)—improve behavior in children with ADHD. Stimulant medications may cause side effects, which include loss of appetite, weight loss, and irritability. However, these tend to fade over time. The American Academy of Pediatrics recommends combining medication with behavioral training for the best results.

Do girls get ADHD?

Yes. Though boys are more than twice as likely to be diagnosed with ADHD, girls develop this condition, too. In the United States, about 4.3 percent of school-age girls have been diagnosed with ADHD, according to the Centers for Disease Control and Prevention. However, some experts believe that the true

figure is probably higher since certain teachers, parents, and clinicians may still consider ADHD a boy's disorder and be less likely to look for it in girls.

☐ ALLERGIES

My new spouse has a cat, but I'm allergic to cats. Is there anything wrong with just putting up with the symptoms?

Exposure to allergens such as pet dander causes the tissues in your nasal passages to become inflamed, which clogs the sinuses, or air cavities around the nose. That can allow bacteria to accumulate, which could cause a sinus infection, or sinusitis. If you have a history of asthma or a significant family history of allergies and asthma, you may also be setting yourself up for a serious asthma attack.

To keep the cat and protect your health, you might consider allergy shots, or immunotherapy, described in "Which dog breeds are hypoallergenic?" below. And keep kitty out of the bedroom.

Which dog breeds are hypoallergenic?

If you are searching for a dog that is 100 percent allergen-free, you might as well quit looking and get a goldfish

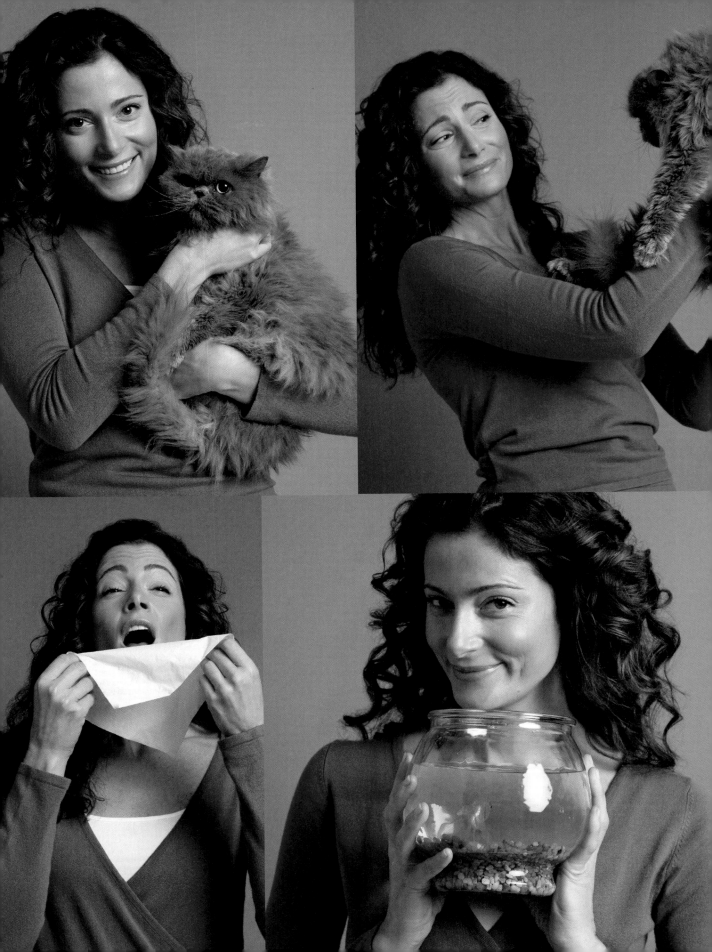

instead. If you are allergic to dogs, any breed—even a Mexican hairless—may cause sneezing, wheezing, and other symptoms. That's because fur itself isn't the problem. The problem is a protein found in a dog's saliva, which is spread by licking its coat and skin. (The allergen is in dog urine, too.) Pet dander, the dandruff-like flakes that dogs shed, carries the protein and causes allergies.

However, certain breeds that don't shed their fur and that produce relatively small amounts of dander may be better candidates for families that include a pet allergy sufferer, according to the American Kennel Club. They include:

- Bedlington Terrier
- Bichon Frise
- Chinese Crested
- Irish Water Spaniel
- Kerry Blue Terrier
- Maltese
- Mexican Hairless
(also called Xoloitzcuintli)
- Poodles (toy, miniature, or standard)
- Portuguese Water Dog
- Schnauzer (miniature, standard, or giant)
- Soft Coated Wheaten Terrier

Some hybrid breeds—so-called designer dogs, such as goldendoodles and cockapoos—may produce less dander, too.

Taking these steps may make life easier if you have a dog allergy: Keep the dog out of the bedroom; bathe and groom the dog once a week; wash your face, hands, and arms after touching the dog; and use a high-efficiency particulate air (HEPA) filter in the bedroom to remove dander from the air. You can also talk to your doctor about allergy shots or immunotherapy. This therapy exposes you to tiny amounts of an allergy-causing protein, or allergen—in this case, pet dander—with the goal of building up your tolerance and reducing your reaction, though the treatment is not always successful.

I've been considering allergy shots, but I can't stand the idea of getting injections for the next couple of years. Is there an alternative?

Yes. Some clinics now offer under-the-tongue drops or tablets called sublingual immunotherapy (SLIT). SLIT not only lets you avoid injections but you may also be able to skip the frequent office visits and administer the treatments yourself at home. The downside? Experts don't know if SLIT is as effective as allergy shots. In the only head-to-head study, which involved patients with birch pollen allergy, shots were better than drops, though the difference was small. Studies are ongoing, and we should know more about needle-free immunotherapy within a few years.

In the United States, the FDA hasn't approved SLIT, but since the drops or tablets contain the same extracts that injections contain, doctors are free to prescribe them.

I'm allergic to mold. What should I do to limit my exposure at home?

Cut down on the population of spores, which are the airborne "seeds" of fungi that produce mold and mildew. The Asthma and Allergy Foundation of America recommends the following steps:

- If possible, install central air conditioning with a high-efficiency particulate air (HEPA) filter.

- If you must use a humidifier, scrub the reservoir twice a week. Be sure to clean air-conditioners and dehumidifiers frequently, too.

- Use a hygrometer to monitor humidity levels in your home. Aim for a number lower than 45 percent; 35 percent is ideal.

- Install an exhaust fan in the bathroom. If that's not possible, open the window after bathing to let damp air escape.

- Repair any plumbing leaks promptly.

- Scrub sinks and tubs with diluted bleach (1 ounce per quart of water) at least monthly.

- Keep garbage cans and wastebaskets clean.

- Clean the refrigerator door gaskets and drip pans.

- Use a dehumidifier in the basement.
- Cover polyurethane or rubber foam bedding in plastic.
- Toss out or recycle old books, newspapers, and clothes.
- Remove leaves from rain gutters and keep them away from the foundation of your house.

☐ **ALZHEIMER'S DISEASE**

Is there anything I can do to prevent Alzheimer's, or is it spelled out in my genes?

It's possible to inherit an increased risk for Alzheimer's disease and other forms of dementia, or the loss of memory and other intellectual abilities. But even if you do, a growing body of evidence suggests that making the right lifestyle choices may offer significant protection. If you are currently taking steps to lower your risk for other major diseases such as heart disease and diabetes by keeping your cholesterol, blood pressure, and blood sugar low, you're already cutting the threat of dementia, too. You know the basics: Don't smoke, keep your weight down, avoid junk food, and eat a balanced diet with plenty of fruits and vegetables, several weekly servings of fatty fish, such as salmon, and olive oil.

You can lower your risk for dementia even further with these measures:

- *Keep your brain on its toes.* Learning new information and acquiring novel skills helps build backup mental power, which scientists call cognitive reserve, that can keep your brain working hard even if some neurons become diseased. A study in the *New England Journal of Medicine* found that people over age 75 who keep their minds active by reading, playing games, and even learning new dance steps cut their risk for developing dementia by 63 percent.
- *Don't be an introvert.* Keeping in touch with family and friends keeps your brain stimulated and energized. Social butterflies may cut their risk for dementia by 26 percent, according to one study.
- *Get regular exercise.* In one study of 2,263 men age 71 and older, inactive volunteers who started an exercise program cut their risk of dementia in half compared to those who did not. In another study, people who exercised just twice a week were half as likely to have dementia 21 years later as those who were inactive, even if they had inherited the gene for late-life Alzheimer's.
- *Be hard-headed.* Wear a helmet if you bike or ski. Serious head injuries may increase Alzheimer's risk by 58 percent.

Should I be tested for the Alzheimer's gene?

Only you can decide. Doctors often discourage patients from finding out whether they carry the ApoE 4 gene, which can increase your risk for Alzheimer's disease up to 15-fold. That's because a positive test doesn't guarantee that you'll develop the disease, and a negative test doesn't mean that you won't. With that uncertainty, why put yourself through so much anxiety?

That said, a 2009 study in the *New England Journal of*

DRUG-FREE FIX

A Saline Nasal Rinse

Clearing mucus from stuffed-up nasal passages with a saline rinse can help relieve congestion from allergies. You can make your own saline at home with ½ teaspoon salt, ½ teaspoon baking soda, and 16 ounces of warm tap water. Pick up a reusable nasal spray bottle or a nasal bulb syringe at a pharmacy. Or you can buy commercial saline nasal spray or mist (Ocean); just avoid products that contain the preservative benzalkonium chloride, which may worsen your symptoms.

Medicine found that most people who learn that they carry ApoE 4 handle the news pretty well and don't become depressed or plagued by anxiety. Other research shows that people who test positive are more likely to eat a better diet, take needed medications, and adhere to other healthy behaviors. However, if you decide to get tested, it's essential that you consult with a genetic counselor before and after to ensure that you understand the implications of your result.

My father has Alzheimer's and he's becoming difficult to manage. Are there strategies that help or does he need to be in a nursing home?

Many hospitals offer training programs for people who care for patients with Alzheimer's disease and other forms of dementia. Learning ways to ease the aggression, agitation, confusion, and other common behaviors in dementia patients can make daily life easier to manage. The Alzheimer's Association recommends these strategies:

- *Maintain a neat, orderly home.* Avoid clutter; it can cause people with dementia to become distracted and upset. Don't rearrange furniture. Make sure rooms are well-lit.
- *Create a soothing atmosphere.* Loud, sudden noises may make a person with Alzheimer's anxious or angry. Play soft music your father enjoys to block sounds from outside. Try giving him a massage.
- *Keep him busy.* Relaxing activities, such as arts and crafts, can help prevent restlessness. Take your father for walks or go for a drive.

When you no longer feel as though you can provide a safe and healthy environment for him, it's time to find a qualified nursing facility.

I'm exhausted and stressed from taking caring of my parent with Alzheimer's and really feel like I need a break. What are my options?

You can't provide the best care if you're exhausted and stressed. The following resources may be able to provide some relief:

- *Friends and family.* Ask a relative or good friend to take over for you for a few hours.
- *Adult day care.* Many communities have day programs for elders; some are designed specifically for Alzheimer's patients. Contact your local council or agency on aging to find one.
- *In-home assistance.* Professionals who provide respite care can offer everything from nursing and personal care to helping with household chores and providing companionship for the patient. Ask around at your community center or church, or contact your local or state authority on elder affairs.

FACT OR FICTION

Aluminum Cookware Causes Alzheimer's

Fiction. Lab animals develop dementia-like symptoms when exposed to large amounts of aluminum. The brains of some, though not all, Alzheimer's patients have unusually large deposits of the metal. But there's zero proof that the tiny amount of aluminum that transfers from pots and pans to food during cooking causes Alzheimer's disease or any other form of damage to the brain. (Where else would the aluminum come from? Drinking water contains trace amounts, which can reach the brain.)

ANEMIA

I'm always exhausted. Should I start taking iron pills and eating more red meat in case I'm anemic?

No, at least not yet. Here are four good reasons why you should always talk to a doctor before increasing your iron intake.

- **You may not be anemic.** Fatigue is a symptom of countless conditions, including sleep disorders, heart failure, diabetes, thyroid disease, and depression. It's also a side effect of some medications. See a doctor and find out what's causing your exhaustion.

- **Consuming more iron may not help.** If you are anemic, that means your blood isn't delivering enough oxygen to cells throughout your body. Iron deficiency is the most common cause, but several unrelated problems can trigger anemia, too.

- **Anemia can be a symptom of another serious condition.** Menstrual problems, pregnancy, an iron-poor diet, and frequent use of ibuprofen and other non-steroidal anti-inflammatory drugs (NSAIDs) can cause iron deficiency. But so can ulcers, colon cancer, certain digestive diseases, rare inherited disorders, and other conditions that need medical attention.

- **You might overdo it.** Your body needs adequate amounts of iron, but too much can be harmful. Hemochromatosis, or the buildup of excess iron in the body, can cause symptoms ranging from weakness and fatigue to "bronzed" skin, as well as lead to the development of other serious conditions.

I've taken iron supplements to prevent anemia for years, but now I've reached menopause. Do I still need them?

You may not, but speak with your doctor before you stop taking them. Doctors prescribe iron supplements to women who become anemic because they lose an unusually large volume of blood during their periods. Since that's no longer a problem, iron supplements may not be necessary. But check with your doc to ensure that there aren't other reasons he wants you to take them. For example, some gastrointestinal disorders (such as celiac disease) can interfere with the absorption of iron.

What's the difference between iron-deficiency anemia and pernicious anemia? Are the treatments the same?

Both disorders result in abnormally low levels of red blood cells, but this problem occurs for different reasons.

- **Iron-deficiency anemia.** Iron is necessary for forming hemoglobin, the protein in red blood cells that carries oxygen. Women are more likely to develop iron-deficiency anemia due to loss of blood during menstruation. Also, a pregnant woman may run low on iron because she must produce red blood cells for herself and the fetus. In most cases, eating more iron-rich foods and taking iron supplements clears up the problem.

- **Pernicious anemia.** Healthy red blood cells also require another nutrient, vitamin B_{12}. Some people don't produce enough intrinsic factor, a stomach protein that allows the body to absorb vitamin B_{12} from food. Along with fatigue, pernicious anemia causes diarrhea, bleeding gums, and other serious side effects. Sufferers require monthly vitamin B_{12} shots.

Blood tests show that I'm low on iron, but I don't feel tired. Should I be concerned?

There's no cause for alarm, but your doctor may suggest iron supplements and diet changes as a preventive measure. You may feel fine now, but having low iron levels means you are a candidate for anemia. Rather than wait for the symptoms to emerge, adding an iron supplement to your daily regimen could keep them at bay.

I was told I can't donate blood because my hemoglobin is low. Does that mean I'm anemic?

Not necessarily. Before you can donate blood, a technician takes a small blood sample (usually by pricking your finger) to measure your hemoglobin, which is the protein in red blood cells that carries oxygen. Low hemoglobin is the most common reason would-be blood donors are turned away. However, it's not proof that you are anemic; you may simply be lower than normal that day. Still, you may want to consider whether your diet is low in iron, an essential component of hemoglobin. Some good sources include:

- Beef
- Whole grains
- Spinach, broccoli, and peas
- Oysters and shrimp
- Rice and potatoes
- Tomatoes
- Watermelon

Note that eating certain foods and drinking certain beverages, including chocolate and caffeinated drinks, interfere with your body's ability to absorb iron, as can consuming very large amounts of fiber and calcium (or antacids containing calcium).

 FACT OR FICTION

If Your Joints Ache, Get Out the Umbrella

Fact. Believe it or not, your grandmother was right: A flare-up of arthritis pain may be able to predict rain. Your joints contain nerve receptors that respond to changes in atmospheric pressure. These receptors are particularly sensitive to falling barometric pressure, which usually means it may rain. People with arthritis have less cartilage to cushion joints, so they're most likely to notice these fluctuations. One study found that changes in the weather worsened symptoms in 83 percent of patients with osteoarthritis.

☐ ARTHRITIS

When is it time to give up on the ibuprofen and glucosamine and have surgery to replace an arthritic knee, hip, or other joint?

If medications, physical therapy, and lifestyle changes can no longer ward off the discomfort, it's time to consider an artificial joint. This doesn't represent a failure on your part or mean that you didn't do the right thing for your aching joint. Arthritis can be a progressive disease, meaning that it often worsens over time. In many people, the tough, slippery cartilage that safeguards the ends of joints eventually wears away altogether. That leads to pain and stiffness as the bones, now exposed and unprotected, rub against one another. As this point, patients with severe knee or hip arthritis may walk with a pronounced limp and have to limit their daily activities. Joint replacement surgery, while a major operation, can eliminate pain and help you resume your normal routine. Arrange to meet with an orthopedic surgeon to discuss whether you're a good candidate.

What about having arthroscopic surgery instead of joint replacement surgery?

Arthroscopic surgery may not relieve your pain, stiffness, and other arthritis symptoms. In arthroscopic surgery, a doctor peers into a joint through a tube-shaped instrument equipped with a light and lens in search of damaged tissue. The instrument also allows the surgeon to trim away or flush out fragments of cartilage and bone, in hopes that removing this debris will relieve arthritis pain.

Arthroscopic surgery is appealing since it only requires a tiny incision, which means the patient can be up on his feet quickly. However, several major studies failed to find any evidence that removing torn cartilage, bits of bone, and other debris eases the pain of knee arthritis. In the most recent study, patients who underwent knee arthroscopy were no more or less likely than others who had fake surgery (the surgeon makes a small incision but doesn't remove any debris) to be pain-free after two years.

Can injections help knee arthritis?

If pain-relievers such as non-steroidal anti-inflammatory drugs (NSAIDs) no longer keep your pain in check, your doctor may inject you with an anesthetic, though that will probably only dull the agony for a few weeks at the most. Chances are, he will inject another drug, called a corti-costeroid, which may temporarily chill inflammation that's fanning the flames of pain. When steroids stop working, many doctors today inject a product called hyaluronic acid, which has an unusual origin: Some prepara-tions are made from rooster combs. All joints, including your knees, are lubricated with

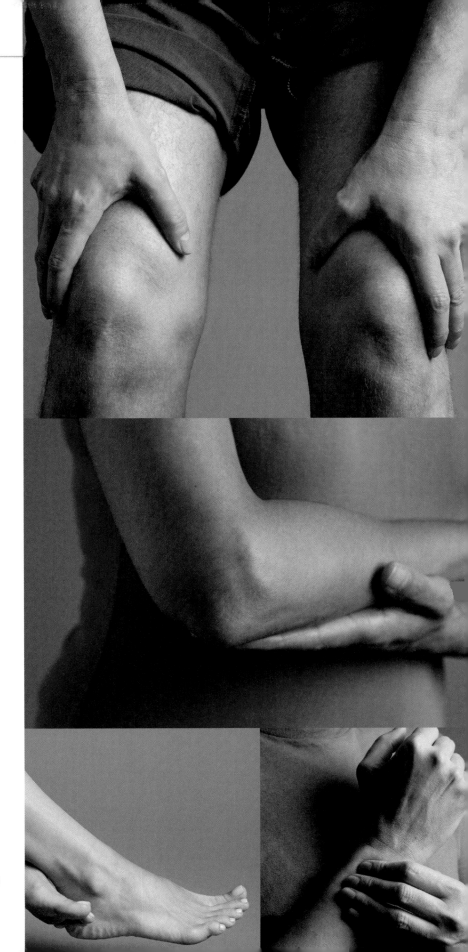

a fluid that contains hyaluronic acid. Levels of hyaluronic acid drop in people with osteoarthritis. Injecting this compound into the knee relieves pain and restores mobility in some, though not all, patients. In one study, up to 80 percent of patients experienced some relief, though other studies have found no benefit at all.

When hyaluronic acid works, it seems to relieve pain for 6 months to a year. While not much is known about long-term use, a few studies show that some patients can benefit from repeated injections.

I have arthritis in my knees and hips. Do I have to give up my weekly tennis match?

Keep your tennis date. Far from off-limits, physical activity is a vital part of managing arthritis. Doctors didn't always know this; in the past, most discouraged arthritis patients from exercising, fearing that too much running around would wear away cartilage and further damage joints. However, experts now know that exercise reduces arthritis pain and stiffness, according to many studies. Working your muscles makes them stronger and better able to act as shock absorbers, which means less strain on the joints. Exercise also helps keep weight under control, reducing the load that joints must bear.

Getting the full benefits of exercise takes more than lacing up your tennis shoes once a week. Aim for at least 30 minutes of aerobic exercise—the kind that gets your heart and lungs working harder—on most days. In addition, perform some type of strength training (such as lifting weights or using exercise bands) at least twice a week, recommends the Arthritis Foundation. Daily stretching can help loosen up stiff joints, too.

There may be days when arthritis leaves you too sore to exercise. That's okay. You may also need to slow down the pace. If tennis is your game, try playing doubles, which requires a player to cover less ground. In general, it's best for people with arthritis to limit their play in sports that involve a lot of jarring and twisting movements. Many find that they prefer low- or no-impact activities such as walking, cycling, or swimming. Talk to your doctor or a physical therapist about what makes sense for you.

I used to crack my knuckles a lot. Will that cause arthritis?

No, but you might want to avoid this habit all the same. Cracking a knuckle can create space between the joints in the finger. That causes air bubbles to form in the synovial fluid, or joint lubricant. When the bubble bursts, it lets out a distinctive popping sound. People who crack their knuckles do not have an increased risk for developing arthritis, several studies have found. However, one study of 300 adults found that knuckle-crackers are more likely to have swollen hands and weak hand grips. Although it hasn't been proven, one theory holds that cracking knuckles weakens finger ligaments.

☐ **ASTHMA**

I've always avoided sports because of my asthma, but I want to start cycling. Is it safe?

Yes, in fact, many successful athletes have asthma. Exercise can cause most people with the condition (and even some who don't) to wheeze, develop chest tightness, and experience other common asthma symptoms a few minutes after they start huffing and puffing. However, some simple steps can help keep you in action.

● *Bring your bronchodilator.* Inhaling short-acting bronchodilator medication 15 minutes before exercise can keep airways clear for 4 to 6 hours in up to 90 percent of people with asthma. Using a bronchodilator can help if you feel symptoms coming on while you're playing or exercising, too.

• *Warm up.* Jogging lightly before you work out may help to prevent tightness.

• *Choose the right sport.* Some people with asthma may find that sports requiring constant movement (such as basketball or soccer) are more likely to trigger exercise-induced asthma. The best choice? Indoor swimming, since warm, humid air is less likely to trigger an attack and being horizontal may help relieve lung congestion.

When and how should I use a peak flow meter?

Use a peak flow meter when you want to find out how well you are managing your asthma. The information it provides can help your doctor make decisions about your medication. A peak flow meter is a small, inexpensive device that measures how well your lungs are working. You blow in one end as hard as possible and a meter measures the force of your exhalation. If you have mild asthma that's generally well-controlled, you may only need to use a peak flow meter if you feel like your condition may be getting worse. However, if you have moderate or severe asthma, your doctor may suggest taking a few readings |daily. In any case, if using a peak flow meter shows that your asthma is not under control, your doctor can increase or change your medication. If your lung function is improving, you may be able to reduce your dose.

Do food colorings cause asthma?

That seems to be a myth, though some still claim it as a fact. The theory that food colorings can trigger asthma attacks dates back to the 1950s. A few studies found that some asthma patients were sensitive to tartrazine, a yellow dye widely used in processed foods, drugs, and cosmetics. However, that research has been criticized as flawed. (In some of the studies, subjects were exposed to tartrazine after being deprived of medication for hours, so it wasn't clear why they suffered asthma attacks.) While there may be a very small number of people who are sensitive to tartrazine, a 2006 review found that there's no reason for most people with asthma to avoid it.

What should I do if I'm at a ball game or concert and I start to develop symptoms but I don't have my inhaler?

It's a nightmare scenario, but these steps can help you regain control and catch your breath:

• *Don't panic.* Emotional stress can worsen an asthma attack.

• *Sit down.* It's easier to breathe when you're in a seated position. Don't lie down.

• *Drink some cola, tea, or coffee.* If you're having a mild attack, consuming caffeine may help; it's chemically related to theophylline, a bronchodilator drug. It may take several cups, however.

• *Get help.* If a mild asthma attack doesn't subside in 15 minutes, go to the stadium or arena's first-aid center, if it has one. If not, go to an emergency room immediately. If you can't speak more than a word or two from shortness of breath or feel like you're about to pass out, have someone call for an ambulance.

□ **BACK PAIN**

Are abdominal crunches the best exercise for preventing back pain? If not, what is?

No. The crunch is a modified sit-up that works muscles deep in the abdomen. You lie down with your lower back flat against the floor, knees bent, and hands behind your neck. Then you slowly use your stomach muscles to lift your upper body off the ground. However, crunches ranked 11th out of 13 in a study of back exercises by researchers at San Diego State University. (Some other experts even believe ab crunches can harm the spine.) What's the best back exercise?

The bicycle maneuver: Lie flat on the floor with your lower back pressed to the ground and your hands behind your head. Raise your knees to a 45-degree angle and pretend to pedal a bicycle. As you do so, touch your left elbow to your right knee, then your right elbow to your left knee.

How likely is surgery to cure my lower back pain?

First ask yourself: Do I really need back surgery? Most people with lower back pain can manage flare-ups with rest, pain relievers, heating pads, ice packs, and other conservative treatments. The anguish usually goes away in a month or so. Surgery is an option for serious low back pain that doesn't respond to nonsurgical therapy and persists for a year or more.

Spinal fusion is the most common type of surgery for chronic low back pain. In this procedure, a surgeon inserts a bone fragment between two vertebrae (spinal bones) to restrict their motion and keep them from causing pain. (Bone fragments are "harvested" from the patient's body, come from a donor, or may be synthetic.) Bone fragments may be held in place with plates, screws, or other hardware. One study found that about two-thirds of patients who underwent spinal fusion believed it improved their symptoms. However, three other studies found no difference between patients who had spinal fusion and others who did back exercises and received psychological counseling about coping with pain.

A growing number of patients who opt for back surgery are choosing to have lumbar disc replacement, which uses artificial vertebrae. Some early research suggests that disc replacement is more effective than spinal fusion, but until longer-term studies are done, it's impossible to say for sure. There is rarely any need to rush into back surgery, so think long and hard and do plenty of research before deciding what's best for you.

My chiropractor wants me to come in several times a week to work on my back pain. Is he just trying to cash in?

Not necessarily. Spinal manipulation can provide mild to moderate relief of back pain, according to studies. That appears to be true for acute pain (the agony you feel right after hurting your back) and chronic pain (the nagging backaches many people live with). However, there is currently no evidence that your back will benefit if you see a chiropractor regularly for longer than 3 months. Furthermore, simpler—and less expensive —measures such as applying heat, exercising, and taking pain relievers may be just as effective as chiropractic, according to some research.

I threw my back out. Should I stay off my feet until it feels better?

No, you'll heal faster if you stay *on* your feet. Doctors used to prescribe several days of bed rest when patients complained of sore backs. But studies show that lying around does not speed up recovery from acute back pain. In fact, pain ebbs sooner if you keep moving, albeit gently. Too much bed rest could even cause muscles to weaken, making you more likely to reinjure your back.

My doctor wants me to try TENS for my back pain. What is it? Will it work?

Don't get your hopes up. TENS stands for transcutaneous electrical nerve stimulation. During a TENS treatment, a small battery-operated device delivers electrical impulses through electrodes attached to the skin. In theory, TENS blocks pain signals from traveling along nerves and reaching the brain. TENS is used to treat many different forms of pain, and some research suggests it might help an aching back. But in one study of 145 patients with chronic back pain, the electrical zaps were of no benefit.

Is yoga good or bad for back pain?

Yoga might help ease chronic back pain, but be sure to choose the right form to get the most benefit—and avoid hurting yourself. Yoga is a workout for the body and mind, combining movement, breathing techniques, and mental focus. There are several forms of yoga, each emphasizing different aspects of the discipline. One study found that patients with chronic low back pain who took a 12-week program of vini-yoga had milder symptoms and were more functional than others enrolled in a back exercise class. Viniyoga is a low-key, relaxed form of yoga that emphasizes moves that lengthen the spine. Less is known about the back benefits of other yoga forms.

☐ BREAST CANCER

My mother and sister both had breast cancer. What's my risk?

Having one first-degree relative who has had breast cancer— that is, a mother, sister, or daughter—doubles your risk. Having two close relatives with the disease increases your risk roughly three-fold. However,

these estimates are only averages and many other factors come into play. For instance, if your relative was over 60 when she developed breast cancer, your risk is somewhat lower. What's more, some key aspects of your personal history, such as the age when you had your first menstrual period or first child, play a vital role, too. The National Cancer Institute has created a Breast Cancer Risk Assessment Tool (www.cancer.gov/bcrisktool) that will show how your risk compares to that of the average woman. Finally, keep in mind that only 15 to 20 percent of women diagnosed with breast cancer have any family history of the disease.

I've been told my breast cancer is in situ, or non-invasive. Does that mean it won't spread?

In situ means "being in the original position." In breast cancer, that refers to abnormal cells that are limited to the site where they began. In other words, they haven't spread deep into the tissue or to other organs but remain confined to the milk-producing glands (lobular carcinoma in situ, or LCIS) or the tubes that carry milk to the nipple (ductal carcinoma in situ, or DCIS). These cancers are referred to as noninvasive, or nonspreading, and are usually very curable. That said, women

with in situ cancers, particularly LCIS, have a greatly increased risk for developing additional breast cancers, which may be invasive. Therefore it's essential that they get mammograms and physical exams regularly.

I have stage 2 breast cancer. Wouldn't a mastectomy be more likely to save my life than a lumpectomy?

No, survival rates among women with your type of cancer are the same for both surgical procedures. In a mastectomy, the surgeon removes the entire breast and, often, lymph nodes under the arm. A lumpectomy, sometimes called breast-sparing surgery, involves removing only the tumor and surrounding tissue. While the more-drastic mastectomy may seem like the safer bet, studies that followed women for more than 20 years have found that lumpectomies are just as effective. Women who undergo lumpectomy usually receive radiation treatments, too, which lowers the risk of a breast cancer recurrence.

Does wearing a bra, getting breast implants, or using anti-perspirant cause breast cancer?

These claims may circulate on the internet, but there's no

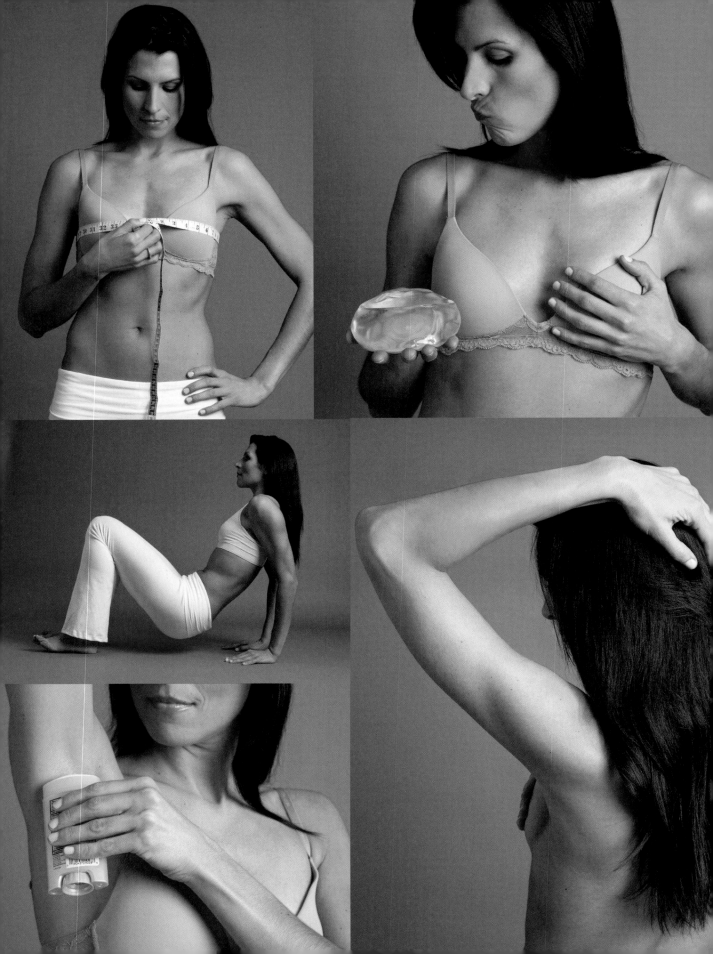

solid evidence that they are true. The idea that bras cause cancer comes from a book titled *Dressed to Kill*. It claimed that bras compress the breast's lymphatic system, causing toxins to back up and poison its tissue. One study did find lower breast cancer rates in women who go braless, but the difference was tiny and could be explained by other factors, the authors said. Likewise, there is no solid proof that breast implants cause breast cancer, though they may interfere with mammograms.

Many antiperspirants contain aluminum, while some deodorants and other cosmetics contain preservatives called parabens. Aluminum and parabens are absorbed through the skin. Both behave like weak versions of the hormone estrogen, which can promote the growth of breast cancer cells. However, a 2008 analysis by French researchers found no reliable evidence that using underarm products increases the risk for breast cancer.

Is 1 week of breast radiation as good as 6?

It seems to be, for certain patients. Current radiation therapy is a huge time commitment: 5 days a week for 6 to 6½ weeks. But studies suggest that new, targeted 1-week radiation techniques are just as effective for early-stage breast

cancer. One example: When 20 women with stage 1 breast cancer tried two daily sessions of proton-beam therapy for just 4 days, researchers at Massachusetts General Hospital in Boston found no cancer recurrence 8 to 22 months later. The side effects of the radiation, such as pain, swelling, or discoloration, lasted for up to 8 weeks afterward. A comprehensive cancer center can offer the best treatment advice.

Cancer treatment has left me drained and fatigued. Can acupuncture help?

It might. Acupuncture seems to help cancer patients cope with nausea brought on by chemotherapy. And it may help with other treatment-related symptoms. A study at Memorial Sloan-Kettering Cancer Center in New York City found that fatigue was reduced by 31 percent in patients receiving chemotherapy who had one or two acupuncture sessions per week. This study was small and preliminary, but it suggests that acupuncture might help you feel more energy. If you decide to try this therapy, be sure the acupuncturist is trained to work with cancer patients. If you have had lymph nodes removed from under an arm, don't allow any needles to be inserted into that arm.

☐ BREAST TENDERNESS

Is breast pain and tenderness a symptom of cancer?

You can probably relax—pain and tenderness are not common symptoms of breast cancer. In most cases, these symptoms are caused by changes in hormone levels. For example, women often develop swollen, sensitive breasts just before or during their menstrual periods. Some women feel breast pain during the first months of pregnancy, and oral contraceptives and hormone therapy can have the same effect. When hormones are the culprit, the pain is usually felt all over the breast. Over-the-counter pain relievers may help for mild pain, though it usually fades on its own.

If you develop persistent pain that's focused in one spot, see a doctor. It could be a cyst, abscess, or infection. Likewise, if your pain is accompanied by nipple discharge, especially if it's bloody, see a doctor.

I've reached menopause and suddenly I've developed breast tenderness. I thought this only happened if you had PMS. What's up?

Breast tenderness is a common symptom of premenstrual

syndrome, but there are several possible explanations for why you have developed the problem in menopause.

- *Hormone therapy.* If you're taking estrogen and progestin to control hot flashes and other menopausal symptoms, breast tenderness is a potential side effect.
- *Other medications.* Some antidepressants have been linked to breast pain, including fluoxetine (Prozac) and sertraline (Zoloft).
- *Trauma.* Have you been in an accident? A blow to the breast can cause lingering pain.
- *Arthritis.* Pain from arthritis in the chest and neck can be felt in the breast.

A friend told me that cutting out coffee will cure my breast tenderness. Is that true?

Cutting back on coffee and other beverages containing caffeine may help. Once again, hormones could be the problem. Consuming caffeine appears to raise estrogen levels and cause other hormonal changes, which may in turn increase the risk for painful breast cysts. The results of studies attempting to prove this theory have been inconsistent, but, anecdotally, some women swear that going caffeine-free relieved their breast pain.

Will vitamin E or evening primrose oil relieve my breast pain?

Not likely. Although some doctors recommend vitamin E to patients with breast pain, several studies have found that taking 600 international units a day for 2 months offers no relief from breast pain. Some experts theorize that breast pain occurs due to an imbalance of fatty acids in the tissue, which is why some sufferers take evening primrose oil (EPO). Overall, however, studies give little reason to think that EPO will help. In one study, the inactive oil used as a placebo was actually more effective than EPO.

□ BRONCHITIS

What's the difference between bronchitis and the cough that comes with a cold?

The coughing in both cases is the body's way of eliminating mucus that's clogging your airways. In bronchitis, the mucus is produced by inflamed membranes lining the tiny bronchial tubes in the lungs. Those membranes may become inflamed by any irritant, be it a virus, smoke, air pollution, or other airborne toxins. In the case of a cold, it's inflamed nasal passages that produce the mucus, which drips down the back of your throat, irritating the airways and causing a cough.

Chronic bronchitis is another story altogether (see the question "I'm constantly coughing and sometimes I'm short of breath. What's wrong?" at right).

The mucus I'm coughing up has gotten thicker and darker. Do I need antibiotics?

Not necessarily. In the early stages of bronchitis, you're likely to cough up small amounts of white mucus. Over time, though, the mucus may become thicker and turn yellow, green, or brown. You may have read or heard that this change means you have

DRUG-FREE FIX

Wearing a Bra at Night

Reducing the movement of your breasts against the chest wall may help prevent breast pain, so wearing a supportive bra may help. Many women find that wearing a snug-fitting bra at night is especially beneficial. If an underwire bra is uncomfortable, try a sports bra.

developed a bacterial infection. But that's not necessarily the case. The change in color and texture comes from the presence of inflamed cells from the lining of your airways. In other words, it's normal.

I'm constantly coughing and sometimes I'm short of breath. What's wrong?

You need a complete medical evaluation to find out for sure, but chronic bronchitis is one possibility. A bout of acute bronchitis, the kind that often accompanies the common cold or flu, usually clears up on its own in a few weeks. However, chronic bronchitis doesn't go away. Over time, inflammation and mucus can narrow the airways. Your doctor may suspect chronic bronchitis if:

● You have had a nasty cough that produces yellow or green mucus for 3 months or more at a time during 2 successive years

● Your cough is worse in the morning

● You frequently feel out of breath

● You smoke

Most people who develop chronic bronchitis are smokers, so the first and most important step is to quit. If your lung function has begun to diminish, a doctor can prescribe an inhaler containing a bronchodilator medication to help open up your airway.

If I have bronchitis and I'm on antibiotics, I'm no longer contagious, right?

That's a common misconception. Most cases of bronchitis are caused by viruses. Antibiotics don't kill viruses (they kill bacteria). That means the pills your doctor prescribed won't stop you from passing the virus on to others—and aren't likely to speed up your recovery, either. Nonetheless, about two-thirds of people who see a doctor for bronchitis in the United States receive prescriptions for antibiotics, possibly because physicians prescribe the drugs to appease patients.

Until your symptoms have cleared up, keep taking steps to avoid spreading germs.

● Wash your hands frequently or use alcohol-based hand sanitizers.

● Avoid touching the inside of your nose or rubbing your eyes.

● Cover your mouth with a tissue when coughing or sneezing. (Coughing into your sleeve is an even better idea.)

□ **BURSITIS**

I thought bursitis was an old person's disease. How come I got it at 45?

Although bursitis is more common among people over 40, anyone can develop it. Some forms, such as hip

bursitis, occur most frequently in active people. (One in 10 serious runners develops hip bursitis, for example.)

Bursitis is inflammation of a bursa, which is a small, fluid-filled cushion that prevents bones from rubbing against skin, muscles, tendons, and ligaments. You have about 160 bursae throughout the body, but the hot spots for trouble are the shoulders, knees, hips, and elbows. A bursa may become inflamed for many reasons. Infections and trauma (such as banging your elbow) can cause bursitis. It may also be a symptom of some types of arthritis, including gout and rheumatoid arthritis. But the most common cause is repetitive movement or persistent pressure during activities such as running, swinging a tennis racket, or kneeling. Even sitting, standing, or leaning on your elbows for long periods can cause a bursa to become inflamed, swollen, and painful. Rest, ice packs, and nonsteroidal anti-inflammatory drugs (NSAIDs) such as ibuprofen are the usual prescription.

If I've had bursitis once, could it return?

Yes, but taking the right steps can help prevent that from happening. If repetitive motions caused your bursitis, the solution is to avoid that activity or find a way to minimize the damage, such as

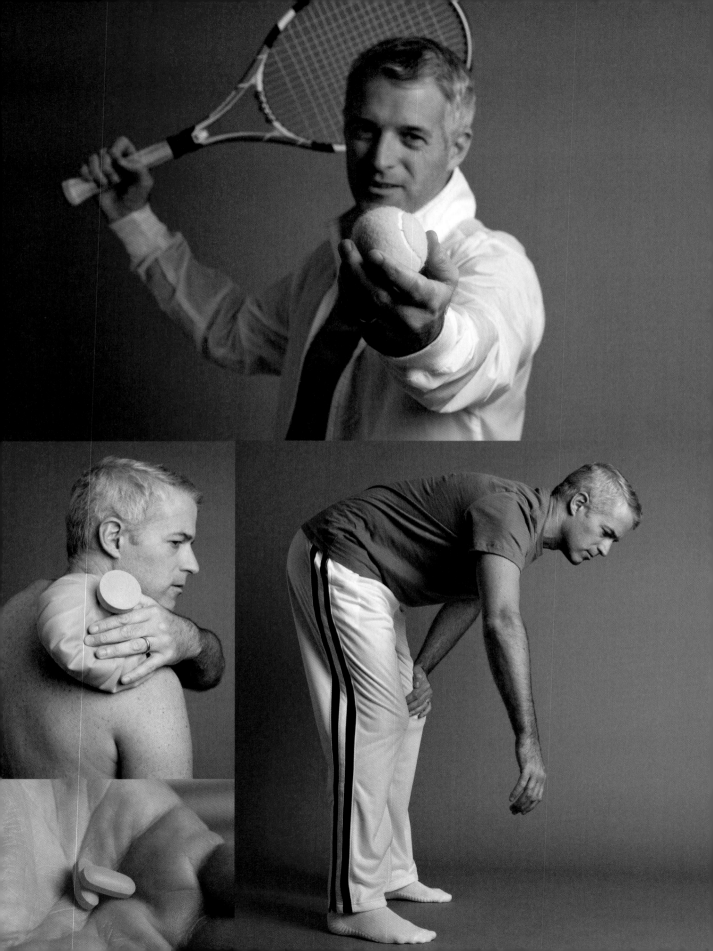

wearing kneepads when you garden to protect the bursa in those sensitive joints. If jogging triggered your hip bursitis, it may help to buy running shoes with more cushioning or to alternate running with cycling or some other lower-impact aerobic activity. Also, ask a fitness trainer or physical therapist about exercises that will increase the strength and flexibility of the muscles that control hip movements.

Other strategies can be even simpler. For instance, if you have bursitis in one knee, sleep with a cushion or pillow between your thighs so that the opposite knee isn't pressing against the injured bursa. Talk to your doctor about other ways to prevent placing further strain on an injured bursa.

Pain relievers and ice aren't helping my bursitis. Is there anything a doctor can do?

Yes, there are several steps a doctor can take that may relieve the pain.

- *Fine needle aspiration.* Your doctor can use a syringe to draw fluid from the inflamed bursa, which may relieve the swelling and pressure.

- *Antibiotics and other medications.* Lab tests of the fluid may reveal signs of an infection, in which case your doctor will prescribe antibiotics. If the fluid contains tiny crystals, gout is likely causing the persistent pain, so your doctor may prescribe a gout medication.

- *Corticosteroids.* An injection should ease the inflammation.

I've always been athletic, but lately I can't even put on a coat without severe shoulder pain. Could surgery help me?

You may be a candidate for surgery if more conservative treatments don't help. People who play sports that involve overhead arm motions, such as swimming and baseball, can develop a condition called shoulder impingement, though the problem can afflict nonathletes, too. Impingement occurs when you raise an arm and part of the shoulder blade presses down on a tendon called the rotator cuff. Inflammation of the bursa lying over the rotator cuff can cause impingement, as can tears or inflammation in the tendon itself.

Impingement often responds well to rest, pain relievers, corticosteroid injections, and strengthening and flexibility exercises. If pain persists for 6 months or more, your doctor may recommend surgery. In the procedure, a surgeon removes or drains an inflamed bursa and may remove a small amount of bone from the front edge of the shoulder blade to allow the arm to move freely.

☐ CANCER

I'm a cancer survivor. Lately I've just had this feeling that the cancer has returned. Should I mention this to my doctor, or am I being paranoid?

You're not being paranoid. Cancer often does recur, of course, so worrying that it could happen to you is perfectly natural. Keep in mind, though, that it's not a sign your cancer has returned every time you feel a little run-down or achy—but if your gut tells you something is wrong, talk to your doctor. Some oncologists recommend using a 2-week rule: If a symptom disappears inside that time frame, it's probably nothing to worry about, but consider reporting any other unexplained pain or complaint. Be sure you talk to your oncologist about the likelihood of a recurrence and what symptoms to look for, and see your doctor for routine checkups.

Our house sits next to power lines. Does that make us more likely to get cancer?

You have little cause for concern. A few studies published in the early 1990s appeared to confirm long-held worries that radiation from power lines cause cancer. However, an investigation revealed that much of the critical data in those studies was fabricated. More than two dozen other studies have failed to show that people living near power lines have an increased risk for any type of cancer.

Is there anything I can do, besides quitting smoking, that will reduce my risk of cancer?

Quitting smoking *is* mandatory, but it's just a start. We now have plenty of research to show that these steps can slash your cancer risk:

• *Eat a healthy diet.* Eating plenty of fruits and vegetables (five servings daily is a good goal) seems to lower the risk for colon, esophageal, lung, oral, and stomach cancer. Choose whole grains instead of refined grains whenever possible. Limit consumption of red meat; don't eat it charred or well-done; and avoid processed meats, such as bologna.

• *Maintain a healthy weight.* Being overweight increases the risk for cancers of the breast (in women who have reached menopause), colon, uterus, esophagus, and kidney. Excess weight may be linked to other types of cancer, too.

• *Exercise.* Getting plenty of physical activity helps keep pounds from piling on your waistline. What's more, studies

suggest that exercise reduces the risk for breast and colon cancer whether you lose weight or not.

• *Keep your alcohol intake in check.* Alcohol abuse increases the risk for cancers of the breast, esophagus, larynx (voice box), liver, mouth, and throat. If you consume alcohol, limit yourself to one or two drinks (for women and men, respectively) per day.

• *Limit your time in the sun.* Overexposure to ultraviolet radiation raises your risk for skin cancer. Use sunblock with sun protection factor (SPF) of 15 or higher and, when possible, avoid outdoor activities between 10 a.m. and 4 p.m. Also, shun tanning beds.

Can a benign tumor turn malignant?

By definition, a benign tumor is not malignant and can not become cancerous. It may grow larger, but a benign tumor

will not spread throughout the body and invade other organs. However, a tumor that is not malignant may not necessarily be benign. "Precancerous," or "premalignant," tumors are growths that have the potential to become cancer. Some (though not all) polyps that are detected by a colonoscopy can develop into cancer, for example. Also, some benign tumors, such as breast cysts, signify that a person has a heightened risk for cancer.

Is there a risk that surgery to remove a tumor could cause the cancer to spread?

For all practical purposes, the answer is no. As far as experts know, there are only a few types of cancer surgery where that's even a theoretical possibility, and surgeons take steps to prevent it from happening. In surgery for testicular cancer, for example, surgeons tie off blood

?? FACT OR FICTION

Avoid Massages if You Have Cancer

Fiction. The concern arises from the idea that increased blood circulation from all that rubbing and kneading could cause cancer to spread throughout the body. There is no evidence that's true, though the American Cancer Society advises instructing a massage therapist to avoid tumor sites and suspicious lumps. A number of studies show that massage may help cancer patients cope with stress, pain, and nausea.

and lymph vessels, which might otherwise allow tumor cells to enter and spread throughout the body. There is also a theoretical possibility that a needle used to take a sample from a tumor for biopsy could carry a few cells along the track of the needle as the needle is withdrawn. But it's extremely unlikely that the cells could implant and grow.

In recent years, some studies have hinted that removal of breast tumors may spark the growth of tumors elsewhere in the breast, though that theory is hotly debated. On the other hand, a common belief that a tumor will spread if it has been exposed to air during surgery is unquestionably false.

I'm getting chemotherapy for my cancer. Is it okay to take antioxidant supplements like vitamin C?

Ask your doctor first. Believe it or not, you could be doing more harm than good. Taking antioxidant supplements protects healthy cells from the toxic effects of chemotherapy, which studies show can help ease side effects. However, research suggests that high doses of vitamin C, beta-carotene, and other antioxidants may protect cancer cells, too, making chemotherapy and radiation less effective. In a few studies, cancer patients who took antioxidant supplements

were more likely to die than others given placebos. Bottom line: Talk to your doctor before taking anything that hasn't been prescribed.

☐ CARPAL TUNNEL SYNDROME

How could I have carpal tunnel syndrome if I rarely use a keyboard?

Working on a keyboard is just one of many activities involving the hands that has been linked to carpal tunnel syndrome (CTS). This disorder affects the median nerve, which enters the hand through a shaft called the carpal tunnel and supplies feeling to the fingers (except the pinky). There are tendons and ligaments in the carpal tunnel, too, and if they become swollen or inflamed, they can cramp the median nerve, resulting in pain, numbness, and tingling in the hand.

Surprisingly, there is not much hard data to prove that any specific job or hobby causes CTS. However, typists and data-entry clerks, as well as assembly-line workers, musicians, mechanics, baristas in espresso shops, and cashiers often complain of wrist pain. Gardening, golf, and other hobbies that involve a lot of hand movement may increase the risk, too. Yet some people appear to develop the problem simply because they

were born with a cramped, narrow carpal tunnel. Injuries can bring on the symptoms, too, as can thyroid problems, fluid retention (due to pregnancy, for instance), and cysts or tumors in the tunnel.

Will wearing a wrist splint cure my carpal tunnel syndrome?

Wrist splints can help control symptoms in mild cases of CTS. They're designed to take pressure off the median nerve by keeping your wrists from flexing. Splints are most likely to help if you have had CTS for less than a year and the tingling and other symptoms aren't too severe. Wearing splints, especially at night, may be most effective when combined with steroid injections, which will bring down inflammation in the wrist.

Do I need to wear my splints only when I work?

No. While some people with CTS wear splints all day, studies show that these wrist stabilizers are most effective when worn at night. Many people sleep with their wrists flexed, which crimps the median nerve. In fact, some sufferers notice the symptoms of CTS for the first time in the morning. Or, if the pain and tingling are bad enough, they may be awakened in the middle of the night,

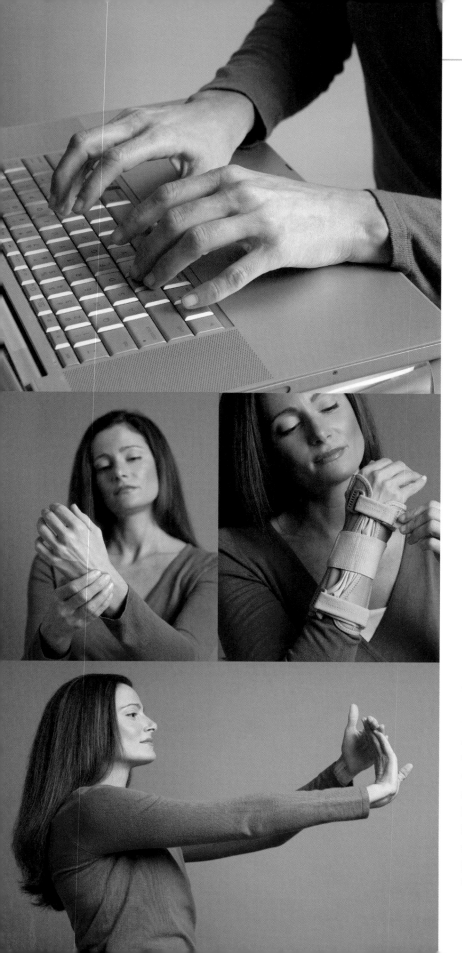

instinctively shaking their hands and wrists for relief.

Should I have custom-fit splints made?

You'll probably do fine with splints purchased off the shelf at a pharmacy or medical supply store. You can seek out an occupational therapist who specializes in hand therapy to have splints made that precisely conform to the shape and size of your hands and wrists. However, a study in the *Journal of the American Medical Association* found no difference in the benefits of custom-fit versus over-the-counter splints.

Surgery seems like a drastic choice. How do I know I need it? Will it help?

If other measures fail and severe pain and other symptoms persist for more than 6 months, surgery is the best choice for long-term relief of CTS. In the procedure, a surgeon pares away the band of tissue in the wrist that's pressing against the median nerve. Carpal tunnel "release" is one of the most frequently performed surgical procedures. Other treatments, such as splints and steroid injections, bring faster pain relief, but studies show that after 1 year, surgery reduces or eliminates pain in more than 90 percent of patients.

☐ **CATARACTS**

If I have a cataract, do I need surgery right away?

Not necessarily. Cataracts occur when protein in the lens of the eye begins to clump together. These clumps prevent light from passing through the lens and reaching the retina, the membrane at the back of the eye that transmits visual information to the brain. As a cataract grows, it can cloud vision or give the world a brown tint.

Simple steps such as getting new eyeglasses or using brighter light around the house often allow people to put off having a cataract removed. Surgery usually isn't necessary until a cataract affects your daily life by interfering with your ability to read, drive, or watch TV, for example. (One exception: A cataract that doesn't impair vision may still need to be removed if it prevents your doctor from performing a thorough eye exam or treating another eye disorder.)

I need cataract surgery. If I'm getting an artificial lens implanted, will I still need glasses after cataract surgery?

You may or may not. In cataract surgery, a doctor uses tiny instruments to remove the lens through an incision in the cornea. In most cases, the lens is replaced with an artificial one that also corrects your vision. A small portion of patients do not receive an artificial lens because either they have some other eye disease or problems arise during surgery. In those cases, a patient needs contact lenses or eyeglasses with high magnification.

The traditional artificial lenses used in cataract surgery, known as monofocal lenses, come in three different varieties: They either allow the eye to focus on objects in the distance, at a middle distance, or nearby. A patient who chooses a distance lens (as most do) still needs reading glasses to view near objects. However, newer multifocal lenses allow the eye to focus for distance *or* near vision. Studies show that more than 80 percent of cataract patients who receive multifocal lenses no longer need glasses. However, some of these patients complain of halos, glare, or poor night vision, though eye doctors say these problems fade over time. People who have a history of detached retinas and other eye problems may not be candidates for multifocal lenses.

If you have an astigmatism (a misshaped cornea, which can distort vision), you will need an additional procedure during cataract surgery and/or toric lenses, which help correct the problem in most patients. No matter what type of lens you receive during cataract surgery, don't be surprised if your vision doesn't improve right away, since it takes a day or two after the procedure for inflammation to subside.

⚠ WHAT YOU DON'T KNOW

Statins May Cut the Risk for Cataracts

People who took statin drugs such as simvastatin (Zocor) and atorvastatin (Lipitor) to lower their cholesterol had a 50 percent lower risk for cataracts in one study by University of Wisconsin researchers. Although more studies are needed, it may be that statin drugs protect the eyes by reducing oxidative (free radical) damage to cells and lowering inflammation. For reasons that aren't clear, simvastatin was significantly more protective than other statins.

My doctor suggested monovision, but won't it give me a headache to have different eyesight in each eye?

Some eye surgeons say an approach called monovision can

restore the full range of vision following cataract surgery in some patients. After removing the natural lens, the surgeon implants a monofocal lens for distance in the patient's dominant eye and a monofocal lens for near vision in the other eye. That sounds like it might make you dizzy or give you a headache, but experts say the brain "decides" which eye to use, depending on whether you need to focus on a distant or near object. Monovision isn't for everyone—some patients find that their vision at one depth or the other is too blurry. But a 2009 study found that more than 80 percent of patients who had the procedure were satisfied.

I had cataract surgery recently and, ever since, I've been seeing "floaters." What should I do?

See an eye doctor immediately. If your physician is unavailable, go to an emergency room. You may have a detached retina, which is a potential complication of cataract surgery and requires prompt medical attention. A detached retina isn't painful but can lead to permanent loss of vision. An eye surgeon can fix the problem using a laser or a technique called cryopexy that "freezes" the retina back into place. The sooner you see a doctor, the more likely the procedure will preserve your vision.

☐ **CELIAC DISEASE**

All of a sudden I can't tolerate wheat products, but I'm over 50, so it can't be celiac disease, can it?

Anyone can develop celiac disease at any age. This uncomfortable condition, which can have serious long-term consequences if not treated, disrupts the body's ability to absorb nutrients from food. The problem starts when the immune system mistakenly attacks the lining of the small intestine, damaging tiny finger-shaped structures called villi that help transfer nutrients from the gut to the bloodstream. These attacks are set off when a person eats food containing a protein called gluten, which is found in wheat, rye, barley, and some other grains. (That includes oats, though some scientists believe its gluten may be safe for people with celiac disease.)

While children can develop celiac disease, it may emerge any time in life. Certain events can trigger it, including surgery, pregnancy and childbirth, viral infections, and severe psychological stress.

What's the difference between celiac disease and gluten intolerance?

Gluten intolerance is 10 times more common than celiac disease. Like celiac disease patients, people who have this condition develop diarrhea and other gastrointestinal symptoms when they consume gluten. However, gluten intolerance is not an autoimmune disease and doesn't cause permanent damage to the gastrointestinal tract. The treatment for both conditions is the same: Eliminate gluten from the diet. However, patients with celiac disease have a greater risk for nutritional deficiencies and other conditions, meaning they require closer medical monitoring.

What are some clues that I have celiac disease and not some other digestive disorder?

The symptoms of celiac disease can vary from one patient to the next but may include bloating, abdominal pain, chronic diarrhea, vomiting, and constipation. A sufferer may lose weight and have stools that are pale brown or gray and have a foul odor. These symptoms can mimic those of other digestive disorders, as well as other conditions such as iron-deficiency anemia and chronic fatigue.

Simply eliminating wheat and other foods that contain gluten to see if your symptoms improve is not enough to diagnose celiac disease. The only way to know for sure that you have it and not some other digestive disorder, such as gluten intolerance, irritable bowel syndrome, or Crohn's disease, is to see your doctor, who can diagnose the condition with a blood test and biopsy.

The doctors will start by testing your blood for high levels of antibodies known as tTG and EMA. But here's something your doctor might not know: He should also have your blood tested for the presence of genes known as HLA-DQ2 and HLA-DQ8, which increase the risk for developing celiac disease up to 31-fold. This gene testing is crucial, since people who abstain from eating gluten may test negative for tTG and EMA antibodies, but still have celiac disease. If any of these tests is positive, a doctor will remove a small tissue sample from your intestine using a slender instrument called an endoscope. A biopsy that reveals damaged villi confirms the diagnosis of celiac disease.

I see more and more gluten-free foods on the shelves. Is celiac disease becoming more common?

It looks that way, though it's not clear why. Doctors once believed that celiac disease was a rare condition in most countries outside Europe. For instance, estimates suggested that only about 1 person in 10,000 had symptoms of the

disease in North America. We now know that the disease is 100 times more common in North America than previously believed, afflicting roughly 1 person in 100. In fact, the prevalence in the United States (based on comparisons of blood samples from different eras) is 4.5 times higher today than in the 1950s.

One reason for this increase may be that children today are exposed to fewer germs. Some scientists believe that exposure to germs in childhood helps the immune system develop properly, making it less likely to mistakenly attack healthy tissue, which is the cause of celiac disease and other autoimmune disorders.

Does celiac disease increase my risk for any other conditions?

Yes. Untreated celiac disease makes you more likely to develop conditions such as anemia, arthritis, diabetes, osteoporosis, liver disease, thyroid disease, infertility, and certain types of cancer. People with celiac disease often complain of depression, fatigue, skin rashes, a tingling sensation or restlessness in the legs, canker sores, fluid retention, and other problems. Avoiding gluten will improve your day-to-day symptoms and may help lower your risk for serious complications.

What is "silent" celiac disease? If I have it, does that mean I'll definitely develop symptoms eventually?

Some people have positive blood tests for celiac disease but don't have damaged villi or show any symptoms. People with silent celiac disease may eventually develop full-blown symptoms, however. You do not necessarily need to follow a gluten-free diet if you have silent celiac disease, though some doctors believe doing so could lower your risk for future complications. At minimum, you should see your doctor for frequent checkups to monitor your status.

☐ CHRONIC FATIGUE SYNDROME

Is CFS real?

Yes. Although some skeptics have questioned whether chronic fatigue syndrome (CFS) is a legitimate medical condition, doctors have recognized various diseases characterized by persistent fatigue since at least the mid-18th century. Anyone can feel tired or burnt out now and then, but CFS has longer-lasting and specific symptoms, beginning with unrelenting fatigue lasting for at least 6 months that interferes with daily activities and isn't relieved by sleep. Other symptoms used to diagnose CFS include:

- Short-term memory problems and poor concentration
- Sore throat
- Tender lymph nodes
- Muscle and joint pain and swelling
- Headaches

In addition, CFS can cause chills and night sweats, chest pain, shortness of breath, irritability, jaw pain, and weight loss or gain.

What causes CFS?

No one knows what causes chronic fatigue syndrome (CFS), despite years of intensive research. Some of the leading theories focus on three possible causes:

- *Infection.* The symptoms of CFS often emerge for the first time on the heels of illness caused by an infection, such as a bad cold or mononucleosis. Some scientists have

speculated that CFS is caused by a virus. Suspects have included the Epstein-Barr virus and a form of herpes, but, so far, no microbe has been conclusively linked to CFS.

- *Inflammation.* The immune systems of some people with CFS seem to behave erratically. That has led to a theory, still unproven, that chronic inflammation in the nervous system causes CFS.

- *Hormones.* Many CFS patients have low levels of certain hormones, including cortisol. This hormone helps produce energy, controls inflammation, and is involved in other important processes. However, studies have so far failed to show that hormone replacement therapy can relieve CFS.

- *Low blood pressure.* Standing for a long period not only

makes many people with CFS tired, but it makes them light-headed. Light-headedness when you stand up is a classic symptom of hypotension, or low blood pressure, leading some scientists to suspect that this problem may be linked to CFS. However, symptoms only improved in some CFS patients who took medication for hypotension.

What's the difference between CFS and fibromyalgia?

Patients with CFS and fibromyalgia have similar symptoms, most notably fatigue and pain. But in fibromyalgia, pain is especially severe and follows a predictable pattern. Patients complain of aches and stiffness in the muscles, tendons, and ligaments. The worst pain tends to be in 18 specific "tender

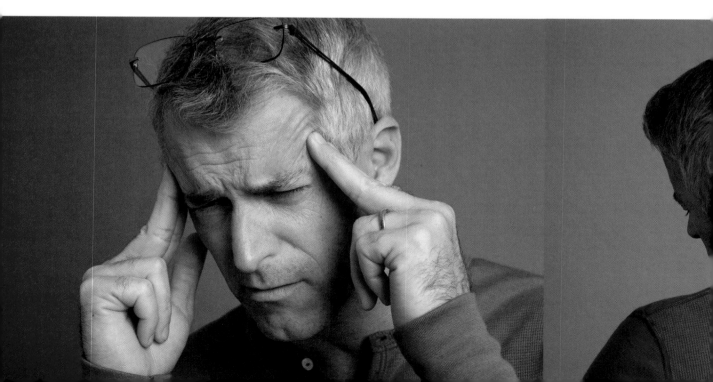

points," which include the shoulders, ribs, knees, neck, lower back, and thighs. Doctors diagnose fibromyalgia if a patient has pain in 11 or more tender points for 3 months or more. Furthermore, certain accompanying health problems, such as irritable bowel syndrome, are more common in fibromyalgia patients.

My doctor prescribed an antidepressant for my CFS. Does that mean I'm depressed?

About two-thirds of people with chronic fatigue syndrome suffer from depression and/or anxiety, so it's not uncommon for doctors to prescribe antidepressant or antianxiety medications. But doctors also

FACT OR FICTION

CFS Patients Shouldn't Exercise

Fiction. A workout may leave you exhausted, but you'll probably feel better in the long run. British researchers asked a group of chronic fatigue syndrome patients to walk or perform some other aerobic exercise at least 5 days a week, increasing their daily activity to a maximum of 30 minutes. After 3 months, these patients were twice as likely as others who took flexibility or relaxation classes to say that their symptoms had improved and that they felt better. A year later, three-quarters of the exercisers had resumed normal daily activities, and some had returned to work.

prescribe antidepressants to ease CFS symptoms. One study found that CFS symptoms improved in patients who took an antidepressant called phenelzine (Nardil), even though none of the participants had been diagnosed with depression. Other antidepressants (including Prozac) have

proven less effective at alleviating CFS symptoms.

How long does CFS typically last? Can I ever expect to feel better?

It's hard to predict how long symptoms of chronic fatigue

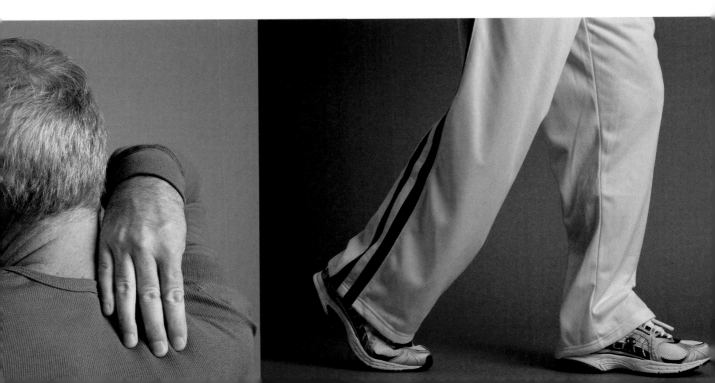

syndrome will last, though you can hope to improve over time. Patience is key. Some people diagnosed with CFS feel better within 6 months, though one study of 144 patients found that, by that time, three-quarters of patients still felt fatigue, pain, and other debilitating symptoms. However, more than two-thirds recovered within 2 to 4 years. If there's any clear-cut good news, it's that CFS is not fatal. Many patients are able to manage symptoms until the condition is resolved.

Why are most people with CFS women?

No one knows. Anyone can develop chronic fatigue syndrome, but women are four times more likely than men to be diagnosed with the condition. Some scientists believe that CFS is caused by a glitch in a part of the brain called the hypothalamus, which controls hormone production by directing the actions of the pituitary gland. Studies show that certain hormones are more likely to behave abnormally in women—but not men—with CFS. For example, in healthy people, cortisol naturally rises in the morning, but one study found that in women with CFS, levels of this hormone remain low upon waking.

☐ CHRONIC OBSTRUCTIVE PULMONARY DISEASE

Can oxygen therapy restore my lost lung function?

Oxygen therapy may help your lungs work better, allow you to cope with other symptoms of chronic obstructive pulmonary disease (COPD), and even add years to your life. COPD is a serious disease caused by chronic bronchitis or emphysema (some sufferers have both disorders) that makes it hard to breathe and can (in chronic bronchitis) trigger a nasty cough. The main cause of COPD is cigarette smoking. Over time, as damage to structures in the lungs worsens, breathing becomes more and more difficult. If your symptoms are severe and tests show that your blood has dangerously low levels of oxygen, your doctor will prescribe oxygen therapy.

Oxygen therapy comes in several different forms, including portable canisters that allow patients to leave home for brief periods. Your doctor may require you to use oxygen therapy only part of the time; some people only need it when they sleep, while others require the therapy only when they're up and moving around. However, most patients with severe COPD fare better—and live longer—if they use oxygen therapy 15 to 24 hours a day, according to two long-term studies.

My doctor suggested pulmonary rehabilitation, but that sounds like a lot of work. What's involved?

A pulmonary rehabilitation program takes a serious commitment, but studies show that chronic obstructive pulmonary disease (COPD) patients who make the effort feel better, have more satisfying lives,

FACT OR FICTION

Only Smokers Get COPD

Fiction. Cigarette smoke is by far the main cause of chronic obstructive pulmonary disease (COPD), but inhaling other irritants can damage the lungs and cause this disease, too. In fact, air pollution appears to be an increasingly common cause of COPD in many countries, some scientists say. Breathing in chemical fumes and dust in the workplace is another potential threat. COPD is rare in people under age 40, but it can occur, often due to a genetic condition called alpha-1 antitrypsin deficiency.

and—in some studies—live longer. Rehab may take place in a hospital or in your home. A typical program has several components.

- *Exercise.* The main focus of exercise training is to build up your endurance so that normal activities don't leave you out of breath. You may be asked to walk, climb stairs, or cycle to develop leg strength. One study found that people with chronic bronchitis who did these types of exercises for 12 minutes a day for 10 months increased the distance they could walk by 24 percent. Exercises to strengthen the upper body, such as weight lifting or wearing a weighted backpack, are critical, too.

- *Breathing retraining.* Rehab specialists teach new techniques that can help you overcome some of the difficulty of inhaling and exhaling. For instance, breathing in through your mouth and exhaling slowly through pursed lips—think of the shape your mouth forms when you whistle—helps slow down your respiration and makes every breath feel more satisfying. Some studies show that learning yoga techniques improves breathing, too.

- *Education.* Most rehab programs also include education in how to manage COPD, emphasizing the importance of quitting smoking, taking needed medications, eating the right foods, and exercising.

I have COPD but I still smoke a few cigarettes a day. How bad could that be?

Bad. One study found that chronic obstructive pulmonary disease patients who continued smoking lost twice as much lung power over an 11-year period compared to others who quit. What's more worrisome, continuing to smoke appears to weaken the immune system and may make your lungs more vulnerable to bacterial infections.

Can't stop smoking? Try combined therapy. Studies suggest that smokers most likely to succeed in quitting use some form of medication, such as nicotine replacement therapy, and receive some form of counseling.

I have COPD and my fingernails turned grayish blue. What does this mean?

It means you need immediate medical attention, so get to a hospital—have someone take you or call an ambulance, if necessary. Blue or gray fingernails or lips are a sign that your blood is very low in oxygen, a symptom of severe chronic obstructive pulmonary disease. Doctors can provide oxygen treatment and other medications to bring your blood's oxygen concentration back

to a safe level. Other signs of severe COPD include difficulty catching your breath or talking, mental fuzziness, and rapid heartbeat.

I have COPD and heard that the inhaled steroid I'm taking could increase my risk of pneumonia. Should I stop taking it?

Don't stop using it if your doctor prescribed it, and it's working. While there are some studies showing a somewhat higher risk of pneumonia with inhaled corticosteroids such as budesonide (Symbicort) and fluticasone (Flovent), other studies show no increased risk. Your best bet for avoiding pneumonia, as your doctor should have already recommended, is a pneumococcal vaccine.

☐ COLDS

How can I stop my cold from turning into a sinus infection?

Colds morph into sinus infections because bacteria and viruses thrive in mucus trapped in swollen sinus passages. Easing the congestion and swelling is the solution. Start at the first signs of a cold, such as a scratchy, tickly throat, runny nose, and/or sneezing. Use a decongestant nasal spray or pills for a few days (follow package directions to avoid "rebound" congestion from sprays). To encourage mucus to drain, add a saltwater nasal rinse using a store-bought or homemade saline solution and a neti pot (available from health food stores), a bulb syringe, or a sinus rinse kit from the drugstore such as the Ayr Saline Nasal Rinse Kit or NeilMed Sinus Rinse Nasal Wash. Applying warm compresses to your cheeks or drinking a cup of hot tea also helps; the warmth seems to help cilia, the tiny whisk broom–like hairs lining your nasal passages, work more effectively at sweeping out mucus, bacteria, and viral particles.

I catch colds all the time. How many per year is normal?

Adults average two to four colds per year; kids get up to a dozen. More than 200 different viruses can cause the common cold, a big reason no one's yet developed a vaccine against it. Different cold viruses are active at different times of the year, so you can catch a cold in any season. Rhinoviruses, responsible for about 30 percent of colds, tend to circulate in spring, summer, and early fall, while colds in the winter and early spring tend to be caused by coronaviruses.

Cold viruses can live on hard surfaces like countertops and door handles for up to 4 hours. Your best defense is regular, vigorous hand washing with soap and water, which can remove 99 percent of virus particles. You can also lower your risk by using a saline nasal spray to moisten your nasal passages. In one study, people who used one daily had 30 percent fewer colds than those who didn't.

Every time I renew my efforts to go to the gym, I seem to catch a cold. Is it all in my head?

You may be on to something. Intense exercise can decrease levels of infection-fighting white blood cells in your body temporarily and boost levels of stress hormones that may interfere with your immune system's ability to fight off cold viruses. Coupled with the possibility that you're picking up germs from gym equipment or in the locker room, your workouts might very well be making you sick.

That doesn't mean that all exercise opens the door to colds. In fact, a consistent, medium-intensity routine is a proven cold-stopper. Taking a brisk, 40-minute walk 4 days a week, for example, can cut the number of colds you experience by 25 to 50 percent and can make the colds you do catch shorter by half, studies show. Moderate exercise boosts the number and activity level of important immune-system players called natural killer cells.

Is there really a wrong way to blow your nose?

Mom was right about this one. Vigorous honking really is counterproductive for two reasons. First, it triggers "reflex nasal congestion"—your nasal passages swell up temporarily, which traps mucus. Second,

FACT OR FICTION

Chicken Soup Clobbers Colds

Fact. There's science behind this age-old comfort-food remedy. When a researcher from the Nebraska Medical Center tested his mother-in-law's chicken soup recipe in a test tube, he found that it could reduce inflammation and congestion caused by virus-fighting immune system agents called neutrophils by about 75 percent. No one to make soup for you? No problem. Canned chicken soup worked, too.

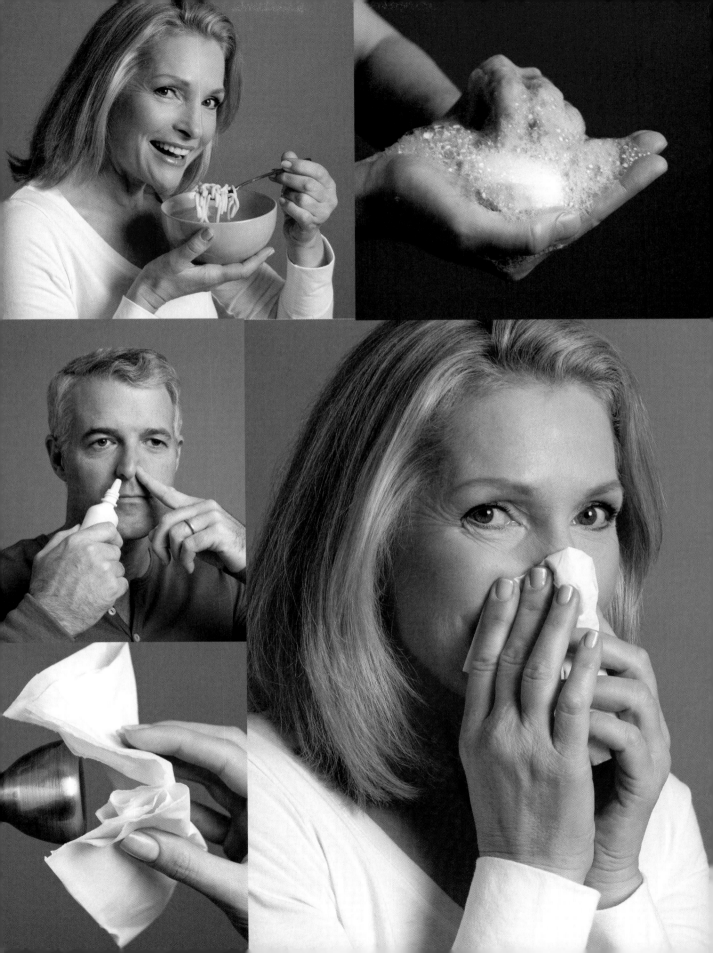

full-force nose blowing creates a vacuum deep in your sinus passages; once you stop blowing, mucus gets sucked backward, deeper into your sinuses. A better way to blow: With a tissue over both nostrils, close one side and gently blow the other for 3 to 5 seconds. Switch sides. It may take several blows, but it works.

☐ **COLON CANCER**

Will eating more fiber cut my risk for colon cancer?

Maybe. Whether fiber prevents colon cancer remains controversial. Some big studies haven't found any benefit (leading to headlines that made dietary fiber sound like a dud). But there's some evidence that it does help, including a National Cancer Institute study of the diet and health of more than 34,000 people. Those who ate the most fiber were 27 percent less likely to have precancerous colon growths called polyps than those who ate the least. Whole grains and fruit offered the most protection, another good reason to enjoy a bowl of oatmeal with berries for breakfast.

Of course, there are plenty of other good reasons to put high-fiber foods on your plate, including weight control, which brings us right back to colon cancer prevention. You can lower your risk for this common and sometimes fatal cancer by keeping your weight within a healthy range. Getting regular exercise can lower your risk by up to 25 percent; a half-hour walk, four times a week, is all it takes. And if you're a regular meat-eater, cutting back on red meats and processed meats such as hot dogs, sausage, and lunch meats can also help. Experts at the National Cancer Institute estimate that people who eat red meat or processed meats twice a day most days increase their cancer risk by 24 percent; eating it once a day raises risk by about 20 percent above normal.

Colon cancer runs in my family. Does that mean I need a colonoscopy before I'm 50?

Absolutely. Most of the time, colon cancer is not hereditary. But 5 to 10 percent of the time it is, and the added risk could be passed down to you. A family history of colon cancer can increase your own risk two to four times higher than average. It may be even higher if several relatives on the same side of the family have had colon cancer, if affected relatives are in more than one generation, or if colon cancer struck early (before age 60).

If there's colon cancer in your family, talk with your doctor about when you should begin getting colonoscopies and how often they should be repeated. Some experts recommend starting 10 years earlier than the earliest known case in your family. And in some cases, you may need annual rechecks.

My doctor found a polyp. Does that mean I'm going to get colon cancer?

No. During a colonoscopy, doctors find the fleshy bumps called polyps growing in the colons of up to 3 out of 10 people. Less than 10 percent would have become cancerous if not removed. But since it's impossible to tell just by looking which polyps could lead to cancer and which won't, doctors tend to remove all of the polyps they find, then send them on to a lab for testing. In general, about 30 percent turn out to be benign growths called hyperplastic polyps, which are like skin tags. Most of the rest are called adenomas. And while most adenomas aren't cancerous, doctors take them seriously because two-thirds of all cancers in the colon and rectum begin inside this type of polyp.

Lab tests will show whether there are precancerous cell changes inside adenomatous polyps. Your doctor will use that information, along with the number and size of polyps she found, to determine how often you should get repeat colonoscopies in the future. If you had just one or two small adenomas with few cell changes, you may need rechecks every

5 to 10 years, for example. But if you have more than three, if polyps are large, or if they show signs of more advanced cell changes, your doctor may recommend rechecks every 3 years or even more frequently.

My doctor removed polyps from my colon. How do I know he got everything that could become cancerous?

Conventional colonoscopy and high-tech "virtual" colonoscopies aren't foolproof, and neither are the doctors who perform them. Studies show that these colon checks, whether done with a tiny video camera attached to a probe or with a CT scanner, miss about 10 percent of polyps. Most often overlooked are polyps hiding near the anus and those near bulges in the wall of the colon. The best way to improve the detection power of your next colonoscopy may be to ask your doctor what her "detection rate" is. Experts say a careful doctor finds polyps in about 25 percent of male patients and about 15 percent of female patients. Doctors who do fast colonoscopies tend to miss more polyps; a slower look that takes 6 minutes or more seems to find more of the growths that could turn into cancer.

WHAT YOU DON'T KNOW

Your Surgeon Should Check 12 or More Lymph Nodes

Colon cancer surgery patients whose doctors check 12 or more lymph nodes for signs that cancer has spread have the best survival rates. Signs of spreading cancer are treated with chemotherapy. But a recent study found that 60 percent of hospitals check fewer than 12 lymph nodes. The work is painstaking and involves removing fat tissue, finding tiny nodes, then checking them carefully for signs of cancer. Ask your doctor to do the 12-node check, and inquire afterward if the pathologist's report has info on the whole dozen.

I'm having surgery for colon cancer. Does this mean I'll have to wear a colostomy bag for the rest of my life?

Most people don't need a colostomy bag after colon cancer surgery. Colostomies are more likely if the cancer is close to your rectum. In this procedure, part of the colon is brought through the abdominal wall, and stool is drained into a bag attached to the opening in the skin. Colostomies can be temporary or permanent. Most are left in place for 2 to 6 months so that the colon can heal from complicated surgery before stool passes through it again. You may need a permanent colostomy bag if your cancer was large or if anal sphincter muscles were removed during the procedure.

My doctor is recommending radiation or chemotherapy in addition to surgery for my colon cancer. Why would I need those treatments after the cancer is removed?

After surgery to remove cancer from your colon or rectum, these additional treatments provide extra protection against cancer's return, guard against its spread to other parts of your body, kill off cancer cells that may be lurking in surrounding tissue, and even shrink tumors in your colon or elsewhere if they couldn't be completely removed.

While early-stage colon cancer usually requires only surgery, more advanced stages often get these add-ons. If you had stage 2 cancer, which has grown through the wall of your colon, you may need radiation in the area where the cancer occurred to prevent regrowth. If your cancer was in stage 3, which means it spread to your lymph nodes but no further, you may need radiation plus chemotherapy. In stage 4 colon cancer, chemotherapy may shrink cancers that have spread to your liver and other places. Chemo and radiation may also help control large tumors in your colon at this stage.

☐ **CONGESTIVE HEART FAILURE**

My doctor wants me to exercise, but I'm scared. How much is okay?

It sounds counterintuitive, but exerting yourself a little can help alleviate some symptoms of congestive heart failure (in which the heart can no longer pump enough blood through the body) and avoid complications. Light exercise can make your heart stronger, improve blood flow, help you feel more energetic, lower your odds for heart failure–related trips to the hospital, and even help you live longer.

Starting slowly is the key. For example, you might do 2 minutes of walking or riding a stationary bike, then rest for a minute, then repeat. Over a couple of weeks, you add more minutes. But everybody is different; talk with your doctor before you begin about the workout length and intensity that's right for you. You may be fine exercising at home, but if your condition is more severe, or you'd just prefer more guidance and company, ask about local cardiac rehabilitation programs—hospital-based exercise programs for people who have congestive heart failure or have survived heart attacks.

Just watch for signs that you should stop, or even call the doctor, such as chest pain, shortness of breath, ankle or abdominal swelling, or a fast pulse when you're resting.

Why does my doctor want me to weigh myself every day?

When your heart cannot pump blood efficiently, fluid may build up in the air sacs in your lungs, a dangerous condition called pulmonary edema. It may also accumulate in your arms, legs, ankles, feet, and abdomen. This can make your heart work harder and even lead to breathing problems that merit a trip to the emergency room.

Most people with congestive heart failure (CHF) take a variety of medications to control fluid retention, follow a low-salt diet, and avoid drinking excess fluids. But you can't assume these strategies will work perfectly all the time. Daily weigh-ins let you spot water retention, a sign of worsening heart failure, quickly. Since water is fairly heavy, even a little water retention will show up on the scale.

Weigh yourself every morning, after you've used the bathroom but before you've had breakfast. Call your doctor right away if you gain 3 or more pounds in a day, or 5 or more pounds in a week, or if you've been slowly gaining weight over the past few weeks or months. Your medication doses may need an adjustment.

Why do I have to take so many different drugs for my congestive heart failure?

It often takes a whole array of medications to tackle the challenges of this condition. Drugs like digitalis can strengthen your heart's ability to pump; beta-blockers help your heart relax and fill completely with blood; nitroglycerin and other medications improve circulation by relaxing blood vessels; diuretics prevent fluid buildup, and calcium channel blockers, ACE inhibitors, and angiotensin II receptor antagonists help reduce blood pressure. Other medications may be used, too, such as drugs to prevent blood clots from forming. Together, these drugs can keep your heart stronger and healthier, help prevent serious complications such as fluid retention in the lungs, and help you feel less tired and more able to do everything from working to cooking dinner to taking the dog for a walk.

Why do I have to avoid ibuprofen, antacids, and decongestants?

Ibuprofen (Advil, Motrin) and naproxen (Aleve) can contribute to fluid retention, which can be a serious problem if you have congestive heart failure. Avoid sodium-containing antacids, such as Alka-Seltzer, for the same reasons. Most decongestants may contribute to elevated blood pressure, which could strain your heart.

I can't breathe when I'm lying down. What will help?

Trouble breathing is a sign that your heart is having difficulty pumping oxygen-rich blood from your lungs out to the rest of your body. Fluid may be building up in your lungs as well. Propping yourself up with an extra pillow or two can help. Call your doctor, however, if shortness of breath seems to be growing worse or wakes you up at night. Go to the emergency room if it doesn't get better when you sit up.

Also go to the emergency room or call 911 if you have congestive heart failure and suddenly have chest pain that's sharp, intense, or occurs while you're resting; if your heart

slows down or speeds up and you feel nauseated, dizzy, or fatigued; if you have sudden numbness or weakness in your arms or legs; a sudden, severe headache; fainting spells; or confusion, loss of balance, or slurred speech.

☐ CONSTIPATION

I'm eating more fiber and drinking more water, but I'm still constipated. What else can I do?

Consider a new fiber strategy. A tablespoon of ground flaxseed powder (available online and in health food stores) three times a day, mixed into juice, yogurt, even sprinkled on a salad, can work wonders. And be sure to take a multivitamin. Getting adequate magnesium may help keep you regular, digestive-health experts say.

Another way to get things moving is to get yourself

moving. Exercise can reduce straining and speed the passage of food through your digestive system. For some people, it cuts the odds of becoming constipated by about 40 percent.

You can also put your digestive system on a training schedule. Sit on the toilet at times of day when a bowel movement is most likely: about a half-hour after you wake up in the morning and 20 minutes to a half-hour after each meal. Your body's natural gastrocolic reflex could take over, pushing stools along and out. If nothing happens after 5 to 10 minutes, no big deal; get up and try again later on.

For severe, chronic constipation that's been a problem over several months, see your doctor. He may prescribe the drug lubiprostone (Amitiza), which boosts the fluid production in your intestines. Another cause of chronic constipation is uncoordinated intestinal muscles—a condition that gets better with a biofeedback program that teaches you how and when to push during a bowel movement.

 FACT OR FICTION

You're Constipated If You Don't "Go" Every Day

Fiction. Moving your bowels anywhere from three times a day to three times a week is considered normal. You may be constipated if your own personal bowel rhythm has changed and you've have two or fewer bowel movements per week, if your stools are lumpy and hard, if you have to strain, or if your bowel movements are incomplete about 25 percent of the time.

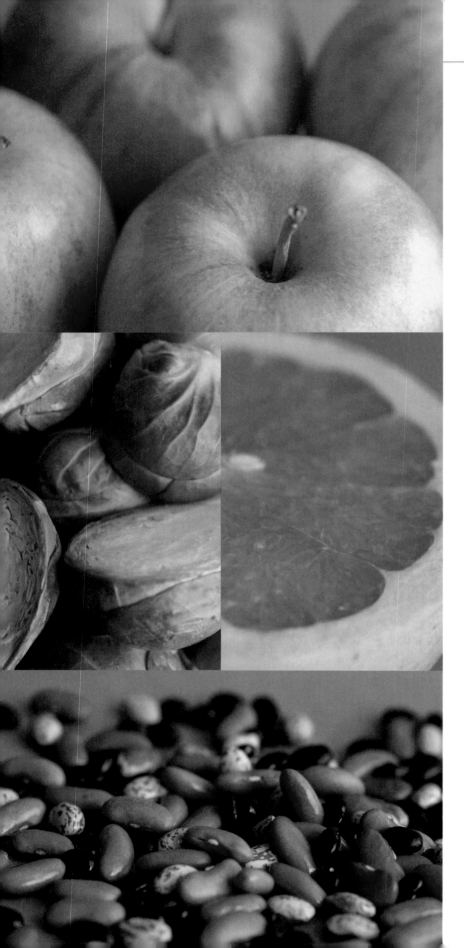

My husband's been very constipated since the doctor changed his blood pressure medicine. Should he ask to have it switched?

Absolutely. Up to 40 percent of constipation may be caused by prescription and over-the-counter drugs. These include calcium channel blockers, diuretics, antacids containing aluminum or calcium, antidepressants, antihistamines, iron supplements, prescription pain relievers called opioids, and pseudoephedrine (found in many cold medicines). Relief could be as easy as getting a different prescription.

Which foods should I avoid if I tend to get constipated?

No single food can cause constipation, but if you eat entire meals that contain no fiber and that are high in fat or sugar, you could be contributing to your bowel woes. Skimping on fluids compounds the problem by making your stools harder and drier. The list of culprits that can lead to constipation, or make it worse, ranges from white bread, rice, and pizza to ice cream, cheese, and processed foods. But you probably don't have to cut these out completely; just keep portions small and pair them with fiber-packed fresh vegetables, fruits, and whole grains. Boosting your daily fiber quotient can cut your odds for developing constipation nearly in half.

When should I resort to an enema, and which kind should I buy?

If you're uncomfortable because you haven't had a bowel movement for several days and over-the-counter fiber laxatives aren't working, a gentle enema might help. Five to 10 ounces of warm tap water in an enema bag may be all you need. But it's easier to buy a ready-to-use enema in a bottle with a long, lubricated spout. Look for an enema containing saltwater (saline) or for a type with mineral oil to help soften your stool and make it more slippery. Follow package directions; it should work in 5 to 10 minutes.

Take some smart safety precautions: Insert gently and slowly into your rectum to avoid damaging delicate tissue inside.

Drink a glass of water afterward; enemas can be so effective that they're dehydrating.

While enema manufacturers say its safe to use one daily for up to a week, doctors say one should be all you need. If the enema doesn't produce a bowel movement, or if constipation continues despite success with your first enema, it's time to make an appointment with your doctor.

☐ **CROHN'S DISEASE**

My doctor has recommended steroids for my Crohn's disease, but I'm worried about the side effects. Do I have other options?

If your Crohn's is mild, you may be able to get away with taking an aminosalicylate drug such as mesalamine (Rowasa) and sulfasalazine (Azulfidine) and/or

an antibiotic such as Metronidazole (Flagyl) or ciprofloxacin (Cipro). Aminosalicylates, related to aspirin but much stronger, control inflammation, while antibiotics knock back intestinal bacteria that help fuel inflammation. Both have been proven to improve symptoms in most people with mild Crohn's, and they help about half go into remission. Combining both antibiotics may be as effective as a steroid.

If you have moderate to severe Crohn's disease, a steroid such as prednisone or budesonide (Entocort EC) is the fastest way to control inflammation, responsible for the pain, diarrhea, and intestinal damage this digestive disorder causes. It usually takes 8 to 12 weeks, at which time your doctor will start tapering your dose until you're off steroids after several more months.

If you cannot take steroids, drugs called immunomodulators, such as azathioprine (Imuran) and mercaptopurine (Purinethol), also can help reduce inflammation, but with these drugs, it could take up to 4 months to put your Crohn's into remission. Another option, usually reserved for people who don't respond to steroids, are new drugs called biologics, including infliximab (Remicade), adalimumab (Humira), and certolizumab pegol (Cimzia). Given by infusion or injection in your doctor's office or at a hospital, these drugs inactivate an immune

 FACT OR FICTION

Stress Causes Crohn's Disease

Fiction. Don't let anyone tell you that the tensions in your life are to blame for Crohn's disease. It's a real, physical illness with a real, physical cause. Stress can make your symptoms worse, however. If you're feeling overwhelmed or have no one to share your experiences with, consider joining a support group online or in your community. A great way to start is with the Crohn's & Colitis Foundation of America.

system protein responsible for much of the inflammation in Crohn's. You may need just one infusion or injection, or more if your Crohn's disease is more advanced and includes fistulas—essentially holes in your intestines caused by Crohn's.

Studies show that biologics can improve symptoms in just weeks for up to 80 percent of people with Crohn's and put people into complete remission about one-third of the time. These drugs are not for people with congestive heart failure and can raise the risk for serious infections. Right now, they are usually not prescribed as first-line treatment for Crohn's, but that could change in the next few years; experts are beginning to think that they should be prescribed for people at high risk for Crohn's complications such as fistulas.

Medicines aren't controlling my Crohn's disease very well anymore. Will surgery "cure" it?

Surgery can't cure Crohn's, but if your condition is no longer responding to medications or if you have complications such as blockages, bleeding, perforations (literally holes), or abscesses in your intestines due to inflammatory bowel disease, surgery may be the right step. It can allow you to avoid chronic pain, stop using steroids if you've become

dependent on them, and live a healthy, active life again.

About three out of four people with Crohn's eventually need surgery. Procedures range from simply draining an abscess or widening areas of the small intestine that have grown narrow to taking out the entire colon. It's major surgery. But if you need it, it's wise to go ahead. These procedures can buy you years of comfort.

You should know that for half the people with Crohn's, symptoms return within 5 years of surgery. About one in four people will need surgery again. After your procedure, your doctor will probably recommend that you take inflammation-cooling amino-salicylate drugs such as mesalamine (Asacol, Pentasa, Apriso, Lialda), olsalazine (Dipentum), or balsalazide (Colazal) to help prevent a return of your symptoms.

☐ **DEPRESSION**

Should I bother with therapy for depression? Isn't an antidepressant my best bet?

An antidepressant can help you feel better in just a few weeks. But adding talk therapy can make you feel even better and increase your odds for staying depression-free in the future. In one analysis of 16 studies, people who took an antidepressant and got 12 weeks or more

of therapy were twice as likely to beat depression as those who just got the drugs.

When it comes to therapy for depression, a practical, problem-solving type called cognitive behavioral therapy seems to get the best results. Unlike classic psychoanalysis, which may take years, cognitive therapy is short-term, usually about 16 sessions. It lifts depression for about 75 percent of people who try it, by helping them recognize and reverse negative and self-critical thoughts (like "I'm so stupid" or "things will never improve"). You'll learn how to break down problem solving into small, doable steps so that everything from cleaning out your kitchen cabinets to finding a new job doesn't seem impossible. And you'll probably be encouraged to start making time for the things you used to enjoy, whether it's going to the movies, baking cookies, or getting back to a hobby you once loved.

I get depressed in winter. Should I buy a light box? Do I need a prescription?

Winter doldrums and full-fledged seasonal affective disorder (also called SAD) come on as days grow shorter and the sun's rays become less intense. Just getting outdoors during the day is enough to lift some people's spirits in the dark of winter. If that's not enough to shake your seasonal

How to Prevent a Return of Depression

If you've had a bout of depression, you may be vulnerable to a relapse. The best ways to protect yourself include some sessions of cognitive behavior therapy, which teaches you how to problem solve and turn negative thoughts around; mindfulness-based stress reduction, which teaches you to release stress; and simply staying aware of the small changes in mood or thinking that signal the start of depression, so you can get the help you need. Taking antidepressants for a longer period of time can also prevent a relapse.

depression, investing in a light box may help.

You don't need a prescription, but you should be on the lookout for the right light box or lamp. They're easy to find online and in drugstores and hardware stores, but not all are equally effective. And at $200 to $500 apiece, this is an investment you'll want to get right. Look for one that delivers light at an intensity of 10,000 lux, the intensity shown in studies to help lift SAD within 3 to 5 days for many people. You should be able to position the box or lamp so that the light comes from above your eyes, not below or at eye level; and your box should deliver full intensity at a reasonable distance from the light, so that you can sit comfortably nearby, not crowded beside the lamp. (Some only provide full light intensity within a few inches of the source.)

Light therapy seems to work by resetting your body clock so that you feel more energetic

and upbeat. The usual "dose" is 30 minutes to 2 hours a day, in the morning. If depression is making it difficult for you to lead your normal life, though, it's smart to talk with your doctor to see if other strategies, such as adding an antidepressant, would help.

I think my spouse is depressed, but he won't get help. What can I do?

If there's depression in your marriage, it's time to act—for your partner, yourself, and your relationship. Waiting it out, hoping it will go away, or hiding it from yourself and others only increases your own risk for becoming depressed and puts greater strains on your marriage.

Your first step is to get help for your spouse. He or she may not realize that depression is setting in. Classic signs include a persistent sad, anxious, or "empty" mood; feelings of hopelessness or pessimism; helplessness or

guilt; loss of interest in activities that once gave pleasure, such as hobbies or even sex; lack of energy; sleep problems; and weight and appetite changes. But you may notice other things: Your partner may be working long hours or calling in sick more often, drinking more alcohol or using recreational drugs, or may seem "worked up" and restless.

Level with him or her, gently. You might say you're concerned about how he or she is feeling and that you'd like to make an appointment with your doctor. Then go together. Your doctor can rule out other medical conditions that look like depression, such as diabetes or heart disease, and check medications with side effects that can also mimic its symptoms, and recommend the best treatment, such as antidepressants and therapy.

But don't stop there. You and your marriage also need support. Seeing a mental health counselor together can help, and take care of yourself by finding a trusted friend in whom you can confide. Also try to find ways to make your daily life easier; the spouse of a person with depression often takes on more and more responsibilities, from bill paying to keeping the house clean. It can be a recipe for burnout and resentment. As your spouse's depression lifts, you can begin working on areas of your marriage that were thrown off-balance.

I want to conquer depression on my own, without drugs. What's the best approach?

Start by being honest with yourself: Depression is a real medical condition that deserves serious attention. We're not saying you definitely need medication or a therapist, but you owe it to yourself to involve your doctor. She can help assess whether do-it-yourself strategies really are lifting your depression so that you feel like your old self again.

One of the most effective drug-free strategies for mild to moderate depression is exercise. A half-hour of brisk activity three to five times a week, such as walking, riding an exercise bike, using a stair-stepper or treadmill, or swimming or working out to an exercise DVD or in an aerobics class, boosted the moods and cut fatigue for people with depression in one University of Texas Southwestern Medical Center study. And there's plenty of other evidence that getting active can help by reducing stress, boosting energy levels, helping you sleep better, and boosting levels of feel-good brain chemicals called endorphins.

Since stress is a potent trigger for depression, learning a stress-reduction technique can also help. One technique, called mindfulness-based stress reduction, is proven to lower anxiety and also to prevent about half of all depression relapses. The soothing art of yoga is another stress-reducer proven to help lift depression and, as a bonus, relieve some of the aches and pains, such as lower back pain, that often accompany depression. You may find that simply releasing stress everyday with quiet breathing exercises or progressive muscle relaxation (tense and release groups of muscles in your body, moving from your toes and feet up to your shoulders, neck, and face) can also help.

☐ DIABETES TYPE 1

How do I know if an insulin pump is right for me?

Tired of insulin shots? The pump, a computerized device no bigger than a cell phone, can be a great alternative because it delivers a tiny dose of insulin continually into your body. It can help you keep blood sugar in tighter control, cutting your risk for complications such as vision loss, kidney damage, and even amputation. And it can make everyday life easier. You can be more flexible about when you eat and exercise and even how much you eat, and you can sleep late without worrying about missing an insulin shot.

But an insulin pump doesn't run itself. You'll still have to test your blood sugar several times daily and calculate extra insulin doses at meals based on how much carbohydrate you're going to eat (from foods like bread, noodles, fruits, even vegetables and milk). And you'll have to learn how to take care of your pump and infusion site, the spot where the tubing enters your body. It can also be expensive, so check how much of the cost your insurance policy will cover. While insurance may pick up most of the average $6,000 price tag for the pump itself, it may not cover supplies such as tubing, needles, and blood sugar test strips, which together can cost up to $500 a month.

My blood sugar is running high even though I use insulin. Am I doing something wrong?

The problem may be pre-meal insulin doses that are too low or mealtime portions of carbohydrates that are too big. If your blood sugar levels are high between meals, you may need to increase the dose of short-acting insulin you take before you eat.

You may also be eating larger portions of carbohydrate foods than you realize, especially if you're eating out. Restaurants are famous—or infamous—for dishing up oversized portions of everything from spaghetti to rolls to dessert, which could lead to higher blood sugar levels than you expected.

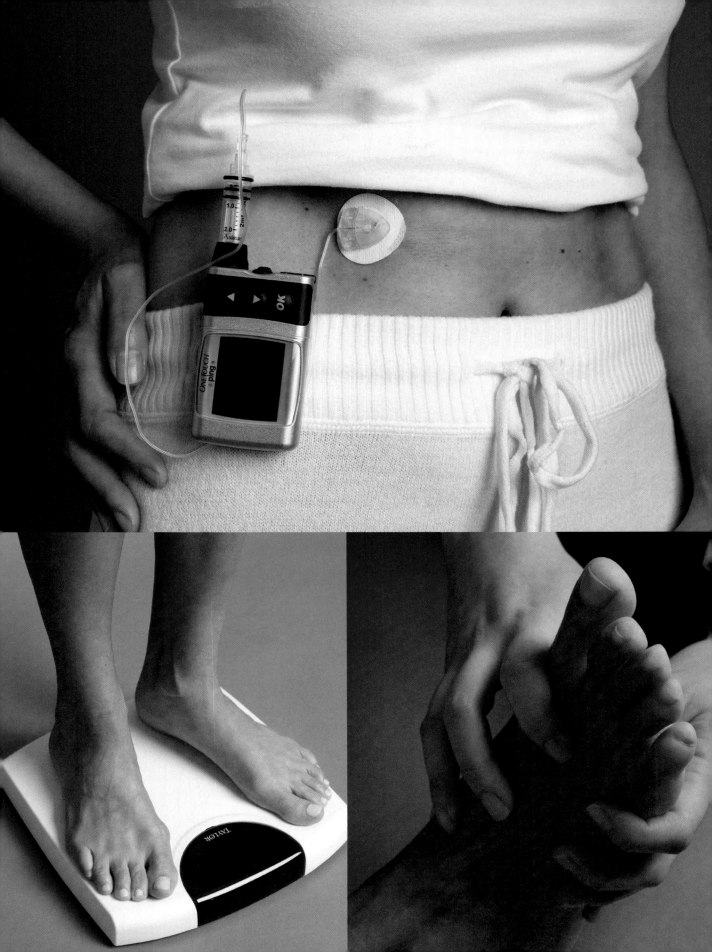

Eyeball portion sizes, or even get out your measuring cups for a day, to make sure that your serving sizes are on track.

If nighttime or morning blood sugar levels are too high, talk with your doctor about adjusting your bedtime insulin dose, too.

I like to run, but I'm afraid my blood sugar will drop too low. How do I prevent that?

Talk with your doctor about whether you can reduce the amount of fast-acting insulin you take at the meal before your workout. This will leave extra blood sugar in your bloodstream to cover your body's needs during exercise. Since medications, doses, and schedules are different for everybody, don't do this on your own.

It's also smart to check your blood sugar before you head out. Have a snack if it's below about 100 mg/dL. If you're starting a new exercise program, stop to recheck during your workout, too. Checking afterward and rechecking every few hours also helps; exercise can keep your blood sugar lower for up to a day after a workout, as your muscles continue pulling extra glucose from your bloodstream. Carry some hard candies or glucose tablets with you to reverse low blood sugar fast, and run with a buddy. Explain the signs of low blood sugar and ask her to help you spot them if they occur.

Signs include nervousness, shakiness, hunger, sweating, lightheadedness, irritability, chills, fast heartbeat, clumsiness, blurred vision, nausea, sleepiness, tingly or numb tongue or lips, headaches, and confusion.

What do I do if I forgot to take an insulin shot?

If that injection you were supposed to take before breakfast, lunch, or dinner slipped your mind, you can usually make up for it with an adjusted dose of insulin later on. Here's how it might work: If you remember your shot immediately after eating, a dose of insulin just one or two units smaller than your full pre-meal amount may be all you need. If an hour or two has passed since your last meal, a half-dose may work. And if it's nearly time for your next meal, adding a few extra units of insulin to this next shot may be your best strategy.

But these are just general guidelines. Since everyone's doses and injection schedules are different, it's important to ask your doctor, nurse, or certified diabetes educator what's best for you. While you're talking about making up for missed shots, be sure to discuss the best way to handle a missed bedtime shot, too. The right strategy depends on the type of insulin you use and when you realize you forgot an injection.

Why does it seem like the more insulin I take, the more weight I gain?

When you use more insulin, your cells absorb more glucose (sugar) from your bloodstream. If that sugar isn't burned for energy, your body stores it as fat. The extra pounds that can come with better blood sugar control can be extremely frustrating. But don't let that stop you from taking good care of your diabetes.

Prevent weight gain by following a healthy eating plan that keeps portions and calories under control. Add regular exercise plus more everyday activity—such as taking the stairs instead of the elevator and playing outside with the kids. Physical activity can help your body burn off blood sugar instead of storing it where you don't want it.

□ **DIABETES TYPE 2**

How possible is it to control diabetes with lifestyle changes alone?

It depends where you are in the course of your disease. At first, eating a healthy diet, getting regular exercise, and losing weight can be quite effective at battling insulin resistance, the metabolic "glitch" behind type 2 diabetes. Insulin tells cells to absorb blood sugar. Staying sensitive to insulin can help delay your need for medication or allow you to use smaller doses.

In one study, people with type 2 diabetes who lost a significant amount of weight—an average of 24 pounds—within 1½ years after their diagnoses were twice as likely to bring their blood sugar levels under control as those who did not. Food choices matter, too. In a recent Italian study of people with type 2 diabetes, 56 percent of those who followed a traditional Mediterranean diet (think fish, olive oil, whole grains, nuts, and vegetables) were still medication-free after 4 years compared to just 30 percent of those on a low-fat diet with the same number of calories. The "good" fats from the Mediterranean diet seem to nurture insulin sensitivity, the researchers say.

Over time, your body may become less sensitive to insulin despite your best efforts. In a British study of 4,075 women and men with diabetes, just 9 percent were still controlling it with diet and exercise after 9 years. If you need it, medication in addition to the right lifestyle can help you stay healthy with diabetes and avoid complications in the years to come.

What's the healthiest number to aim for on an A1C test?

An A1C test reveals your average blood sugar level for the

How A1C Translates to Blood Sugar Numbers

Hitting your A1C target reduces your risk for diabetes complications. But until recently, it was nearly impossible to compare your A1C number with the results of daily blood sugar checks because these tests measure blood sugar in completely different ways. That meant it was nearly impossible to know whether you were on track to reach your A1C goal. Now, thanks to an American Diabetes Association translation of A1Cs into average daily blood sugar levels, it's easier than ever to work toward healthy blood sugar levels.

IF YOUR A1C IS ...	YOUR AVERAGE BLOOD SUGAR LEVEL IS ....
6%	135 mg/dL
7%	170 mg/dL
8%	205 mg/dL
9%	240 mg/dL
10%	275 mg/dL
11%	310 mg/dL
12%	345 mg/dL

past 2 to 3 months. It can pick up high blood sugar trends you might miss in daily testing, so this check is a great way to see whether your diabetes management plan is really working. The American Diabetes Association recommends aiming for a level below 7 percent because studies show this reduces your risk for blood sugar–related damage to eyes, kidneys, and nerves. The American College of Endocrinology recommends a lower target of 6.5 percent.

Talk with your doctor about whether going even lower than 6.5 percent is a smart strategy for you. Experts say an A1C below 6.5 percent may help protect against heart attacks as well as other complications, especially for people who've been recently diagnosed with type 2 diabetes. But there's evidence that in people who've had diabetes for many years, it may not help. A recent study of 10,251 people, average age 62, who'd had type 2 diabetes for at least 8 to 10 years found that those who tried to push their A1Cs below 6 percent with medication and lifestyle changes had a 22 percent higher risk of dying than those who aimed for the usual target. The study was stopped early as a result. Experts are still trying to find an explanation. The bottom line for now? It may be better to aim for an A1C of 6.5 and 7 percent and take other steps to protect your heart, such as keeping your blood pressure and cholesterol levels in healthy ranges.

I have a lot of pain in my feet from nerve damage. What can I do to relieve it?

A pain reliever like acetaminophen (Tylenol), aspirin, or ibuprofen (Motrin, Advil) may be all you need. Try to take it before pain becomes severe for best results. If you need more relief, try a capsaicin cream, which contains hot capsicum pepper. It may make your pain somewhat worse at first, but after 3 to 4 days, it begins blocking pain signals. It can cause skin irritation, so try it on a small spot first. If these don't work, and if nerve pain is interfering with your everyday

life, your doctor may recommend a tricyclic antidepressant, such as amitriptyline (Elavil) or desipramine (Norpramin). These seem to work by helping you pay less attention to the pain and are especially helpful at night, when pain can keep you awake. Epilepsy drugs such as gabapentin (Neurontin) may also help, but can leave you feeling dizzy, confused, and sedated. Gels and patches containing the numbing agent lidocaine can also reduce pain.

For some people, vitamin deficiencies contribute to pain. Ask your doctor about tests to see if you're low in vitamins B$_6$ and B$_{12}$; if you are, a supplement may help. Nondrug solutions include acupuncture, which cut pain for 77 percent of the people who tried it in one small study, and a TENS unit, which controls pain by sending a low-level electrical current through your skin.

How can I avoid gaining weight now that I'm taking diabetes medication?

It's a frustrating fact of life for many people with type 2 diabetes: Your doctor may be recommending that you lose weight to improve your blood sugar levels and your health, but at the same time, she's prescribed oral medications such as rosiglitazone (Avandia), pioglitazone (Actos), glimepiride (Amaryl), glipizide

(Glucotrol, Glucotrol XL), glyburide (Diabeta, Micronase, Glynase), or insulin injections that contribute to weight gain.

Start by asking your doctor about drugs that don't seem to increase weight. These include sitagliptin (Januvia), exenatide (Byetta), and metformin (Glucophage). Taking in fewer calories and getting more exercise will help, too. Consider joining a weight loss program, such as Weight Watchers, or working with a dietitian so you'll have some structure, accountability, and support.

Losing weight is definitely worth the effort it takes. In one study of 5,000 people with type 2 diabetes, those who followed a weight loss diet that emphasized portion control and who exercised for a year lost nearly 9 percent of their body weight (18 pounds for someone weighing 200 pounds); as a result, their blood sugar levels were lower, they needed less medication, and they felt more fit and energetic than those who didn't follow a weight loss plan.

I found a blister on my foot. What should I do?

See your doctor right away. Poor blood flow to the feet is common in diabetes and means even a small cut, scratch, sore, or blister could become infected and difficult to heal. Once infected, the extra glucose in your blood (if your blood sugar is elevated) could feed bacteria, making things worse. If an infection isn't treated quickly, there's a small risk of gangrene and even amputation.

Pat yourself on the back, too, for catching this problem early. When you have diabetes, it's important to carefully wash and dry your feet every day and to spend a few minutes checking for cuts, sores, blisters, calluses, or ingrown toenails. Protect your tootsies by always wearing shoes and socks—don't go barefoot or wear sandals.

I get a lot of yeast infections. Is it because of diabetes and, if so, what can I do about it?

Diabetes can dampen your immune system's ability to fight off infections. If your blood sugar is high, sugar levels in vaginal secretions may also be high and can feed an infection. Your best strategy: Redouble your efforts to keep your blood sugar under control. Talk to your doctor about whether you should use an over-the-counter yeast cream or take a prescription anti-yeast medication. Use the medicine for as long as your doctor recommends. It may take longer for you to fully fight off a yeast infection than it would for a woman without diabetes. If you're using a drugstore cream, for example, you may have to use it for 2 weeks to be sure you've cleared up the infection.

☐ **DIARRHEA**

What should I drink to replenish fluids if I get diarrhea?

Water's not enough. In addition to the fluids you've lost, diarrhea reduces levels of salts and minerals called electrolytes that play a role in thousands of cellular functions, including keeping muscles and kidneys healthy and controlling your body's fluid balance. To replace electrolytes, you could sip fruit juice, broth containing sodium, or eat soft fruit such as bananas. But it's easier to reach for a rehydration drink such as Pedialyte, Ceralyte, or Infalyte. Some are even available as ice pops, and they aren't just for kids. Sports drinks and oral rehydration salts, which you mix with water, also work.

You can make your own electrolyte drink by mixing into 1 quart of water the following: 2 tablespoons of sugar, ¼ teaspoon of table salt, and ¼ teaspoon of baking soda (if you don't have baking soda add an extra ¼ teaspoon of table salt). Adding ½ cup orange juice or a mashed banana will improve the taste.

Sip small amounts of your chosen drink every half-hour when you have diarrhea. If you have signs of dehydration, such as thirst, less urge to urinate, dark-colored urine, tiredness, or lightheadedness, drink more. If dehydration symptoms persist,

or if you have diarrhea for more than 3 days, call your doctor.

When is dehydration an emergency?

An adult should call the doctor or go to the emergency room immediately if he has diarrhea and feels faint when standing up; has a fever over 101.5°F; passes little or no urine; or has a fast heart beat. Call the doctor or take a child with diarrhea to the emergency room if she has signs of dehydration such as dry mouth and tongue; no tears when crying; no wet diapers for 3 hours or more; sunken abdomen, eyes, or cheeks; a high fever; is irritable or listless; or has skin that doesn't smooth out after it is gently pinched and released.

I'm going on a cruise. What can I do to prevent diarrhea?

Nasty norovirus is an infamous cruise ship stowaway responsible for ruining many a vacation with days of diarrhea and stomach cramps. The virus actually causes trouble on dry land, too, but cruise ships are an especially perfect environment for its spread because they keep groups of people in close proximity for days on end. If the virus sneaks on board, it can run wild. Norovirus lives on hard surfaces and even on upholstery for up to 3 days. People who've been sick are contagious for 2 to 3 weeks afterward. And it takes just a few virus particles to spark a raging infection that could put a big dent in your vacation.

To protect yourself, wash your hands often. There's some evidence that people on ships who get the bug are the ones who don't practice tip-top hygiene in restrooms and who don't use hand sanitizers after an outbreak. Instead of shaking hands with your shipmates, use this jaunty alternative recommended by cruise lines: Knock elbows.

For advice on using Pepto-Bismol to help prevent traveler's diarrhea, see page 108.

□ **DIVERTICULITIS**

I've had one "attack." How can I avoid another?

Fortunately, three out of four people who've had one bout of diverticulitis never have another. You can increase your odds for being a member of this lucky club by following the liquid diet and taking the full course of antibiotics prescribed by your doctor right after an attack, so that inflammation and infection can heal fully.

When you're ready for normal food again, slowly increase the fiber in your diet by choosing whole grains instead of refined grains and by getting more fruits, vegetables, and beans at mealtime. In one British study of 56 people with diverticulitis, just 8 percent of those who increased their fiber had further complications or needed surgery, compared with 30 percent of those whose meals were low in fiber. Aim for at least 30 minutes of exercise five times a week, too. It one University of Washington study, exercise cut the risk of bleeding related to diverticulitis by 46 percent.

Fiber and exercise may help because they ease constipation.

Experts now suspect that straining to have a bowel movement damages little pouches in the lining of your gastrointestinal tract, leading to the inflammation and infection of diverticulitis.

If I get pain or bleeding, can I just put myself on a liquid diet and wait it out at home?

Don't try to handle a diverticulitis attack on your own. Your doctor can rule out other conditions that cause pain and/or bleeding such as food poisoning, appendicitis, inflammatory bowel disease, hemorrhoids, or even uterine fibroids or colon cancer. She can also determine how severe your diverticulitis is and decide on the best treatment strategy. Most of the time, that means bed rest, pain relievers, antibiotics to knock out the infection, and a liquid diet to let your intestinal lining heal. If your pain is severe, or if you're vomiting, have a fever over 100°F, or experience signs of serious infection such as a high white blood cell count, your doctor may recommend a few days in the hospital so that you can receive antibiotics and nourishment intravenously for optimal recovery. In rare cases, surgery is necessary if bleeding is severe, or if there's a hole, an obstruction, or abscess in your intestines.

FACT OR FICTION

You Should Avoid Nuts and Seeds If You Have Diverticulosis

Fiction. Fears that small, hard foods could lodge in diverticula—pouches in the intestinal wall—and trigger an infection have led doctors to warn people with diverticulosis to stay away from high-fiber nuts, seeds, popcorn, and corn for decades. But a recent University of Washington study of 47,288 men found that these foods don't cause trouble. In fact, men who ate them at least twice a week had 20 percent fewer attacks of diverticulitis (infected diverticula) than those who ate them less than once a month.

Foods Trigger Adult Eczema, Too

Doctors and parents have long known that eczema can flare up in babies and toddlers who've had milk, eggs, or wheat products like bread and noodles. Now, evidence is mounting that adults with eczema may react to foods, too. Researchers have found that one in four adults with severe eczema have food allergies. Culprits in one small Italian study included nuts, tomatoes, milk, eggs, and grains. Don't cut out foods on your own; work with your doctor to see if foods are affecting your skin and eliminate one at a time.

My doctor recommends surgery for my diverticulitis. Do I have any other options?

If a stay in the hospital with intravenous antibiotics to fight infection hasn't improved your diverticulitis, surgery is probably your best bet. Removing the part of your large intestine that's infected can help you avoid life-threatening complications such as a rupture, the development of holes called fistulas (which drain infection and stool from your intestines into your bladder), an infection of your entire abdominal cavity, inflammation of nearby organs such as your uterus or bladder, or a blockage in your intestines.

About 20 percent of people with diverticulitis ultimately need surgery. Your doctor may even recommend it if you're age 50 or younger and have had just one serious attack of diverticulitis; new thinking suggests that removing problem areas early may be the best way to avoid complications later on. For a few, however, there may be an alternative. In one study from Beth Israel Deaconess Medical Center in Boston, just 36 percent of people with small abscesses due to diverticulitis needed surgery if they received antibiotics and had the abscesses drained.

☐ **ECZEMA**

Will sitting in the sun or using a tanning bed improve my eczema?

A little. You may get better results, with less risk for sunburns, wrinkles, and even skin cancer, however, if you go the medical route and see a dermatologist for phototherapy using a special sun lamp or booth. There are three types of phototherapy: broadband, which requires three to five treatments per week; the more effective narrowband UVB therapy, which takes two or three sessions per week; and PUVA, which involves the skin-sensitizing drug psoralen, administered topically or orally, with exposure to UVA rays.

Ultraviolet rays improve eczema by damping down immune system reactions that cause itchy, dry, red rashes and by discouraging skin infections. In one German study of people with severe eczema, 80 percent saw an improvement, and some no longer needed other treatments. Why bother seeing a doctor? Medically supervised light therapy is better than just sitting in the sun. In one study, 12 weeks of narrowband therapy improved itching and rashes by 28 percent, while natural sunlight got just a 1.3 percent improvement.

What's the best moisturizer for my skin?

The one you like best. The more moisturizer you use and the more often you use it, the better your skin will look and feel.

That said, there are some guidelines. It's wise to steer clear of moisturizers with drying, irritating, or potentially allergenic ingredients such as alcohol and fragrances. And while thick, greasy ointments may be best at trapping moisture in your skin, you may not want to use one all over your body. Try keeping two types on hand: A lighter cream or lotion for your face and arms, for example, and a heavier version for extra-dry spots, for overnight use, and for less-visible areas of your body such as your feet and knees.

How you moisturize matters as much as what you use. Aim to slather within 3 minutes of bathing. Get out of the tub or shower, pat yourself dry leaving some water on your skin, then moisturize immediately. Experts say trapping moisture this way can improve eczema dramatically. Studies show that it does raise moisture levels in the skin and can even reduce the amount of medication, such as steroid creams, that you'll need.

Using a mild soap or a soap-free cleanser such as Cetaphil or Eucerin may help your body retain its own natural moisturizers. Avoid liquid soap products that are strong detergents.

I've heard that prescription eczema creams cause cancer. Are they dangerous?

For severe eczema, the immunomodulator creams tacrolimus (Protopic) and pimecrolimus (Elidel) can bring relief when moisturizers and steroid creams can't. But in 2006, black-box warnings about skin cancer and lymphoma risk were added to these drugs. The warnings were based on animal studies showing higher risk for cancer development when high doses were used,

AVOID THIS MISTAKE

Stopping Your Medication

Don't skimp on eczema medicine. In one study, researchers found that about 65 percent of parents stopped applying prescription ointments to the skin of kids with eczema just 3 days after it was prescribed. To get the most out of your eczema treatment, use it exactly as your doctor prescribes.

and on a few reports of cancers in people using them. So far, according to the FDA, there's no direct evidence that the creams actually cause cancer in people.

Should you worry? The American Academy of Dermatology and the Canadian Dermatology Association both say these drugs are safe when used as directed. The drugs are FDA-approved for eczema in people over age 2 and shouldn't be used more than twice a day or for more than 6 weeks. These drugs do work: In a review of 31 studies involving more than 8,000 people with eczema who used these drugs, British researchers found that they eased itching, oozing, crusty skin, and rashes by about 50 percent.

☐ **FLU**

I've had seasonal flu once this year —can I get it again?

It's unlikely, but it can happen. The one upside to catching the flu is that most people develop some immunity against future

infections. Protection is strongest against the specific virus you caught. In one study of 35 people who had the influenza A virus in the previous 4 years, new exposure to the same virus didn't make any of them sick. In another study of 306 people during an outbreak of the A/Victoria/75 flu, a new strain that struck in the 1970s, those who'd had other types of flu in the previous 7 years had some protection: 18 percent of them caught the new bug compared with 27 percent of people who hadn't had the flu in recent years.

If you caught seasonal flu or H1N1 swine flu a year ago, however, it's still a good idea to get vaccinated this year, and every year. That's because strains can change genetically and leave you susceptible to new infections.

I had the flu 2 weeks ago and am still exhausted. Is something wrong?

Probably not. It can take up to 10 days for your immune system to fight off the flu. You'll need an additional

10 days to shake off the fatigue; the virus itself as well as immune-system chemicals called cytokines can make you feel profoundly tired.

The best way to overcome flu fatigue is old-fashioned self-care: Get plenty of sleep, eat well, and avoid overtiring or overstressing yourself. For example, it may be fine to take a short walk around the block, but you might want to post-pone exercise routines that will take a lot out of you. Monitor your symptoms, and call your doctor if you also have a high or prolonged fever, difficulty breathing, pain or pressure in your chest, dizziness or confu-sion, or even if flu symptoms like body aches, fever, and cough improve, but then return.

How long should I stay home from work or school when I have the flu?

At least until your fever has been gone for 24 hours without the use of aspirin, ibuprofen, or other fever-reducing drugs. Longer may be better, how-ever. While fever may come down in 3 to 4 days, you can shed viral particles when you cough or sneeze for 5 to 10 days. If you work in health care or with young children, the elderly, or other people with reduced immunity, it may be wise to stay home for at least 7 days or until your symptoms are gone, whichever is longer.

☐ GALLSTONES

My doctor says I don't need drugs or surgery for my gallstones, but I'm worried. What can I do to prevent an attack?

If your doctor has discovered that you have "silent" gall-stones, time is on your side. Over the next 5 years, you have a 90 percent chance of having no gallstone-related problems at all. But it's important to take action, because your odds for an attack rise to one in four over the next 10 years.

Aging, genetics, and your sex (women get more gallstones) all raise your risk, as does car-rying extra pounds. Be sure to lose pounds slowly; rapid weight loss—dropping more than 3 pounds a week, for example—slows the flow of bile out of your gallbladder. When bile sits, it hardens and forms stones. Slow weight loss, of 1½ pounds per week or less, seems safe.

Aim for 30 minutes of exercise five times a week, too; in one Harvard School of Public Health study of more than 45,000 men, those who got that much exercise reduced their risk for gallstone attacks by 20 percent or more. Exercise is especially important if you, like most people, have a desk job or spend a lot of your time sitting. Harvard researchers have found that sitting at work and in the car for more than 40 hours per week increases your odds of an attack by 42 percent; sitting for more than 60 hours per week more than doubles them. And if you're a woman using hormone replacement therapy (HRT) to control menopausal hot flashes, consider using a patch instead of pills. In a British study of more than one million women, HRT pills increased the risk for winding up in the hospital with a gallstone attack by 74 percent; a skin patch increased it by 17 percent.

DRUG-FREE FIX

Coffee

Drinking four or more cups of caffeinated coffee a day could cut your risk for gallstones by 45 percent, report Harvard School of Public Health researchers who tracked the health and beverage habits of 46,000 men. Tea and caffeinated soda didn't help; the higher caffeine levels in coffee stimulate contractions of the gallbladder, which keeps bile moving so stones can't form.

I'm scheduled for gallbladder surgery. Will removing my gallbladder have serious side effects?

For most people, it won't. You can live without this little organ because your liver produces bile, a digestive fluid that breaks down fats from the foods you eat. Normally, the bile is stored in your gallbladder and gets squeezed into your intestines after you eat a meal. Without it, your liver will pump bile directly to your small intestine. Since it may pump out more bile more often than your gallbladder would release, about 1 in 100 people do notice that their bowel movements become softer and more frequent after a cholecystectomy, the medical term for gallbladder surgery. If this happens to you, talk to your doctor about medications and dietary changes that might help.

You should also know that if you have other digestive system disorders, such as irritable bowel syndrome, you're at higher risk for chronic abdominal pain after gallbladder surgery.

Is it possible to get rid of gallstones without taking out my gallbladder?

Yes, but if your doctor thinks you're a good candidate for

surgery, go for it. If other medical conditions make surgery too risky, you may be able to take the drugs ursodiol (Actigall) or chenodiol (Chenix), which slowly dissolve small gallstones. Your doctor may also be able to inject a chemical into your gallbladder to do the same thing. It's not ideal. There's a 50-50 chance that stones will return. And these techniques work only for gallstones made of cholesterol, the most common type, not for those made of bilirubin.

You may have heard about shock-wave therapy to pulverize gallstones. This procedure is rarely used these days because it can leave behind bits of gallstones. Nearly half of the people who've had it ultimately need gallbladder surgery anyway.

☐ **GOUT**

Which foods should I avoid so I don't have another gout attack?

The culprits are purines. Your body needs some purines; they're an important part of the chemical architecture of genes in plant and animal cells. Purines also break down into uric acid, which your body uses to keep the linings of blood vessels healthy. But too much leads to the accumulation of needlelike uric acid crystals in tendons and joints, and to painful gout. Foods

DRUG-FREE FIX

Water

Sipping five to eight glasses of water every day could cut your risk for a gout attack by an impressive 57 percent. Boston University researchers who checked up on 535 gout sufferers found that attacks were more likely in people who skimped on H_2O, getting zero to four glasses of water a day.

highest in purines include anchovies, sardines, meat or poultry gravy, liver, mussels, and sardines. Foods moderately high in purines include many high-protein foods such as beef, chicken, turkey, pork, fish, and seafood.

Beer, liquor, and soft drinks sweetened with high fructose corn syrup can also increase your odds for an attack by boosting uric acid production and making it more difficult for your kidneys to eliminate it.

The good news is that some foods protect against attacks. Milk-drinkers were 43 percent less likely to develop gout in one large Harvard School of Public Health study. And in a recent British study, drinking a single glass of skim milk lowered uric acid levels in the blood of study volunteers by 10 percent. Yogurt seems to help, too. And snack on cherries. This home remedy for gout has been proven to lower uric acid levels in the bloodstream.

Can gout permanently damage my joints?

Yes. If your gout has been acting up for years without treatment, uric acid crystals can build up to the point where they form hard lumps in the linings of joints or in bone near the joint, making movement difficult and painful and even deforming the joint. Crystals usually form first in cooler parts of your body that are farthest from your torso, such as your toes (the big toe is a classic gout spot) and fingers. But over time, you may have damage in your knees, wrists, elbows, and, indeed, any joint.

If you have gout, it's important to see your doctor. He may order tests to check for the presence of crystals in joint fluid and of uric acid levels in your bloodstream. He may also ask you to follow a low-purine diet, cut back on alcohol, and lose weight, and he may prescribe medications to lower levels of uric acid in your body. He should also ask about any medicines you take; drugs such as thiazide diuretics, nicotinic acid, and high doses of aspirin can also cause gout.

Will I need gout medicine for the rest of my life?

During and after an attack, doctors recommend nonsteroidal anti-inflammatory drugs such as ibuprofen, or prescribe the anti-inflammatory medicine colchicine or steroids to ease gout pain and inflammation. But if you continue to have two or more gout attacks per year; if your attacks are extremely painful despite a low-purine diet, weight loss, and cutting back on alcohol; or if you have signs of joint damage or nodules called tophi, you may need to take uric acid–lowering drugs. One type, called allopurinol (Zyloprim, Aloprim) or a newer drug febuxostat (Uloric), reduces your body's production of uric acid; another, probenecid (Benemid, Probalan), prompts your kidneys to eliminate more uric

acid. You'll take these drugs for life. They're proven to cut your odds for painful attacks dramatically and will help protect your joints against further buildup of damaging uric acid crystals.

□ **HEARTBURN**

Do I really have to give up pizza and chocolate? They don't seem to set off my heartburn.

In the past, doctors handed out long lists of forbidden foods to people with heartburn. Chocolate, mints, and pizza were at the top. Today, research is catching up with what millions of heartburn-sufferers have discovered firsthand: Everybody's food triggers are unique. In one study, Stanford University researchers who reviewed 100 heartburn studies concluded that no single food triggered that gnawing pain for large groups of people. If you can eat a slice or two at your

favorite pizzeria followed by a little mint chocolate-chip ice cream without getting heartburn afterward, go ahead and enjoy!

But figure out your own personal triggers and avoid those. Common culprits include citrus fruits, chocolate, coffee and tea, drinks with caffeine or alcohol, fatty and fried foods, fizzy drinks, garlic and onions, mint flavorings, spicy foods, and tomato-based edibles like spaghetti sauce, salsa, chili, and, yes, pizza.

It's also important to eat in moderation so that you can maintain or get back to a healthy weight. Carrying extra pounds increases your odds of developing heartburn pain dramatically. If nighttime heartburn bothers you, it's also smart to finish dinner at least 3 hours before bedtime. In one Japanese study, heartburn was 7.5 times more common in people who went to bed soon after eating closer to lights out than in those who waited 3 hours.

My husband has been popping antacids every day for years. Shouldn't he see a doctor?

Yes, he should. It's fine to treat occasional heartburn with antacids, but stubborn, chronic heartburn can cause damage to the esophagus that could lead to cancer. Heartburn that lasts for weeks, months, or even years can also leave you with a chronic sore throat,

DRUG-FREE FIX

Fiber

Eating high-fiber bread—with at least 3 grams of fiber per slice—and choosing more fruits, vegetables, and whole-grain side dishes like brown rice, whole-grain pasta, and quick-cooking barley could ease your heartburn. In one study, people who ate the most fiber were 20 percent less likely to have heartburn symptoms as those who ate the least. Fiber may help by soaking up stomach acids before they can cause trouble.

cough, wheezing, laryngitis, and nausea.

See a doctor if heartburn occurs more than two or three times a week or has been an on-and-off problem for months or years, or if you've been taking antacids regularly for more than 2 weeks or have been increasing the amount of other heartburn drugs you take. Also pay a visit to your doctor if nothing's working. He can recommend medications that suppress acid production and protect your esophagus, as well as lifestyle changes that can help turn off the problem.

For more cautions about using over-the-counter antacids, see page 99.

What's safe to take for heartburn during pregnancy?

Hormonal changes during pregnancy can weaken the ring of muscles that normally keeps stomach acids from splashing back up into your esophagus; a growing baby contributes to the problem by pushing on your stomach and putting pressure on this "valve" at the top of your stomach.

Start with nondrug fixes. Eat small meals throughout the day rather than three large ones; eat slowly; drink fewer fluids with meals; and don't lie down after eating. If you need more relief, check with your doctor to see if you can take an antacid such as Tums or Maalox. Antacids are generally considered safe at the doses recommended on the package for pregnant women and their babies. You may find that liquid antacids provide more relief than chewable tablets because they coat and protect your esophagus, too. If antacids aren't enough, talk to your doctor before trying any other drugstore heartburn remedies.

My heartburn keeps me awake at night. What can I do?

Avoid any foods that trigger your heartburn, wait at least 3 hours after a meal before lying down in bed, and try raising the head of your bed. Experts recommend using bricks or wide wood blocks to elevate it by as much as 11 inches. Lying on your left side, which reduces the pressure on the muscular valve between your stomach and esophagus, can help, too.

Is low-acid coffee better for avoiding heartburn?

"Stomach-friendly" coffees have been available in Europe since the 1920s and are catching on in the United States now, too. They promise to deliver the flavor and caffeine boost (if you choose caffeinated types, though decaf is also available) of regular coffee, with less of the acid that manufacturers claim could make heartburn worse. The coffees—with names like Simply Smooth, Gentle Java, and Puroast Low Acid Coffee—haven't been studied in heartburn patients, so the only way to find out if they help is to try them.

☐ **HEART DISEASE**

Can you have a heart attack and not even know it?

Yes. Silent heart attacks don't cause pain, at least not the intense, chest-crushing type most of us expect. And they may not even show up right away on an electrocardiogram, a test of electrical activity in the heart that can detect muscle damage caused by conventional heart attacks. But an estimated 200,000 people in the United States alone may have one each year. People with diabetes are at higher risk because high blood sugar levels can damage nerves that would normally transmit pain signals during an attack. Having heart disease, of course, also increases a person's risk. In fact, when Duke University cardiologists used magnetic resonance imaging to check the hearts of 185 people with heart disease, they found that 1 in 3 had signs of a history of silent heart attacks. Over the next 2 years, the people who'd had a silent heart attack in the past were 17 times more likely to die from heart disease as those who hadn't had what doctors call unrecognized myocardial infarctions.

Some people experience atypical symptoms during a heart attack, including unusual tiredness, indigestion, and a burning, tingling, or full feeling in the chest, and they might not recognize these as heart attack symptoms. If you think you might be having a heart attack, call 911 right away.

My Dad had a heart attack in his forties. Will I have one, too?

Early heart disease in your family—in men before age 55 and women before 65—increases your risk two to nine times higher than average. But family history isn't limited to your parents. A brother or sister's heart disease may raise your risk even higher: four times higher than a parent's.

If heart disease is a family legacy, make a commitment to a heart-healthy lifestyle: Maintain a healthy weight; aim for a half-hour of exercise at least five days a week; eat a diet rich in produce, whole grains, lean protein and with moderate amounts of "good" fats like nuts and fish; and limit the amount of saturated fat from sources such as whole milk, full-fat cheese, ice cream, and hamburger meat. Keep blood pressure, cholesterol, and triglyceride numbers in check. Be sure to tell your doctor about your family history; the information could be a tiebreaker in deciding if you need

cholesterol medication and if you need advanced heart tests such as a coronary calcium scan to look for signs of plaque in the arteries of your heart.

Can you have a heart attack even if your cholesterol level is normal?

Yes. In fact, up to half of all heart attacks happen to people who have normal cholesterol levels. That doesn't mean cholesterol is unimportant, just that other factors also play key roles. One of the most important is chronic low-level inflammation in the body. Such inflammation can be the result of too much fat deep in your abdomen; too much sitting in front of the TV or computer (in other words, lack of exercise); a diet high in saturated fat and low in fruits, vegetables, whole grains, and beans; and even ongoing low-grade infections such as sinusitis and gum disease. Inflammation is the result of extra immune cells circulating in the bloodstream in response to a perceived threat. Even your arteries can become inflamed when they're under attack by cholesterol particles. This inflammation damages artery walls and leaves them more vulnerable to the buildup of artery-clogging plaque. And if the plaque ruptures, it encourages the formation of heart-threatening blood clots.

A blood test for C-reactive protein (CRP) can gauge your

inflammation level. Be sure you get an hs-CRP (short for high-sensitivity) test, which detects CRP in low ranges, from 0.5 to 10 mg/L. A result under 1.0 mg/L is considered low risk for cardiovascular disease; 1 to 3 mg/L is considered average; and over 3 mg/L is considered high risk. In a recent Harvard Medical School study, people over age 60 with high CRP who took a cholesterol-lowering statin drug saw inflammation cool and their heart attack risk fall by 80 percent. Some cardiologists are beginning to recommend these tests for people over age 60, and for some younger people at high risk for heart attacks. They're even suggesting statin drugs for older or at-risk people with normal cholesterol levels because these drugs reduce inflammation.

Whether or not you go for the test and the drugs, it makes sense to cool inflammation by exercising, maintaining a healthy weight, getting plenty of sleep, eating a heart-healthy diet, and clearing up ongoing, low-grade infections like gum disease (see your dentist).

My husband has been depressed since surviving a heart attack last year. What's wrong?

Your husband is not alone. About 65 percent of heart attack survivors experience depression, and about one in five of

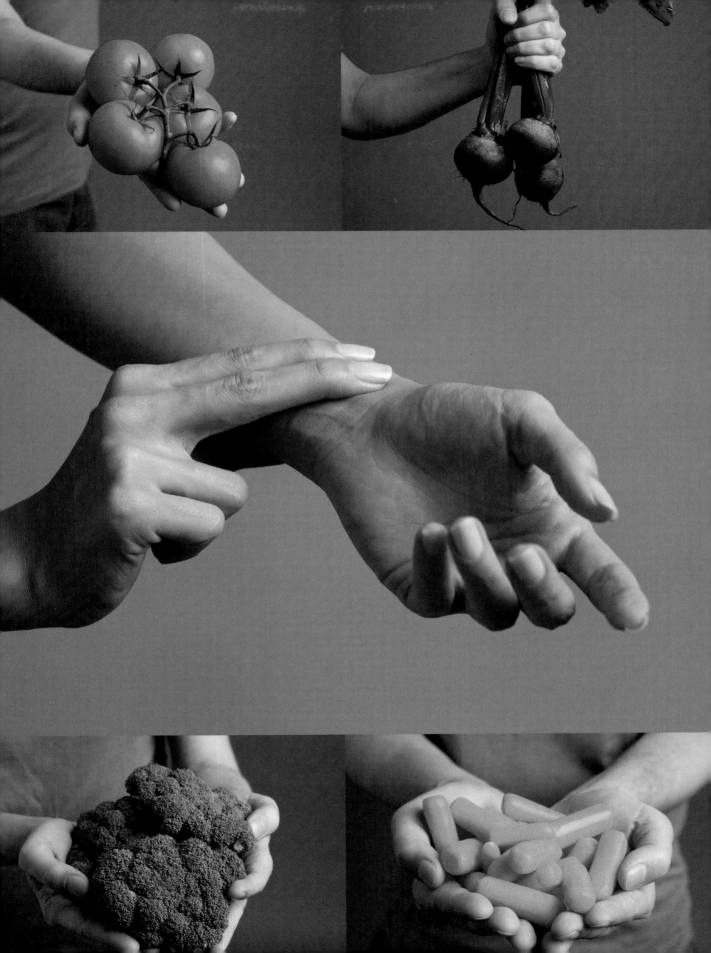

those develop major depression. But patients and their doctors may overlook it because depression and the healing process look similar: Both can leave you tired and anxious, and make sleep difficult.

Experts aren't sure why depression often occurs after a heart attack; it may be because of changes in blood flow to the brain for people who are put on a pump (a heart-lung machine) during surgery or from chemical changes in the body or even an emotional reaction to a frightening brush with mortality…or something else. Whatever the cause, it's important that your husband get help. That's because depression raises a person's risk for future heart problems. People with depression have a tougher time sticking with medication regimens and healthy lifestyle changes. Their blood may be more likely to clot and their hearts more prone to dangerous, off-beat rhythms. Have your husband see his doctor and ask about depression treatment. If he balks, tell him that depression is a common medical side effect of a heart attack and not a sign of mental weakness.

My doctor says I need a nuclear stress test. Is it better than a plain exercise stress test?

Both tests measure your heart's capacity to work hard and can reveal problems such as a lack of blood flow to heart muscle or a tendency to develop off-beat rhythms when your ticker's under stress. For a regular exercise stress test, electrodes from an electrocardiogram machine are attached to your chest; your doctor watches your heart's electrical activity and monitors your blood pressure while you walk or run on a treadmill or pedal an exercise bike. For a nuclear stress test, a tiny amount of radioactive dye is injected into your bloodstream after you've begun exercising. Your doctor can then watch blood flow in your heart, spotting areas that aren't getting extra blood as you boost your activity level.

Which test is right for you? A nuclear test can show whether you have narrowed arteries in your heart that restrict blood flow during activity. Your doctor may recommend one if you've already had a heart attack, had bypass surgery, or are having chest pain, shortness of breath, or other symptoms of heart disease. A regular stress test may be all you need, however, if you're generally healthy and your doctor wants to check your stamina before you begin an exercise program, check your heart health before you undergo surgery, check to see if artery-opening surgery such as angioplasty or stenting is working, or use it as a first step in checking heart disease symptoms.

I'm out of shape. Won't an exercise stress test be dangerous for me?

Talk with your doctor if you're worried. Throughout a stress test, technicians will monitor your heart rate, blood pressure, heart rhythm, and breathing. They'll also ask how you're feeling. They'll stop the test if they notice anything unusual of if you tell them you have pain or discomfort in your chest, arms, or jaw or feel dizzy or light-headed or if breathing becomes too difficult.

Stress tests can also be performed without any exercise at all; about 40 percent of people who undergo these heart checks get a medicine called a vasodilator to increase their heart rate because their doctors have determined that hopping onto a treadmill or exercise bike might not be safe or would be too hard on their joints.

I've heard that stents are dangerous, but my doctor says I need one. Should I say no?

The bottom line: Discuss the risks and benefits with your doctor, and never hesitate to get a second opinion before undergoing any invasive procedure.

If an artery in your heart narrows due to a buildup of gunky plaque, you can have chest pain, shortness of breath, or even a heart attack. Stents are tiny metal tubes that hold open a narrowed artery so it doesn't become blocked and cause a heart attack. Some stents are coated with medicine to prevent plaque and scar tissue from growing right over the stent. But scary headlines several years ago warned that drug-coated stents actually increased heart attack risk by encouraging blood clots to form. Two large studies since then suggest that drug-coated stents are better than baremetal stents at preventing the renarrowing of arteries—but that risks do exist. Canadian researchers who tracked 6,440 stent recipients found higher death rates after 3 years for those who got the drug-coated type. Drug-coated stents may still be the better choice if you're willing to take anticlotting medication for a year or longer after you get the stent.

Why does my doctor want me to have open-heart bypass surgery instead of something less invasive?

Coronary artery bypass surgery uses healthy blood vessels, taken from your lower leg or inside your chest wall, to replace blocked arteries in your heart. It's usually performed during open-heart surgery, with a heart-lung machine to keep

your blood oxygenated and circulating through your body while your heart is stopped. Bypass is major surgery that can keep you in the hospital for a week or more—but for some people, it's a better choice than less-invasive artery-clearing procedures like angioplasty and stenting.

During angioplasty, a balloon-like device is threaded into an artery to flatten plaque and thereby open up the artery. Often, the doctor then inserts a metal tube called a stent to keep the artery open. There's no real surgery involved, just a few small incisions in your groin so that tools can be pushed through the artery in your groin and into the heart. But some areas of the heart can't be reached with these techniques; and even those that can may close up again months or years after angioplasty and stenting.

In contrast, bypass usually keeps arteries open longer because you have brand-new blood vessels supplying blood to your heart muscle. It's often recommended for people who have severe blockages, multiple blockages (up to four can usually be fixed during one bypass procedure), or for those with a heart-threatening condition such as type 2 diabetes or congestive heart failure. Angioplasty and stenting may be appropriate if the blockage is less severe and is in a place that can be reached by the surgeon's tools.

□ **HERPES AND COLD SORES**

Can a cold sore cause genital herpes, too?

Yes. Cold sores around your mouth are usually caused by a type of the herpes simplex virus called HSV-1. Most genital herpes is caused by HSV-2. But you can have either type in either location. Oral sex with someone who has cold sores can cause genital herpes, and oral sex with someone who has genital herpes can lead to cold sores. That's why it's smart to skip sexual activity if you or your partner has any signs of a genital outbreak—even just the tingling or itching that often precedes an outbreak—and to avoid kissing and oral sex when one of you has a cold sore.

I haven't had an outbreak of genital herpes in years. Should I tell my partner I have herpes?

Take a deep breath and let your partner know. (You'd want to know, wouldn't you?) The virus may stay dormant forever, but you should know that sometimes herpes reactivates without causing blisters and can be passed to your partner even if you have no symptoms. If you've had herpes in the past and you and your partner are concerned, you could talk with your doctor about taking an antiviral drug to prevent outbreaks and viral shedding. You may also want to practice safer sex techniques such as using a condom or dental dam during oral sex.

I'm pregnant. Can my baby catch herpes from me?

Yes, but don't panic. A history of herpes in your past really doesn't raise the risk of passing it to your baby. In fact, up to one in four pregnant women have had genital herpes at some point before they became pregnant, but very few babies contract genital herpes before or during birth. Only if you develop herpes for the first time during your pregnancy or if you have an active outbreak when you go into labor is there real cause for concern.

If you've ever had genital herpes, tell your obstetrician. She will do an exam when you

go into labor to look for any signs of active infection. If you have an infection, your doctor will recommend a Caesarian section to avoid exposing the baby.

To prevent a new herpes infection while you're pregnant, be sure to practice safe sex. Tell your doctor right away if you contract herpes for the first time while you're pregnant. If you've never had herpes before, your own body won't have antibodies to help fight it off and your baby will be at higher risk for catching the virus, too.

Are prescription antiviral creams as good as pills for cold sores?

Pills work far better. The prescription antiviral pills acyclovir (Zovirax), famciclovir (Famvir), and valacyclovir (Valtrex) can stop cold sore and herpes outbreaks even before blisters form. It's important to start

taking them as soon as you notice the first signs of an outbreak, which may be a warm, itchy spot; a small, red bump; or tiny blisters. If you get frequent cold sores, you can even take antivirals regularly to prevent an outbreak. In one State University of New York, Stony Brook, study, people with recurrent cold sores who took valacyclovir daily for 4 months had half as many outbreaks as those who took a placebo.

□ **HIGH BLOOD PRESSURE**

Is it true that salt doesn't really affect blood pressure?

Controversy rages about "salt sensitivity," with the salt industry on one side, claiming that sodium affects just a few people, and researchers on the other, saying that too much sodium can raise virtually anyone's blood pressure. It's interesting that sodium intake and rates of high blood pressure have both increased by 50 percent in the past 40 years, and that studies consistently show that eating a healthy diet low in sodium lowers blood pressure.

Too much sodium forces the kidneys to pump more water into the bloodstream in order to dilute it, increasing the blood's volume and therefore your blood pressure. It can also stiffen arteries. Salt's effects may be magnified if you're not

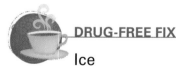

DRUG-FREE FIX

Ice

If you feel a cold sore coming on and don't have a prescription antiviral pill on hand, reach for an ice cube. In one small study, people who applied ice as soon as they felt the tingling, itching signs of an impending blister got just small bumps that disappeared within 2 days. Those who waited until blisters had formed got no relief. Wrap ice cubes in a towel to avoid skin damage and be patient; successful study volunteers kept ice on trouble spots for up to 2 hours. (Take 15-minute breaks every 15 minutes.)

getting enough calcium, potassium, and magnesium—minerals that help regulate blood pressure.

People who are genetically sensitive to salt may see their blood pressure levels rise even if they're consuming only moderately high levels of sodium. For the rest of us, blood pressure may rise if we're overdoing it. And these days, most of us get about three times more sodium than the experts recommend.

Aim for less than 2,400 milligrams of sodium a day if your blood pressure is normal, below 1,500 milligrams if your blood pressure is beginning to rise. To get there, choose low-sodium versions of soups and other processed foods, cut back on fast food and restaurant meals, and choose more fresh foods like salads when eating out. And make sure your diet contains plenty of mineral-rich fruits, vegetables, and low-fat or fat-free dairy products.

Should I test my blood pressure at home?

If you have high blood pressure, home checks are a great way to keep this important health indicator in the safe zone. Home checks can show whether lifestyle changes and medications are doing their jobs, and since blood pressure changes are often impossible to feel or see, can help you spot upward or downward trends quickly so that you and

your doctor can fix them. If you have normal blood pressure but tend to get high readings in the doctor's office (called white coat hypertension), a home monitor can reassure you and your doctor that all is well, too.

Look for a monitor that you can operate with confidence, even if it means spending a little bit more money. Inexpensive manual versions may require you to inflate an arm cuff, slip a stethoscope under it, listen to the sound of your pulse, and keep your eye on a dial or digital display. That's not easy. An automatic monitor that inflates the arm cuff for you, then displays your blood pressure numbers on a digital screen will be simpler to operate, so you'll be more likely to use it more often.

I've had healthy blood pressure for decades, but now it's creeping upward. My doctor wants me to take medicine. Aren't there drug-free ways to lower it?

If you're willing to lose some weight and cut back on sodium, you may be able to put a lid on rising blood pressure. And even if you ultimately do need drugs, these important strategies could allow you to take a lower dose.

First, work toward a healthy weight. If your blood pressure

is in the "prehypertension" range (120–139/80–89 mmHg), losing 10 pounds might be enough to bring it back down below 120/80. Studies show that losing weight can lower your blood pressure by up to 20 points. Next, slash your sodium intake and fill your plate with produce, whole grains, low-fat or fat-free dairy products, and lean protein. In a Duke University study of people with high blood pressure, 77 percent of those who made these two diet changes brought their blood pressures down to normal.

Sometimes, though, only medication will get the job done. Not to worry: There are safe, well-studied medications for this purpose.

My blood pressure is only high at the doctor's office. Does this mean I have nothing to worry about?

In the past, experts thought white coat hypertension was benign. But there's new evidence that if your blood pressure goes up when you're feeling anxious in the examining room, you may be at higher risk for real high blood pressure later in life. When Italian researchers tracked the health of 1,412 people, they found that 40 percent of those with white coat hypertension went on to develop high blood pressure within 10 years, compared to

15 percent of those who started out with normal blood pressure. If your blood pressure jumps to a point between 140/90 and 160/99 mmHg at the doctor's office, talk with him about taking readings at home to track any changes. Learning a stress-reduction technique, such as meditation or deep breathing, could help, too.

Are drugstore blood pressure machines accurate?

Probably not. One study by the Canadian Medical Association found that these devices are unreliable. Most give readings 4 to 8 points too high, but in some cases give normal readings for people who actually have high blood pressure. Getting an automated pressure check is an entertaining way to kill some time while you're waiting for a prescription to be filled at the pharmacy, but it shouldn't replace checks at your doctor's office and/or at home.

□ **HIGH CHOLESTEROL**

Is it smart to check my cholesterol with a home test?

Home cholesterol tests really aren't helpful. While home cholesterol tests are extremely accurate, the most affordable types measure only total cholesterol. They don't provide information about "bad" LDL cholesterol, "good" HDL cholesterol, or triglycerides. You and your doctor need to know all three readings to make decisions about your heart health. And while more expensive home cholesterol-testing devices do check all three of these blood fats, you'll still need to discuss the results with your doctor.

Home testing probably won't save you any money, either, because most of us need cholesterol checks just once every 5 years. If your doctor orders more frequent tests, it's to see whether healthy lifestyle changes or medications are

improving your levels—situations where you'd need a lab test and a doctor's appointment anyway.

Can I change my diet instead of taking a statin to lower my cholesterol?

Maybe. Your "bad" LDL cholesterol is considered high if it's over 100 to 130 mg/dL, or over 70 to 100 mg/dL if you have diabetes or a history of heart disease. If that's you, eating more fiber and adopting other heart-healthy lifestyle changes should be your priority whether or not you take cholesterol-lowering drugs. If you have extra heart risks such as diabetes, your doctor may want you to add medication right away. If you don't have extra risks, it might be okay to give healthy living a try for a few months first. It might be all you need.

Your strategy should include reaching a healthy weight, exercising regularly, and reining in saturated fat, found in whole milk, full-fat cheese, ice cream, butter, fatty meats, and tropical oils. (Your body uses saturated fat to manufacture cholesterol.) Bumping up your daily intake of soluble fiber can help, too. Found in beans, barley, oatmeal, fruits such as pears and apples, and in fiber supplements such as Metamucil and Citrucel, this fiber forms a gel in your intestinal tract that traps cholesterol-rich digestive fluids

 WHAT YOU DON'T KNOW

How to Get the Most Accurate Blood Pressure Reading

For the most accurate reading, avoid exercise, caffeine, cigarettes and cigars, and nasal decongestants for at least a half-hour beforehand; all can temporarily boost blood pressure. Be sure that you're sitting with both feet on the floor, with your back supported, and that the arm used for the test is supported on a table, on the arm of a chair, or by the health-care practitioner doing the check.

and whisks them out of your body. A big bowl of oatmeal for breakfast or a daily half-cup of beans can lower LDLs by 7 to 8 points; two large fiber servings a day can drop it by 17 percent (about 34 points if your LDLs are now at 200).

Soluble fiber can also help you avoid the need for higher doses of cholesterol-lowering statin drugs. In a Robert Wood Johnson Medical School study of 68 people with moderately high LDL levels (from 161 to 186 mg/dL), those who took 10 milligrams of the drug simvastatin (Zocor) and got 3 teaspoons of ground psyllium (the main ingredient in Metamucil) per day lowered their cholesterol levels just as much as people who took a 20-milligram dose of the drug.

My doctor says my HDLs are too low and my LDLs are too high, but my total cholesterol is under 200. Isn't that a healthy number?

Your doctor's right; it's more important to look at your HDLs and your LDLs. Focus on total cholesterol and you might miss trouble brewing. There's plenty of evidence that you need low LDLs *plus* high HDLs for optimal heart health. Every 1-point rise in your HDLs and every 1-point drop in your LDLs reduces your risk for a heart

DRUG-FREE FIX

Walnuts and Avocados

Packed with LDL-lowering fiber and healthy monounsaturated fats, walnuts and avocados can dial back "bad" LDLs and may even boost "good" HDLs, according to some studies. In one study, eating just 14 walnut halves a day for 6 months helped women lower LDLs by 10 percent and boost HDLs by 18 percent.

attack by 1 percent. Most of us should aim for LDLs below 100 mg/dL; 50 to 70 mg/dL if you've already had a heart attack or are considered at high risk (because you have a combination of risk factors such as high blood pressure, diabetes, a family history of heart disease, or overweight). Women's HDLs should be over 50, men's over 40; but higher is better.

Are margarines and orange juice that promise to lower cholesterol worth buying?

If you want to nudge your LDLs a little lower, yes. Margarine and orange juice fortified with natural compounds called sterols and stanols can reduce your "bad" LDLs by 7 to 11 percent if you use them as recommended for at least 3 months. Sterols and stanols work by blocking cholesterol absorption; since they can also lower absorption of healthy nutrients called carotenoids from produce, eat an extra serving a day of a red, yellow, or orange fruit or vegetable so you're not missing out.

I want to save money by switching from a brand-name statin to a generic. Will it work as well?

That depends on how much cholesterol-lowering power you need from your statin. Generic lovastatin or pravastatin may work for you if your "bad" LDLs need to be reduced by less than 30 percent; generic simvastatin may work if you need a larger reduction. But if you need to lower your LDLs by 40 to 60 percent, you may need a brand-name drug such as atorvastatin (Lipitor) or rosuvastatin (Crestor). Generic versions of these potent statins aren't yet on the market, so prices are higher for now.

Most statins are available in several strengths. You can save money by asking your doctor for a dose that's twice what you need and using a pill splitter to cut the pills in half. Take half of a pill as your dose. If you'd like to save money with a

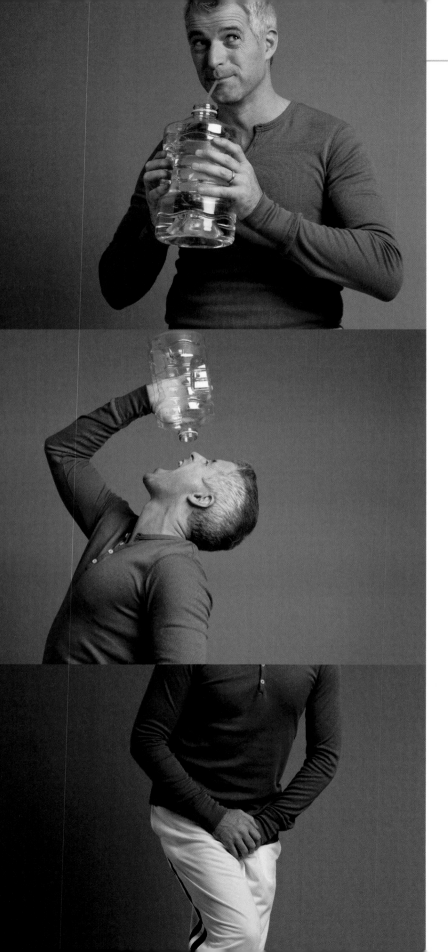

generic, or if your insurance company wants you to go that route, set up a 6-week trial, then have your cholesterol levels rechecked to see if the new drug is working for you.

☐ **INCONTINENCE**

How can I tell if I'm doing Kegel exercises the right way?

Kegels strengthen your pelvic-floor muscles and can reduce urine leaks by up to 60 percent. They work by keeping your urethra, the tube that drains urine out of your bladder, closed tightly. Stronger pelvic-floor muscles will also make it easier for you to hold urine in when you sneeze, cough, lift, or jump.

To do Kegels, use only the muscles that would stop a stream of urine, not those in your abdomen, buttocks, or thighs. To be sure you're using the right ones, do one of these checks. For women, lie down and insert a finger into your vagina; when you tighten your pelvic muscles, you should feel the vagina tighten around your finger. For men, stand in front of a mirror and tighten and relax your pelvic muscles. If your penis moves up and down, but the rest of your body doesn't move, you've found them.

Ready for a workout? Tighten your pelvic muscles as you count to 3, then relax completely as you count to 3 again. Build up to 10 to 15 repetitions and to holding each one for a count of 10. Remember to always do Kegels with an empty bladder.

My doctor recommends surgery for my incontinence. Which type is best?

The "sling" has a slightly better track record than the "suspension" procedure, but be sure to consider side effects and recovery time when making your choice.

The sling uses a strip of your own tissue or a mesh ribbon called tension-free vaginal tape to support your urethra, the tube that drains urine out of your bladder. It's usually an outpatient procedure done under local anesthesia. Suspension procedures usually require a hospital stay and involve attaching tissues that support the urethra and neck of the bladder more firmly to your public bone or to sturdy ligaments.

In one landmark study of 655 women who'd had one of these procedures, incontinence was completely fixed for two-thirds who'd had the sling and for half of those who'd had the suspension surgery. There were trade-offs, however. Women who opted for the sling had more urinary tract infections and problems with urge incontinence, a sudden, overpowering need to urinate, than those who got the suspension procedure.

Vaginal Weights Can Help with Kegels

Inserting weighted cones into the vagina before performing Kegel exercises can make the exercises easier and more effective for women. They can help you isolate the right muscles and give them a better workout. Used twice a day, cones improved incontinence for 70 percent of women in 4 to 6 weeks in one manufacturer-sponsored study and "cured" stress incontinence for 38 percent after 3 months. An independent review of 15 vaginal cone studies, by researchers from New Zealand's University of Otago, confirms that vaginal cones can be effective, too. Several brands, including FemTone and AquaFlex, are available online.

My wife doesn't want to go out for the evening anymore because she gets these sudden urges to use the bathroom. What would help her?

She should start by avoiding foods and beverages that can irritate the bladder and trigger muscle contractions responsible for those unwelcome urges. These include carbonated drinks, acidic foods like citrus fruit and juices, and anything spicy. Go easy on caffeinated drinks like coffee and tea, too. Sipping beverages throughout the day, rather than downing a whole glass at once, may also help quiet an overactive bladder and make any accidents smaller. As a backup, wearing absorbent pads when going out is a good idea.

It's also smart to talk with a doctor. A bladder infection, bladder stones, nerve damage, and other medical problems may be the cause of this type of incontinence. And it can be made worse by medications such as diuretics for high blood pressure or an underlying medical condition such as an overactive thyroid or diabetes. Medications such as tolterodine (Detrol) and extended-release oxybutynin chloride (Ditropan XL) can help by preventing unexpected contractions of bladder muscles. So can bladder retraining, in which you work to ignore the urgent urges to "go," and use the bathroom only when your bladder truly feels full. In one Virginia Commonwealth University study of 123 women with incontinence, 3 out of 4 said this strategy cut their accidents in half.

☐ **INSOMNIA**

I don't want to take sleeping pills. What else will help me get a good night's sleep?

Start with a brisk half-hour walk in the morning or afternoon. Physical activity can be as effective as sedative sleeping pills like Valium and Ativan. Problem sleepers who added 30 minutes of exercise, like walking, just 4 days a week fell asleep 15 minutes faster and enjoyed an extra hour of sleep per night in one study. Just be sure to finish your exercise a few hours before bedtime so that you're not so energized that you can't sleep.

Also, wake up and go to bed at the same time 7 days a week. Putting yourself on a sleep schedule programs your internal clock to wind down and snooze at the right time. Establish a wind-down routine: Turn off the TV, take a warm shower, and slide into comfy pajamas. Then listen to your favorite relaxing music, do some relaxation exercises, or meditate; all are proven to improve sleep. Make sure your bedroom is cool, dark, and free of stress-boosters like unpaid bills and unfinished work projects.

You can also take steps during the day to help you sleep better at night. Open the curtains first thing in the morning; a growing stack of research suggests that early-morning light reprograms your body clock in ways that promote better slumber.

I'm in menopause. I wake up in the middle of the night now and can't get back to sleep for hours. What will help me?

Cool down your bedroom to 64°F or lower. Menopause experts say that this is the magic number that reduces disruptive nighttime hot flashes and night sweats. Wearing pajamas made of a wicking fabric that draws perspiration away from your skin can help, too. You'll find this nightwear for sale online from several companies; search for "menopause pajamas."

If sleep problems persist, ask your doctor whether you're a candidate for a sleep clinic evaluation. In a recent Wayne State University School of Medicine study of 102 midlife women with sleep problems, 53 percent had sleep apnea, restless legs syndrome, or both. Sleep apnea can be fixed by sleeping with a continuous positive airway pressure machine, which gently pushes air through a mask to keep your airways open at night. Exercise, a hot bath (avoid if you get hot flashes), and massage can all help restless legs syndrome, as can medications your doctor can prescribe.

My husband's a big coffee drinker, and, lately, he has trouble getting to sleep. Shouldn't he cut back on caffeine instead of taking sleeping pills?

Caffeine blocks adenosine, the brain chemical that builds

DRUG-FREE FIX

Cognitive Behavior Therapy for Insomnia

Working with a trained cognitive behavioral therapist for just 8 weeks was better than prescription sleeping pills in one Harvard University study of 63 people with stubborn insomnia. CBT for insomnia teaches you better sleep habits, helps you overcome self-defeating attitudes and anxious thoughts that can keep you awake, and gives you an arsenal of skills for nights when sleep is elusive, such as getting up and reading a boring book for awhile. Ask your doctor for a referral to a therapist trained in cognitive behavioral therapy.

up during the day until it eventually makes us nod off at night. Since caffeine can linger in your bloodstream for 7 hours or more, swigging a cup or two during that mid-afternoon slump could leave you wide awake at midnight. Tapering off coffee, cutting back to one morning cup, or switching to decaf could all help your husband get better sleep without resorting to medication.

If he's not convinced, tell him this: In one large Australian study, people who drank just two cups of java a day were 40 percent more likely to have insomnia than those who drank one cup or none. And in a Japanese review of caffeine studies, researchers concluded that laying off the java helped people fall asleep faster, stay asleep longer, and get deeper sleep.

□ IRRITABLE BOWEL SYNDROME

Which foods trigger IBS?

Different foods cause trouble for different people, so it's important to track down your own personal culprits. Keep a symptom and food journal for 2 weeks, then go back and sleuth for connections. Do you always have diarrhea, constipation, gas, bloating, or pain a few hours after eating a particular food? If so, cut out the suspected problem food and see if your symptoms improve. If your main irritable bowel syndrome

DRUG-FREE FIX

Yogurt

Snacking on yogurt with live active bacteria cultures, or taking a probiotic supplement, could ease irritable bowel syndrome (IBS). In one study, pain and cramping were reduced by 50 percent in people with IBS who took a supplement containing *Lactobacillus acidophilus* and *Bifidobacteria infantis*, the same cultures found in yogurt, for a week. They may work by improving the balance of healthy bacteria in the digestive system.

symptom is diarrhea, foods to watch out for include alcohol, chocolate, caffeinated beverages such as coffee and sodas, medications that contain caffeine, dairy products, and sugar-free sweeteners called sugar alcohols, such as sorbitol or mannitol. If gas and bloating bother you, pay attention to "windy" foods such as beans, broccoli, cabbage, and cauliflower. Meanwhile, high-fat foods may intensify bowel pain.

Why is the high-fiber diet my doctor recommended making things worse?

Fiber can help ease diarrhea and improve constipation. But if the nerves in your digestive system are sensitive, the extra bulk may make you feel uncomfortable, especially if you boost your fiber quotient too quickly or with too many gas-promoting foods such as beans, broccoli, cauliflower, and cabbage.

If these foods are bothering you, scale back. The gentlest

way to add fiber to your diet for IBS relief may be a soluble fiber supplement you can mix with water such as Metamucil or Citrucel. In one recent study from the Netherlands, people who added a teaspoon of ground psyllium seed (the main ingredient in Metamucil) to yogurt twice a day saw pain and discomfort improve significantly; people who took a bran supplement got less relief and were more likely to drop out of the study.

I get terrible cramping with my IBS. Do I need medication?

If changing your diet isn't enough, an antidepressant may work by interrupting pain messages from your digestive system to your brain. In one study from Belgium, people with irritable bowel syndrome (IBS) who took citalopram (Celexa) reported that abdominal pain and bloating improved significantly in 3 weeks. Many other antidepressants have similar effects on pain, but the one you choose could help other symptoms as well. Selective serotonin reuptake inhibitors such as paroxetine (Paxil), sertraline (Zoloft), and fluoxetine (Prozac) seem to help ease constipation, while tricyclic antidepressants such as amitriptyline (Elavil), imipramine (Tofranil), and desipramine (Norpramin) may work better if diarrhea is a problem for you. The antispasmodic drugs hyoscyamine (Levsin) and dicyclomine (Bentyl) can also ease pain and cramping by relaxing the intestinal walls.

It's worth asking your doctor about the antibiotic rifaximin (Xifaxan), usually prescribed for traveler's diarrhea, too. Studies suggest that it stays in your intestines instead of being absorbed into the bloodstream and can wipe out an overgrowth of bacteria in the small intestine—the bacteria digestive-health experts suspect could be responsible for IBS symptoms. Getting rid of it has improved IBS symptoms by 36 to 75 percent, and benefits lasted for at least 10 weeks.

☐ **KIDNEY STONES**

Why is it important to collect a kidney stone when it passes?

Finding out what type of kidney stones you have will help your doctor decide what you should do to avoid the next one.

WHAT YOU DON'T KNOW

Some Drinks Can Increase Kidney Stone Risk

These include apple, cranberry, grapefruit, and orange juice, all of which can increase levels of stone-forming oxalates in urine. Skip sodas, too. Drinking about three 12-ounce cans per week can increase stone risk by 15 percent.

Calcium oxalate stones, the most common, may be the result of a high-salt diet, an overload of vitamin D, or even drinking too much soda. Struvite stones usually form in women with ongoing urinary tract infections. Uric acid stones may be the result of a high-protein diet. And rare cystine stones, caused by a hereditary condition, might be prevented if you drink a lot more water.

Doctors hand out collection kits with strainers to people waiting for the exit of a kidney stone. If you don't have one, use a cup or tea strainer every time you visit the bathroom so you don't lose an important piece of evidence.

I've had kidney stones in the past. Should I avoid dairy products?

It's a myth that dairy products boost kidney stone risk, so go ahead and enjoy low-fat or fat-free milk, yogurt, and cheese in moderation. There's some evidence that calcium from food may actually reduce your odds for new stones by binding with stone-forming substances in urine, called oxalates, and

whisking them out of your body. Talk with your doctor before taking calcium supplements, however. It's not clear whether they help or hurt. And steer clear of calcium-containing remedies, like antacids made with calcium carbonate (such as Tums).

Any other dietary advice for avoiding kidney stones?

If you're stone-prone, cut back on sodium; too much boosts urine levels of calcium enough to trigger stone growth. The best way to reduce sodium is to eat more fresh food and avoid processed items, fast food, and restaurant fare.

If tests show that your urine is extremely acidic, you may have to cut back on meat, fish, and poultry. Meat-heavy diets boost levels of stone-creating oxalates and uric acid in your urine and reduce levels of protective substances called citrates. If you get calcium oxalate stones, the most common type, it's also smart to skip high-oxalate foods such as rhubarb, spinach, beets, Swiss chard, wheat germ, peanuts, okra, and even chocolate and black tea.

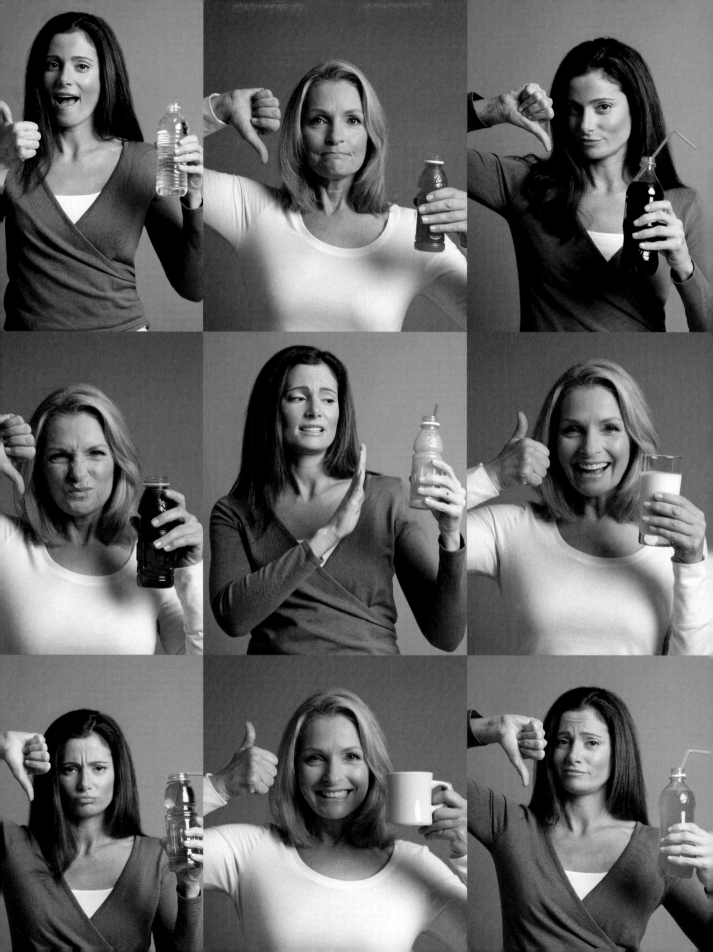

Be sure to drink about ten 8-ounce glasses of fluids a day, at least half of them as water. Drink a glass with every meal. Your doctor may even recommend getting up at night for another cupful. If you're prone to cystine stones, you'll need at least 16 glasses a day to stay stone-free.

How much water does it take to wash out a kidney stone? How soon should it pass?

Sip, gulp, or chug 2 to 3 quarts a day to wash a stone away. About 85 percent of stones will pass in 2 to 3 days.

I have a kidney stone right now. If it doesn't pass on its own, what should I do?

Most kidney stones flush themselves out of the body. Yours may need more help if it's big enough to get stuck in your plumbing, or if it prevents urination, triggers a chronic urinary tract infection, or damages your kidneys.

Problem stones can be blasted into smithereens with x-rays or sound waves in an outpatient procedure called extracorporeal shock wave lithotripsy. Big stones may require percutaneous nephrolithotomy, a surgical procedure in which the doctor makes a tiny incision in your back, then uses a special tool to locate and remove or break up the stone; this surgery requires a hospital stay. If a stone is lodged in the lower half of a ureter (the tube from your kidney to your bladder), your doctor may use a thin, lighted probe called a ureteroscope snaked through your bladder and into the ureter to find it. He may then pull it out or use shock waves to break it up.

☐ LUNG CANCER

My wife has never smoked, but now she has lung cancer. How is this possible?

About 1 in 10 men and 1 in 5 women with lung cancer have never lit a cigarette in their lives. Nonsmokers who develop this cancer may have a genetic vulnerability that leads to the development of cancer. What you breathe in matters, too. Many studies show that nonsmokers exposed to secondhand smoke at home or on the job are at significantly higher risk for lung cancer than those whose lives are relatively smoke-free. Regular exposure to radon gas, from decaying uranium in rock deep below the soil, can increase risk by as much as 12 percent. Air pollution, asbestos, and breathing in fumes from industrial solvents may also increase risk.

The good news: Nonsmokers who develop lung cancer tend to live longer with their illness than smokers do. Certain drugs that treat lung cancer, such as the epidermal growth factor receptor (EGFR) inhibitors erlotinib (Tarceva) and gefitinib (Iressa) also seem to be more effective in some nonsmokers with lung cancer.

My husband is a lifelong smoker. Can any foods help protect him from lung cancer?

Nothing you eat can erase tobacco's damaging effects, but vegetables, tea, and wine might protect him a little. Smokers who ate three or more servings of vegetables per day were 41 percent less likely to develop lung cancer than those who rarely ate produce, reported University of California, Los Angeles, researchers in a study of 1,395 smokers. Sipping a cup of black or green tea daily lowered risk by 21 percent, and having one glass of wine a day cut it by 24 percent (more than one drink a day raised cancer risk). All of these foods and drinks contain flavonoids, antioxidants that may protect against cell damage, prevent the growth of blood vessels that feed tumors, and encourage damaged cells to die.

In another study, smokers who ate raw cruciferous

vegetables like cabbage, cauliflower, and especially raw broccoli lowered their cancer risk by 20 to 55 percent.

I'm a former smoker and lately I've been coughing a lot and feel very tired. Should I be checked for lung cancer?

A persistent cough or wheeze, chest pain, weight loss, loss of appetite, an unexplained fever, coughing up blood, and feeling short of breath can all be symptoms of lung cancer. But they could also be signs that you have another medical problem, so it's smart to see your doctor right away. Based on your examination, she may order a chest x-ray. If it reveals any potential problems, she may order a CT scan to look for any unusual spots on your lungs. Your doctor may even use a bronchoscope to look into your airways and take a tissue sample for testing.

I have emphysema. Does it cause lung cancer?

No. Smoking and repeat lung infections can weaken and break down tiny air sacs in your lungs, leading to the coughing, breathing problems, weight loss, and fatigue of emphysema. This lung damage doesn't directly cause lung cancer. But if you smoke, you're at high risk for both emphysema and lung cancer. Since the signs of emphysema and lung cancer are similar, it can be difficult to tell them apart. Talk to your doctor about whether you should be screened for lung cancer and how to monitor your symptoms.

My husband was exposed to asbestos on the job years ago. Should he be checked for lung cancer?

When microscopic asbestos fibers accumulate in the lungs, they can cause scarring and inflammation that raise the risk for lung cancer, mesothelioma (a cancer of the thin membranes lining the chest and abdomen), and other cancers. It can take 10 to 40 years for cancer to develop. Your husband should tell his doctor that he may have been exposed to asbestos dust and ask whether he needs a chest x-ray or has any signs of an asbestos-related health problem. Stay alert for symptoms, too. These can include shortness of breath, wheezing, hoarseness, a chronic cough that grows worse, blood in the mucus coughed up from the lungs, chest pain or tightness, difficulty swallowing, fatigue, appetite loss, and swelling of the neck or face.

☐ LUPUS

My doctor *thinks* I have lupus. Why isn't he sure?

Unfortunately, there is no simple blood test or x-ray that can definitively diagnose lupus. Plus, commons symptoms such as fever, fatigue, and weight loss mimic dozens of other diseases. Some symptoms, however, are more specific for lupus, such as a rash that gets worse when you're in the sun, painful joints, ulcers in your mouth or throat, protein in your urine, and serositis, an inflammation of the membrane surrounding the heart or lungs. Other symptoms include easy bruising, nerve damage in your hands or feet, hair loss, and anemia. Your age provides another clue, since lupus is most commonly diagnosed in women in their twenties and thirties.

The most important blood test for lupus is the antinuclear antibody test, or ANA test, which measures levels of autoantibodies in your blood. Autoantibodies are immune system proteins that attack and destroy your own cells, leading to the devastating heart, kidney, and other organ damage of lupus. In a perfect world, high ANA levels would be all your doctor needs for a lupus diagnosis; however, several other autoimmune conditions, such as scleroderma, rheumatoid arthritis, and Sjögren's syndrome, also cause high ANA results. Even people without any disease can have a positive ANA test. So the test is just part of the overall evaluation required to diagnosis lupus.

In the end, your doctor has to rely on a combination of science and the art of medicine to diagnose lupus. Often, how you respond to lupus treatment helps your doctor make the definitive diagnosis.

I have lupus. Is it okay to get pregnant?

Only your doctor can answer that since it depends on your overall health. While lupus won't make it harder to get pregnant, it can make it more difficult for you to deliver a healthy baby. About 13 percent of women with lupus develop pre-eclampsia during pregnancy compared to about 3 to 5 percent of women without lupus. Preeclampsia, marked by high blood pressure, swelling, and protein in the urine, can be very dangerous to both you and the baby.

Women with lupus are also more likely to miscarry, have heavy bleeding after delivery, develop blood clots, and deliver their babies early. Also, about 2 percent of infants born to women with lupus develop a condition called neonatal lupus. Most babies recover fine within the first year, but a small number develop an abnormally slow heart rate called heart block and need a pacemaker.

The following steps can improve your chance of a healthy pregnancy:

● Delay your pregnancy until your disease is in remission for at least 6 months.

● Stop taking methotrexate, azathioprine, mycophenolate mofetil, and cyclophosphamide at least a month before you try to conceive to reduce the risk of birth defects. Talk to your doctor about the risks and benefits of halting other medications, including steroids, before you conceive and while you're pregnant.

● Get tested for antiphospholipid antibodies, immune system proteins that interfere with normal blood vessel

function. Studies find that women with these antibodies are more likely to miscarry. Low-dose aspirin or the anticlotting drug warfarin (Coumadin) could significantly reduce that risk.

I've had lupus for 2 years. Now my doctor says my kidneys are showing signs of damage. What does that mean?

It means that you're developing a condition called lupus nephritis. This kidney disease occurs in nearly half of all people with lupus within the first 2 years of diagnosis, eventually affecting 70 percent or more and causing kidney failure in up to one-third. Lupus nephritis occurs when antibodies and cellular debris build up on the kidneys, damaging cells and interfering with the organ's ability to strain out toxins. Lupus nephritis is a "silent" disease with few symptoms. That's why regular urine tests to screen for protein in the urine, an early sign of lupus nephritis, are so important.

Once you're diagnosed, your doctor should start treatment immediately to reduce the risk of kidney failure. The disease has traditionally been treated with a highly toxic, although very effective, drug called cyclophosphamide, but today a less dangerous drug called mycophenolate mofetil is often used.

DRUG-FREE FIX

Diet and Exercise

Don't rely on medication alone to reduce your risk of heart disease if you have lupus. The classic cholesterol-reducing diet (high in fruits, vegetables, and whole grains and low in red meat and other sources of saturated fat) works just as well in people with lupus as in everyone else.

Could vitamin D supplements help with my lupus?

They might, in theory, help with several issues related to your lupus. Recent research has revealed that vitamin D may play a major role in the development of lupus and other autoimmune diseases. And women with lupus generally have low blood levels of the vitamin. That's partly because they are told to avoid the sun (our primary source of this important vitamin). Yet a study of 92 people with lupus living in sunny Spain found that 75 percent had low blood levels of vitamin D despite the fact that some were already taking D supplements. The lower the women's levels, the more exhausted they felt.

Women with lupus who have low levels of vitamin D are much more likely to have high blood pressure, high cholesterol, "sticky" blood that's more likely to clot, and other risks for heart disease, which is already very high in people with lupus.

Although there aren't any studies yet showing that supplementing with vitamin D improves lupus, most experts recommend that women with lupus take the supplements anyway, if only to help counteract the increased risk of osteoporosis caused by steroids and the disease itself. (Vitamin D, paired with calcium, is critical for bone health.) Talk to your doctor about the right dose for you.

Why do I have to take Pravachol even though my cholesterol and blood pressure levels are just a little high?

Because women with lupus are up to 50 times more likely to develop heart disease than women without the disease, even if they don't have any other heart disease risk factors, such as high cholesterol. This means that your risk of angina, stroke, heart attack, and sudden death are sky-high compared with other women your age.

Unfortunately, a lot of doctors who treat lupus don't understand how massive the risks are, even in women like you with normal blood pressure and cholesterol. You're very lucky that your doctor does and has prescribed a statin. Besides lowering cholesterol, statins also reduce inflammation, which is high in people with lupus and significantly increases heart disease risk. That's why statins are the cholesterol-lowering drug of choice for lupus. There's even evidence that statins can reduce signs of heart disease in people with lupus who have normal cholesterol levels, leading some doctors to prescribe them regardless of cholesterol levels. In addition, hydroxychloroquine (Plaquenil), an antimalarial medication often prescribed for lupus, may also decrease the risk for heart disease.

☐ **LYME DISEASE**

How do I know if the tick bite I got was from a deer tick?

The ideal thing to do is to save the tick in a jar or a ziplock plastic bag and take it to your doctor if you develop any symptoms of Lyme disease (see page 62). Or you can take the tick to your doctor within 72 hours of being bitten so that he can prescribe a single preventive dose of antibiotic.

How long do I need to take antibiotics for Lyme disease?

It depends on how early you started treatment. The Infectious Diseases Society of America recommends treating people with early Lyme disease for 10 or 21 days, depending on the type of antibiotic used. If you're starting treatment later in the course of the disease, after symptoms like arthritis have appeared, you'll likely need treatment for 28 days with oral antibiotics. If you still have symptoms after that, another 2 to 4 weeks of treatment is typical. If there is evidence of neurological problems, you may need oral antibiotics for up to 28 days or intravenous treatment for at least 14 days.

I've been through two courses of antibiotics for my Lyme disease, and I still have symptoms. Shouldn't my doctor continue treatment?

No. Three large studies found no evidence that long-term antibiotic therapy made any difference in people who still had Lyme disease symptoms after initial treatment. In fact, about one-quarter of the people who received the additional treatment developed side effects, some of which were life threatening; they included blood clots, allergic reaction, severe abdominal pain, and gallbladder obstruction requiring surgery.

Is it true that once you have Lyme disease, it stays in your system forever?

The idea of "chronic" Lyme disease, infection that doesn't improve with antibiotics, is highly controversial. Most mainstream doctors reject it. The majority of cases of Lyme disease that are caught early are cured with a single course of oral antibiotics. Some people who are treated late in the game, however, may continue

to have symptoms, such as fatigue, muscle and joint pain, nerve pain and tingling, insomnia, headaches, and problems with memory and concentration, after treatment. (If you have Lyme-related heart or neurological problems, you may be treated with IV antibiotics.) But studies find that even these stubborn symptoms eventually disappear in most people without additional courses of antibiotics. In people with ongoing Lyme-like symptoms, laboratory testing shows no evidence of continued infection.

Some people who believe they continue to have Lyme disease symptoms for months or even years may not have had Lyme at all; they may have been misdiagnosed in the first place (Lyme symptoms can be similar to those of fibromyalgia or chronic fatigue syndrome, for instance). Or they may have recovered from Lyme but developed a different illness.

I think I have Lyme disease but my doctor doesn't. How can I know for sure?

If you have the classic bullseye rash and flulike symptoms such as fever, headache, and fatigue, your doctor may diagnose and treat you for Lyme without any blood tests, if you've been somewhere deer ticks live. If you don't have the bulls-eye rash (only about 70 percent of people with

confirmed Lyme disease develop it) but you do have Lyme-like symptoms, your doctor should order a blood test to confirm the diagnosis. Your symptoms could be caused by two other, rarer, infections carried by the deer tick: human granulocytic anaplasmosis (HGA) and babesiosis.

The Centers for Disease Control and Prevention recommends starting with an ELISA (enzyme-linked immunosorbant assay) test to detect the presence of antibodies to the Lyme bacterium in your blood. Nearly everyone with Lyme—as well as some people without the disease—will test positive. (The ELISA test has a high rate of false-positive results.) If the ELISA is negative, it's almost certain that you don't have Lyme, and no further testing is recommended. But if it's positive or not quite clear, your doctor may order a second test, called the Western blot, to confirm the results. The Western blot also tests for antibodies to the bacterium that causes Lyme but is much more sensitive, meaning it is unlikely to be positive unless you definitely have the disease. These two tests are the only ones recommended by major medical organizations.

Note that if you get tested right away for Lyme, in the first days or weeks after the rash appears, the ELISA test may not be reliable since your body may not have had time to form the antibodies the test recognizes.

In this case, your doctor should test you again if you're not already taking antibiotics. Also, if you are put on antibiotics before you're tested, the drugs may stop the body from making enough antibodies for the test to detect.

My husband has Lyme disease and lately he's been very depressed. Could the two be related?

Yes. Changes in mood, including depression and anxiety, as well as sleeping habits, can be a symptom of late-stage Lyme disease. Your husband's depression should ease once the infection is adequately treated. If it doesn't, he should talk with his doctor.

☐ MACULAR DEGENERATION

What is the difference between "dry" and "wet" macular degeneration?

Age-related macular degeneration (AMD) is a progressive eye disease in which the vision in the central part of the eye (the macula) disappears. It's as if someone painted a grayish spot or wavy lines in the middle of a window and you can only see around the edges. Most people develop the dry kind, in which

DRUG-FREE FIX

Quitting Smoking

Although there is no treatment for the dry form of macular degeneration, quitting smoking can dramatically reduce the speed of vision loss. Smoking not only doubles the risk of getting the dry form of macular degeneration but also smokers develop the disease about 5 years earlier than people who never smoked, and they progress to the advanced phase of the disease 43 percent faster.

the retina thins, most likely as a result of deposits—called drusen—that develop under the macula. The good news is that the dry form progresses very slowly and may not entirely destroy your vision; the bad news is that there is no cure.

Wet AMD occurs suddenly when abnormal blood vessels growing under the macula leak fluid and fat, eventually scarring the retina. It can be treated with drugs and surgery, although it tends to recur, requiring multiple treatments. In addition, many people with wet macular degeneration go on to develop the dry type over 5 or more years, while some people with the dry form can also develop the wet form.

I have dry AMD and my doctor has prescribed a mix of antioxidants. Will this cure me?

No. It won't bring back any eyesight you may have lost, and it won't "cure" the disease. But if you have moderate (not early-stage) dry AMD, it could lower your risk of advanced AMD—and significant vision loss—by about 25 percent. The supplement mix, known as the AREDS formulation, consists of 500 milligrams of vitamin C, 400 international units of vitamin E, 15 milligrams of beta-carotene (often labeled as equivalent to 25,000 IU of vitamin A), 80 milligrams of zinc oxide, and 2 milligrams of copper as cupric oxide. The copper is included because taking a lot of zinc can otherwise cause copper deficiency anemia. You can purchase the formulation at drugstores (brands include PreserVision) or buy individual supplements and take them together.

If your eye doctor has recommended the AREDS formulation, be sure to tell your other doctors that you're taking it. People with certain conditions, including cancer, should not take high doses of supplements without the okay of the doctor treating them for that condition.

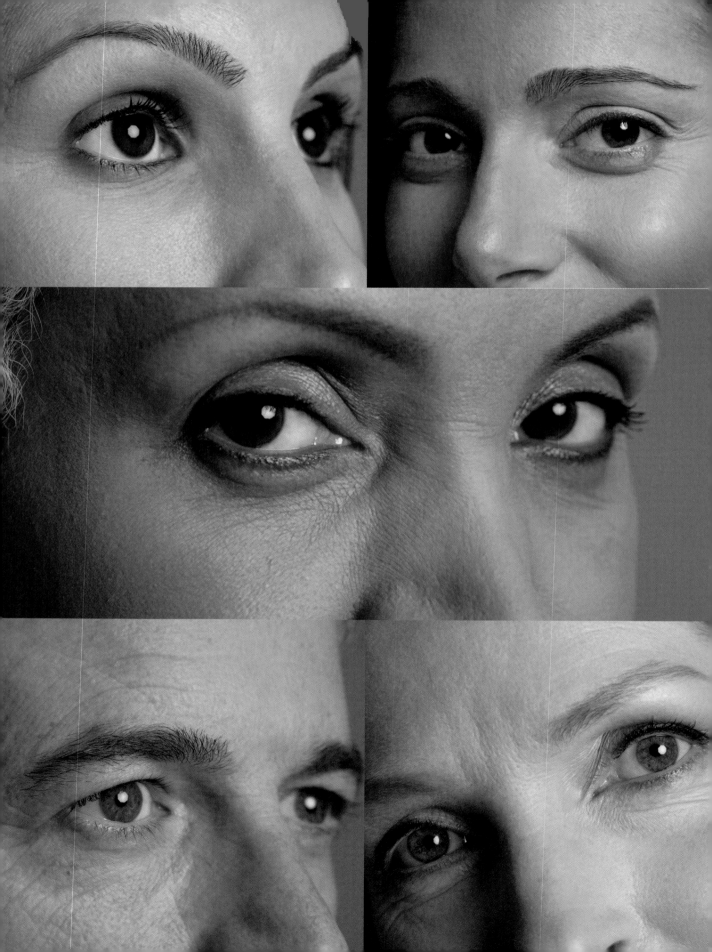

There's no evidence that the formula provides any benefit to people with early-stage AMD.

Should I stop taking my multivitamin if I'm taking the AREDS formulation?

Talk with your doctor and show him your multivitamin bottle. Multis contain important vitamins and minerals that the AREDS formulation doesn't, such as vitamin D, so you doctor may want you to keep taking one. On the other hand, they may also double you up on the AREDS nutrients. As long as the multi doesn't contain more than 100 percent of the recommended daily allowance of any vitamin or mineral, though, it may be okay to keep taking it.

What types of treatments are available for "wet" macular degeneration?

New medications originally developed to treat cancer are now being used for the "wet" form of macular degeneration. These drugs, which include ranibizumab (Lucentis), pegaptanib (Macugen), and bevacizumab (Avastin), target a protein that plays a pivotal role in the abnormal blood vessel growth. They are injected into the eye, usually every month. Side effects include pain and discomfort,

headache, increased sensitivity to light, discharge from the eye, bleeding, or infection from the injection. There is a slightly higher risk of stroke with Lucentis.

Laser surgery used to be the only treatment for this form of macular degeneration, but it had a high risk of damage to the retina resulting in a permanent blind spot. It is rarely used today.

I heard that my risk of heart disease increases if I have macular degeneration. Is that true?

It may be. Researchers followed 3,654 Australians with macular degeneration up to 10 years and found that those who developed the eye disease when they were between age 49 and 75 were twice as likely to die from cardiovascular disease over the next 10 years, regardless of any other heart disease risks. If they developed the wet form of the disease, their risk of dying from heart disease was 5 times higher and they were 10 times more likely to die from a stroke than people who didn't have macular degeneration. The link may be related to inflammation and oxidative stress, both of which damage blood vessels, leading to heart disease and stroke.

The message for you? If you developed macular degeneration before you turned 75, you

should be extra-vigilant about following a heart-healthy lifestyle and reducing your overall risk of heart disease and stroke. That includes getting regular exercise and following a diet high in fruits and vegetables and low in saturated fat, as well as regularly monitoring your cholesterol and blood pressure levels as well as your levels of C-reactive protein (CRP), a marker of inflammation, which raises heart disease risk.

☐ MENOPAUSE
I'm having terrible hot flashes but I don't want to take hormones. What other options do I have?

Hormone replacement therapy is the most effective treatment, and it's relatively safe if you use the lowest effective dose for the shortest time possible. If you don't want to go that route, however, you can try simple lifestyle changes, such as dressing in natural fabrics and layers, putting cold washcloths on the back of your neck (try keeping damp washcloths in the freezer for instant cooling therapy), and sleeping on natural-fiber sheets with a fan blowing over you. Avoid hot foods and drink, which can trigger flashes. And practice breathing slowly and deeply whenever you feel a flash coming on. In three well-designed clinical trials, women who learned to breathe this way slashed their hot flashes in half.

Another approach is to take low doses of certain antidepressants. Oddly enough, drugs such as venlafaxine (Effexor), fluoxetine (Prozac), citalopram (Celexa), and especially paroxetine (Paxil) seem to help against hot flashes. Studies show that women who took Paxil had 44 percent fewer hot flashes a day on average. Other medication options include the blood pressure drug clonidine (Catapres) and the antiepileptic drug gabapentin (Neurontin); these seem to work best for women taking the breast cancer drug tamoxifen.

Unfortunately, none of the herbs or supplements commonly used for hot flashes appear to work very well.

Now that I'm in menopause, I have vaginal dryness. My doctor prescribed Estring, but sex is still painful. Why?

Estring is a ring that you insert into the vagina, where it releases a low dose of estrogen for 3 months. It provides the estrogen that vaginal cells need in order to remain supple and moist. But if your pain occurs on penetration, the problem may be with the entrance to the vagina, which is not dependent on estrogen for its health. You may have better luck with an over-the-counter vaginal lubricant. If not, it's time for a visit to your doctor.

Could menopause be the reason I can't remember anything?

It's awfully tempting to think so, but it's probably not the case. Although about 60 percent of women complain of memory problems in the months or years leading up to menopause, a large study of about 1,600 women found no connection between estrogen levels and performance on memory-related tests, suggesting that some other factor is at work. This time of life is often stressful for women, who find themselves juggling teenage children, aging parents, and career and relationship issues. Those stresses could be responsible for memory problems, as could plain old fatigue, if you're having a lot of night sweats that keep you up. Still, it's a good idea to check with your doctor to make sure nothing else is going on medically.

I'm 52 and still haven't gone through menopause. Is something wrong with me?

No. The average age of menopause in the industrialized world is around 51. That's the *average* age, meaning some women reach menopause in their forties and others don't hit the big M until they are nearly 60. Family history, smoking, and weight can all affect menopause timing, with smoking leading to earlier menopause and being overweight leading to later menopause.

How will I know when I've reached menopause?

If you've gone 12 months without a period, you're officially postmenopausal, meaning that your periods have permanently stopped. Menopause symptoms actually tend to be most intense during the time known as perimenopause, the months or even years leading up to menopause (your last period) and the year after your last period. This is when hormone levels swing up and down, bringing on symptoms like hot flashes. Once you're postmenopausal, you can look forward to a gradual tapering of your symptoms as your body adjusts to the new reality.

Will yoga help with my menopause symptoms?

Maybe—maybe not. A review of seven studies looking at yoga and its effects on mood changes, hot flashes, and other menopause symptoms found mixed results. The best-designed studies that randomly assigned women to yoga, no treatment, or a waiting list for yoga, or that compared yoga to walking or other exercise, found no benefit. Four other less-rigorously designed studies showed some benefit. However, since yoga is a great way to improve flexibility and strength, not to mention maintaining a sense of calm, saying "Om" certainly won't hurt.

☐ **MENSTRUAL PROBLEMS**

Since I turned 40, my periods are so heavy I can barely leave the house. What can I do?

Heavy periods in middle-age are quite common. Thank those fluctuating hormone levels that herald the menopausal transition. However, several medical conditions can also cause heavy bleeding, including fibroids (noncancerous uterine tumors), abnormal thyroid levels, and bleeding disorders. Assuming your doctor has ruled out these conditions, you have several options to stem the bleeding:

● *Birth control pills.* Studies find that oral contraceptives, no matter what type, can slash heavy bleeding by half. You can also talk to your doctor about continuous birth control pills that limit periods to four or fewer a year.

● *Non-steroidal anti-inflammatories (NSAIDs).* Taking a drug like ibuprofen (Advil, Motrin) or naproxen (Aleve) for a couple of days before your period could lighten the bleeding by blocking production of prostaglandins—hormonelike substances that dilate blood vessels. Check with your doctor about the right dose (and don't exceed the dosing recommendations on the label) as there is some evidence of heart-related risks from these drugs. Prescription NSAID options include diclofenac (Cataflam) and mefenamic acid (Ponstel).

● *Tranexamic acid (Cyklokapron).* This drug works by preventing the breakdown of fibrin, a blood-clotting enzyme. One study in 40 women who received the drug for 5 days beginning on the first day of their period showed it helped: The percentage of women who were unable to follow their normal routine during their period dropped from 60 percent before treatment to less than 5 percent after 3 months of treatment.

● *Intrauterine device.* Minerva is an IUD that releases tiny amounts of progestin. Studies find that it can reduce monthly bleeding up to 90 percent or even stop periods altogether.

The main side effects include some breakthrough bleeding during the month and some breast tenderness.

● *Endometrial ablation.* In this outpatient surgical procedure, the doctor uses hot water, radio-frequency waves, or freezing to destroy the lining of your uterus. There are few side effects. Some women stop bleeding altogether, while most find their periods much lighter. This is not the option for you, however, if you plan to get pregnant.

● *Hysterectomy.* Heavy bleeding used to be the main reason for hysterectomy. Today, however, it is used as a last resort when nothing else helps.

Recently I lost a lot of weight by dieting and exercising. I haven't had a period now in 6 months, and I'm not pregnant. What's going on?

Losing as little as 15 percent of your body weight is enough to trigger hormonal changes that

FACT OR FICTION

A Diet High in Soy Affects Your Periods

Fact. Soy contains hormonelike compounds known as isoflavones that may affect your cycle. According to a British review of studies published in 2009, women whose diets were rich in soy foods increased the time between periods by about a day.

cause your period to stop, a condition called amenorrhea. You say you're not pregnant, but your doctor will want to do a blood test to make sure, as well as tests to check your hormone levels. While your amenorrhea is likely related to your weight loss and exercise, your doctor should rule out other causes, such as a pituitary tumor or low levels of thyroid hormone.

The cramps I get every month are just killing me. Will going on the pill help?

It should. A review of 10 studies evaluating different types of birth control pills for cramps found that women's cramps improved by about a third when they took the pill, no matter what type. Of course, using one of the newer birth control pills that limit you to one to four periods a year will *definitely* cut down on the cramps. If the cramps continue after you start taking the pill, you may have endometriosis, a condition in which uterine tissue grows outside the uterus. It can cause horrible pain with periods and is treated with medication or surgery.

My period comes about every 40 days. Is that okay?

It depends on your age. While the average woman's cycle is 28 days, that can fluctuate 5 or

so days in either direction. Menstrual cycles are most erratic 2 years after you start menstruating and 3 years before menopause. So if you're well under 45 with menopause far in your future, it's worth getting checked out by your health-care professional.

Are there any natural ways to reduce PMS symptoms?

There is no one surefire solution, though the supplements below could help some women. Check with your doctor before starting any of the supplements except calcium. Also see "Evening Primrose Oil" on page 178.

● *Calcium supplements.* Calcium levels may be lower the week before menstruation than the rest of the month. That could explain why one study of 400 women found that supplementing with 1,200 milligrams a day of elemental calcium in the form of calcium carbonate

for 3 months reduced pain, depression, bloating, and cravings by nearly 50 percent compared with a one-third improvement in a placebo group. In fact, it's possible that your PMS may actually be an early warning sign that you're not getting enough calcium and/or vitamin D, the vitamin needed to help your body use calcium effectively.

● *Magnesium.* This mineral plays a role in the activity of brain chemicals related to mood, as well as in other processes involved in many PMS symptoms. A handful of small trials found that supplementing with 200 to 400 milligrams a day could reduce a variety of PMS symptoms, including menstrual migraine, bloating, and mood changes.

● *Vitamin E.* There is some evidence that supplementing with 400 international units a day could significantly reduce the physical and emotional symptoms of PMS. Check with your doctor before taking vitamin E, though; it thins the

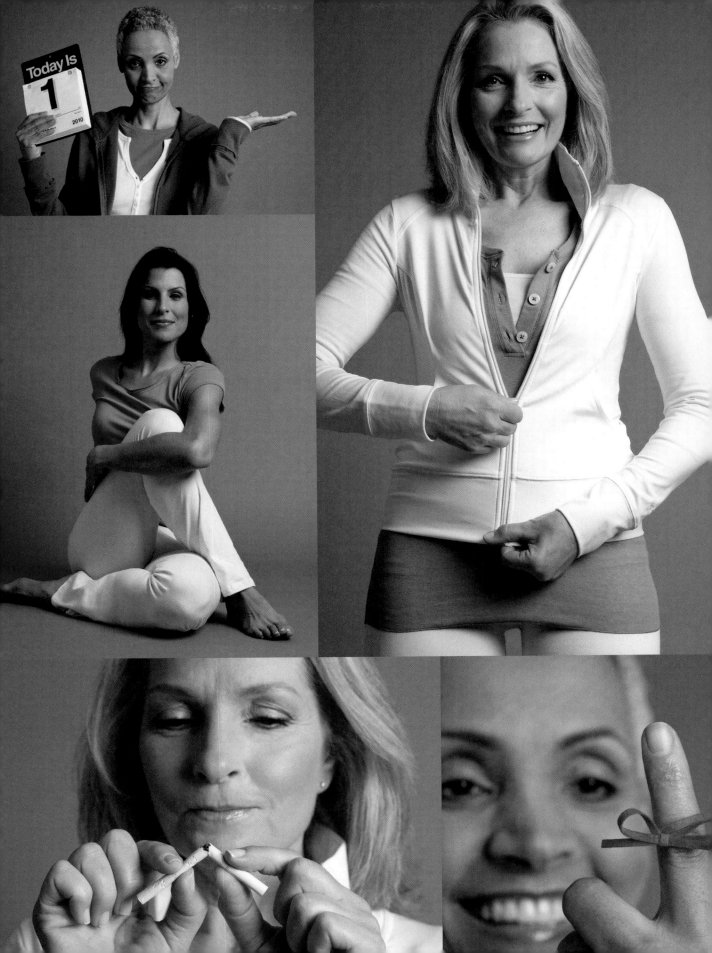

blood, and large doses may increase the risk of heart disease. Some experts recommend natural vitamin E (look for "d-alpha-tocopherol" on the label) over synthetic vitamin E.

☐ METABOLIC SYNDROME

My doctor says I have metabolic syndrome. What's the cure?

Metabolic syndrome isn't a single disease but a constellation of problems that often go together: abdominal obesity, high blood pressure, high triglycerides, low HDL cholesterol (the "good" cholesterol), and high insulin levels due to insulin resistance, the inability of cells to process insulin effectively. Metabolic syndrome dramatically increases your risk of heart disease and diabetes. It's most common in overweight people but can occur even if you're carrying only a little extra weight (in which case your insulin resistance could be hereditary).

While you can take pills to improve your blood pressure, insulin resistance, and triglyceride level, the two best strategies for improving all aspects of metabolic syndrome are diet and exercise. They work best at reducing the excess fat in organs such as the liver that are the underlying cause of the syndrome. The diet to aim for is rich in omega-3 fatty acids (from fatty fish like salmon and some nuts and seeds) and monounsaturated fats (think olive oil and avocados), fruits and vegetables, whole grains for their fiber, and oats, apples, berries, beans, and lentils for their soluble fiber. Sound familiar? It's the Mediterranean diet. In one study of 103 people with metabolic syndrome, just 57 percent of participants still had the condition after 2 years on a Mediterranean diet compared with 87 percent of those who followed a low-fat diet. The worst thing you can eat if you have metabolic syndrome? A diet high in refined carbohydrates, such as white rice, white bread, mashed potatoes, cookies and baked goods, and sugary drinks.

How much exercise you need isn't clear yet, but, as one expert noted in an editorial about exercise and metabolic syndrome: "A little is good, more is better." Aim for at least 30 minutes a day most days of the week—more if you can swing it.

I'm not fat, but I have a big waistline. Why does that matter?

A large waistline is an indication of visceral fat, the stuff deep in the abdomen that surrounds the internal organs and releases inflammatory chemicals that contribute to insulin resistance and heart disease. Generally, experts say you should worry if your waist (measured at the belly button) is 40 inches or more for men or 35 inches or more for women. (The cutoff points for non-Caucasians may be different; talk with your doctor.) Your waist size alone doesn't mean that you have metabolic syndrome, but even if you don't have other signs of the syndrome, visceral fat on its own increases your risk of death from any type of heart disease even if you aren't overweight.

I have sleep apnea and my doctor says that I'm at risk for metabolic syndrome. What's the connection?

Sleep apnea is often seen in people with other signs of metabolic syndrome. One study found that people with sleep apnea were almost 40 percent more likely to have metabolic syndrome than those without. It's no surprise, really, since obesity contributes to both problems. Treating the sleep apnea not only reduces blood pressure (an effect of both metabolic syndrome and sleep apnea) but also increases insulin sensitivity, reducing the risk of cardiovascular disease and metabolic syndrome. The message? If you have sleep apnea, do whatever you can to treat it. It could save you more than a sleepless night; it could save your life. (See "Sleep Apnea" on page 295.)

☐ MIGRAINES

My daughter gets migraines but sometimes she gets some tingling or even numbness in her arm and face. Are the two related?

Most likely. Many people experience a migraine warning called an aura in which they see lines or flashes, smell certain scents, or experience physical sensations, such as tingling in the arms or legs or even numbness on one side.

Can a bad migraine trigger a stroke? Sometimes I get migraine symptoms that seem like stroke symptoms.

Doctors know that migraine results from problems with the brain's ability to control the elasticity of its blood vessels. We also know that women who have migraines with aura have up to twice the risk of ischemic stroke, the type caused by blood clots, than women without migraine. Researchers don't know why. What is clear is that you're not likely to have both a migraine *and* a stroke at the same time.

While the symptoms of stroke and migraine aura may be similar (numbness, tingling, vision changes, speech problems), with a migraine, these symptoms usually disappear before the headache hits, while a stroke often occurs with no headache and with continuing symptoms. In addition, while vision problems in migraine tend to be zigzagging lines and flashing lights, a stroke often causes partial vision loss. Plus, stroke symptoms tend to hit suddenly, while those of a migraine come on more slowly.

If you are ever in doubt about whether you're having a stroke, call 911 and get to the nearest stroke center in your area or, if there isn't one, the closest emergency department.

Why do I get migraines just before my period?

Premenstrual migraine is a well-defined condition that peaks in women in their forties and fades away almost entirely after menopause. In fact, menstruation is one of the most common migraine triggers. The culprit? Low estrogen levels that occur just beforehand. While this type of migraine is less likely to involve an aura, it's otherwise a typical migraine and should be treated the same way.

If you tend to get these headaches every month, talk to your doctor about preventive options; she may advise one of the approaches below.

- Take 550 milligrams of naproxen (Aleve) twice a day, starting 7 days before your period is due. Don't do this on your own, however, without first checking with your doctor. High doses of drugs like Aleve can increase the risk of heart problems.

- Take a triptan drug such as sumatriptan (Imitrex) three times a day starting 2 to 3 days before the migraine typically hits and for 5 days after. In one study, this cut the risk and intensity of menstrual migraines in half.

- Take 360 milligrams a day of magnesium on the 15th day after your last period started and continue until your next period starts. In one study, this reduced the number of days of menstrual migraine.

- Take oral contraceptives, which a study of 229 women with menstrual migraines found reduced or prevented the headaches 81 percent of the time.

Why do I get migraines only when I travel?

Because travel is the perfect storm when it comes to migraine. There's the stress, the change in your normal routine, including your sleeping and eating patterns, and if you travel on a plane, low oxygen levels and air pressure changes. All are migraine triggers. Assuming that you still want or need to travel, talk with your doctor about options to prevent travel-related migraine. See the Prescription Drugs chapter, beginning on page 148, for information on drugs that help prevent migraines.

☐ NAIL FUNGUS

I am prone to toenail fungus. What can I do to avoid it?

The best way to prevent nail fungus is to keep your feet clean and dry. Start by thoroughly drying your feet and toes after bathing. If your feet sweat, apply an antifungal spray or powder (not cornstarch, which can make the fungus grow). Wear socks made of natural fibers designed to wick away moisture and allow air to circulate, and change your socks frequently if they get damp. The same goes for your shoes; it's a good idea to let them air out for a day between wearings. (If you can't, put them in front a fan or stuff them with newspaper overnight.) Make sure your shoes fit properly, allowing you room to wiggle your toes. Shoes that are too tight around the toes not only cause your feet to perspire but can damage the nail, providing a toehold for fungus spores. Avoiding nail damage is the reason you should cut your nails straight across and keep them short.

Wear sandals or water shoes when using a shared bathroom and when in the pool or other damp areas. And make sure to clean your bath mat and tub regularly to avoid transferring an infection to someone else in your family. For the same reason, don't share shoes or toenail or fingernail clippers.

If you already have toenail fungus, see "Toenail Fungus" on page 47 for information on treating it.

Are fungal infections of the toenails serious or will they go away on their own?

Fungal infections of the nails don't have to be treated unless you have immune system problems such as HIV infection, cancer, conditions that require immune-suppressing drugs, diabetes, or reduced circulation to your feet or hands, or you have had a bout of cellulitis (inflammation of the skin and underlying tissue) on your leg in the past. In these instances, an untreated fungal infection can lead to cellulitis, foot ulcers, or other serious complications. Your doctor should also treat the infection (usually with oral antifungal medication) if it hurts or has spread to your skin, causing athlete's foot. If the infection is severe, you can have a podiatrist remove the infected nail so that a new nail can grow in its place, though this may take up to a year. Otherwise, while nail fungus can be ugly and embarrassing, mild infections tend to eventually clear up on their own.

☐ OSTEOPOROSIS

I have osteoporosis and vertigo. Are the two related?

They may be. A study published in the spring of 2009 in the journal *Neurology* found that people with osteoporosis were three times more likely to have benign paroxysmal positional vertigo, an inner ear condition that causes dizziness and can contribute to falls. The connection may be a problem with calcium metabolism. Calcium, of course, is necessary for strong bones. It also plays a role in vertigo. Calcium carbonate crystals in the inner ear tubes help us orient ourselves in space and provide us with our sense of balance; if the crystals are loose, balance is affected.

Falling is a bad thing no matter who you are, but if you have osteoporosis, it can be deadly. Each year, more than 15,000 people over age 65 who have osteoporosis and fall die as a result of their injuries. If you feel any dizziness, tell your doctor. Vertigo can often be treated with a simple series of head movements.

I have osteoporosis and my doctor told me to take 3,000 IU of vitamin D. Isn't that too much?

Although current recommendations call for an upper limit of

2,000 international units of vitamin D a day, many experts agree that figure is too low given what is now known about the so-called sunshine vitamin. In fact, experts find that you would need to take more than 10,000 IU a day before experiencing any problems due to overdose. So if your doctor recommended 3,000 IU a day, that's fine.

That said, don't start taking massive doses of vitamin D without first checking with your doctor. Certain medical conditions, such as kidney disease, high calcium levels, hardening of the arteries, or a disease called sarcoidosis can make you more sensitive to the vitamin, meaning it could take less to trigger toxic effects. Symptoms of vitamin D toxicity include loss of appetite, nausea, vomiting, weakness, nervousness, and excessive thirst and urination.

My doctor says I have osteopenia and wants to put me on medication. Is that really necessary?

It may not be. Osteopenia is a fancy word for bone density that's somewhat low but not low enough to constitute osteoporosis. If you have osteopenia *and* other major risk factors for osteoporosis, such as advanced age, a history of smoking, a family history of osteoporosis, a small frame, or a history of

You Shouldn't Exercise If You Have Osteoporosis

Fiction. While it's true that you have a much higher fracture risk than someone with healthier bones, it shouldn't stop you from exercising. Just avoid exercises that could lead to tripping or falls or that directly impact bone, such as high-impact aerobics, kickboxing, or running on uneven surfaces. Stick with walking, bicycling, and strength training, preferably under the supervision of a personal trainer or physical therapist. Make sure your shoes fit properly and are designed for the type of exercise you're doing.

corticosteroid use, your doctor may want to start you on medication to prevent or slow any further loss. But otherwise, you may not need it.

Osteopenia is diagnosed with a bone mineral density test called DXA, a type of x-ray. The results are reported as T-scores, which indicate how much (in standard deviations) your bone density differs from that of a healthy 30-year-old white person of your gender. A T-score between 0 and −1 is considered normal; that of −2.5 or less gets you a diagnosis of osteoporosis. Anything in between means osteopenia.

There's a catch, though. The T-score was developed to assess bone density in women in their sixties and older—not in the younger women who are increasingly getting tested today. The younger your bones, the stronger they are regardless of your T-score. There's also a growing understanding

that bone strength isn't related just to density; in other words, if you have a low T-score, it doesn't necessarily mean that you have a higher risk of a bone fracture.

A better indicator of your risk if you're under 60 is bone densitometry (DXA) plus FRAX, the Fracture Risk Assessment Tool. The FRAX was developed by the World Health Organization. The tool uses your age, weight, height, ethnic background, history of smoking and alcohol use, medical history, bone mineral density score, and other factors to figure out your 10-year risk of having a hip or vertebral fracture. Your doctor should use both the FRAX and the DXA to determine if you need treatment for osteoporosis. National Osteoporosis Foundation guidelines recommend medical treatment for postmenopausal women or men age 50 and older whose DXA score is −1 to −2.5 and

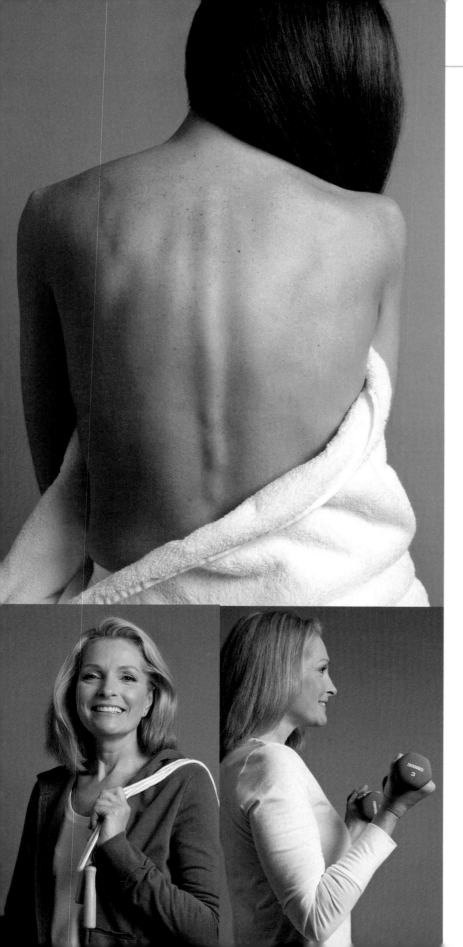

who have a 10-year risk of hip fracture greater than 3 percent on the FRAX, or whose FRAX score is more than 20 percent, regardless of their DXA score.

Whether or not you start taking medication, you should view a questionable T-score as a reminder to do what you can on your own to strengthen your bones, including getting adequate amounts of calcium and vitamin D from diet and supplements, engaging in some form of weight-bearing exercise several times a week. Higher-impact activities such as dancing, hiking, jogging, jumping rope, climbing stairs, or playing tennis are best. (Even just hopping up and down appears to work very well). And if you smoke, quit.

My doctor suggested vertebroplasty for the fractures in my backbone. Will it really help?

Vertebroplasty is a procedure in which the surgeon injects bone cement into fractured vertebrae to strengthen the bone. It can help—but not more than medication, exercise, and physical therapy according to two large studies that compared the surgery to nonsurgical treatments. And of course, undergoing surgery poses greater risks. Given these two studies, doctors are moving away from vertebroplasty.

Some doctors are turning to vesselplasty instead, in which they insert a porous balloon into your vertebrae, expand the balloon, then fill it with bone cement. However, the procedure is new and there are few studies attesting to its effectiveness or safety.

If you opt against the surgical route, talk to your doctor about taking calcitonin (Calcimar, Miacalcin), a synthetic hormone used to treat painful vertebral fractures.

☐ PARKINSON'S DISEASE

The doctor says my husband has Parkinson's disease but he doesn't shake or move slowly. How can the doctor be so sure?

Even though you might think of people with Parkinson's disease as shaking uncontrollably, the reality is that early symptoms don't include much in the way of tremors or shaking. While there are no specific, widely available tests to diagnose Parkinson's, a medical evaluation and medical history would have provided your doctor with the necessary clues. For instance, have you noticed your husband talking less? Does his face seem more expressionless? Is his voice softer, more muffled?

These are all signs of early Parkinson's. Other signs include moving more slowly and having problems completing normal activities, like brushing your teeth, cutting food, or even stirring a pot.

Do you find that your husband swings just one arm when walking and has stopped using his hands when he talks? Has he lost his sense of smell? All Parkinson's signs. Also, look at his writing. People with Parkinson's write progressively smaller. After assessing your husband for these and other symptoms, and conducting a couple of simple movement-related exercise tests, your doctor was able to diagnose your husband.

My doctor suggests that I have brain surgery for my Parkinson's. But I'm scared to have someone drill into my brain! How safe is this surgery?

It depends which surgery your doctor is talking about. Pallidotomy and subthalamotomy, in which the surgeon drills into the brain to create lesions in the areas related to the tremors of the disease, are rarely performed these days. Instead, your doctor was likely suggesting deep-brain stimulation,

recommended for people whose symptoms can no longer be adequately controlled with medication.

In this procedure, the surgeon drills a small hole in the skull through which to pass an electrode, which is implanted into the area of the brain responsible for many Parkinson's symptoms, such as tremor, rigidity, and slow movement. A neurostimulator, a sort of pacemaker for the brain, is implanted under the collarbone (it's about the size of a half dollar). Finally an extension wire is implanted under the skin in the shoulder and collarbone to connect the device to the electrode in the brain. The neurotransmitter sends electrical impulses to the electrode to block the transmission of abnormal electrical signals that cause Parkinson's symptoms.

Studies find that the deep-brain stimulation works much better than medication alone and for longer periods of time. (Patients who have the surgery often decrease the amount of medicine they take.) Of course, surgery carries a higher risk of complications, including infection, headache, and bleeding. There's also no information yet on how people who have it fare over the long term.

☐ PNEUMONIA

How do I know if what I have is pneumonia or bronchitis?

Only your doctor can diagnose which respiratory infection you have. Both are caused by viruses or bacteria and often stem from something simple like a cold. But bronchitis is inflammation of the bronchi, the tubes leading from your trachea to your lungs, while pneumonia is an infection in the air sacs in the lungs, which fill with fluid or pus, making breathing difficult. Other differences:

● *Phlegm.* Bronchitis usually involves clear, green, or yellow phlegm; pneumonia phlegm is often dark green and may be flecked with blood.

● *Fever.* It's more common and much higher (above 101°F) with pneumonia.

● *Chills and shaking.* This is a pneumonia-only symptom.

● *Shortness of breath.* A hallmark of pneumonia, it's rarely seen with bronchitis.

● *X-ray.* Clear for bronchitis; shows areas of inflammation and fluid-filled air sacs with pneumonia.

How do I know when a case of the flu has turned into pneumonia?

Every year, an estimated 46,000 people in the United States—mostly older folks— die from influenza-related

DRUG-FREE FIX

Wii

Playing your kids' or grandkids' Wii—the Nintendo video game system in which the users move around as if actually playing various sports—could improve some symptoms of Parkinson's disease. In one study, 20 people with the disease played Wii tennis, bowling, and boxing an hour a day, 3 days a week for 4 weeks. After the 4 weeks, the participants moved more easily, their fine motor skills improved, and they had more energy. Scores on a depression test also dropped to zero. The benefit may come from increased levels of dopamine released during exercise and while playing video games. Dopamine is the chemical lacking in the brains of people with Parkinson's.

pneumonia, and thousands more are hospitalized. Even people who normally weather the flu just fine—healthy young people— may develop pneumonia after an infection with the H1N1 flu.

If you or someone in your family with the flu develop any of the following symptoms, get to your doctor or the emergency room immediately:

● Difficulty breathing or chest pain

● Purple or blue discoloration of the lips

● Vomiting, being unable to keep liquids down

● Signs of dehydration such as dizziness when standing, absence of urination, or in infants, a lack of tears when crying

● Seizures (for example, uncontrolled convulsions)

● Confusion or being less responsive than normal

I'm going into the hospital for surgery. How can I reduce my risk of catching pneumonia while I'm there?

Hospital-acquired pneumonia is a potentially serious complication after surgery, especially in seniors. About 25 to 50 percent of people who develop it die from it because they were already compromised to begin with and because the bacteria present in hospitals are resistant to many types of antibiotics. To reduce your risk, start by making sure the nurse brushes your teeth three times a day if you have to be on a mechanical ventilator. One study found this slashed the risk of pneumonia in half by preventing normally harmless mouth bacteria from getting sucked into the lungs. Even though nurses in intensive care units are supposed to brush patients' teeth, the study found that less than half did.

Even if you never set foot into intensive care, your risk of hospital-acquired pneumonia or other infections is still high. To protect yourself:

- *Get your shots.* Make sure you're up on all your vaccines, including a pneumococcal vaccine if you're age 65 or older or have a chronic heart or lung condition, at least 2 weeks before the surgery.

- *Be assertive.* Insist that anyone who enters your room wash his or her hands. Be vigilant and get your family members to be vigilant.

- *Watch your blood sugar.* If you have diabetes, make sure your blood sugar is controlled while hospitalized. Too often this small but important detail gets overlooked. Having high glucose levels increases your risk of infection.

- *Stay clean.* Get the nurse to change your gown and sheets if they become soiled and wash your own hands often (or use a hand sanitizer).

- *Watch your catheters.* Make sure the skin around the dressing for any IV catheters (such as those that make it easier to draw blood and provide medications) is clean and dry. If the catheter becomes loose or the dressing becomes loose or wet, tell the nurse immediately.

☐ PROSTATE CANCER

My husband was just diagnosed with prostate cancer. His doctor says we don't have to do anything, just watch and wait. Isn't this dangerous?

Probably not. So-called watchful waiting means closely monitoring your husband's cancer, primarily with blood tests, but not treating it until there are signs that the cancer has grown or spread. A similar concept is called active surveillance, in which the plan is to take action when there is a change but before there is time for the cancer to spread. This might sound counterintuitive to how most of us want our cancer treated (get it out, now!), but numerous studies find this approach is a good one for many prostate cancers, especially ones that are very small, not aggressive, and not causing any symptoms. That's because most prostate cancers grow very slowly. They tend to occur in older men, and the men often die of something else unrelated to the cancer before they ever need treatment. Since cancer treatment is never pleasant and is always expensive, there's no need to treat a cancer that isn't going to hurt you.

In one large study of 3,331 men diagnosed with prostate cancer, 10 percent took a "watchful waiting" approach. Of those men, about half remained untreated throughout the study (an average of 7.7 years). The rest were treated an average of 3.9 years after their diagnoses. (The younger the men and the higher stage and grade of their cancer, the more likely they were to begin treatment earlier.) No difference was found in terms of when the cancer spread or in cancer deaths between men who began treatment immediately and those who waited.

I have prostate cancer and my urologist recommended surgery. I don't want to become incontinent or impotent, though. What do I need to know?

Your doctor wants you to undergo a radical prostatectomy, in which the prostate gland is removed in order to prevent the cancer from growing or spreading. It's sometimes recommended for otherwise healthy men who are likely to live for 10 or more years. The risk of incontinence is pretty low these days, since surgical techniques have improved over the years. If you do experience incontinence, there's a good chance it will disappear gradually over several weeks or months.

To increase the chances that you'll still be able to have erections after your surgery, most surgeons today perform the nerve-sparing form of the procedure, which preserves the nerves that feed into the penis. However, even with a "perfect" nerve-sparing prostatectomy, you can still experience some difficulty following the surgery. The younger you are, the more likely that this type of surgery will keep you working the way you want in the bedroom. But be patient; it may take months after surgery before normal erections return. If you're over age 70, the chances that you won't be able to regain potency after nerve-sparing surgery are higher than if you're under 60.

The best outcomes following radical prostatectomy are seen with highly experienced surgeons. Look for one who has performed at least 250 nerve-sparing surgeries. Studies find lower complication rates as well as a lower risk of cancer recurrence in men whose surgeries were performed by such highly experienced doctors. The jury is still out on whether or not the robotic radical prostatectomy results in better erections than the standard operation.

Unfortunately, if the cancer has spread outside the prostate, the nerves may need to go and you will lose potency. You can still obtain an erection with the use of medications, injections, or a vacuum pump or similar devices.

I am taking hormone therapy for my prostate cancer and the hot flashes are killing me! What can I do?

Now you know how the other half feels during menopause! But seriously, the hot flashes from the hormone therapy, designed to provide a medical "castration" by dramatically reducing testosterone levels, can be, as you say, killer. Many of the same lifestyle changes recommended for menopausal women in "Menopause" on page 275 will work for you. Other options you and your doctor might consider include:

- *An estrogen patch.* One study found that 83 percent of men who wore the patch cooled down. A few side effects worth noting, however, included breast swelling and nipple tenderness.

- *Synthetic progesterone.* After taking megestrol acetate (Megace) twice a day for 4 weeks, men had far fewer hot flashes than those who got a placebo. There were no major side effects.

Although estrogen and megestrol acetate show the greatest benefit in reducing hot flashes, other medications that may help include:

- *SSRI antidepressants.* A couple of small studies found that paroxetine (Paxil), one of the antidepressants known as selective serotonin reuptake inhibitors (SSRIs), can reduce hot flashes in men.

- *The antidepressant venlafaxine (Effexor).* One small trial in 16 men found that the average number and intensity of hot flashes dropped by more than half after 4 weeks on this drug.

- *The antiseizure medicine neurontin (Gabapentin).* Four weeks of high doses (900 milligrams a day) cut the average number and intensity of hot flashes 25 percent more than a placebo in one study.

My dad died from prostate cancer. What can I do to reduce my own risk?

Family history is one of the risk factors for prostate cancer, and some professionals recommend screening exams starting at age 40 if you have a relative with the disease. For more on prostate cancer screening, see "Prostate Exams" on page 331.

Other than getting screened regularly, start by cutting back on red meat and dairy, both of which are linked with an increased risk of prostate cancer. At the same time, boost the amount of cooked vegetables (especially broccoli) and fatty fish you eat and the green tea you drink. One study found that men who drank three cups of green tea a day cut their risk by a whopping 73 percent.

In terms of medications, drugs used to treat prostate enlargement such as finasteride (Proscar) and dutasteride (Avodart) have been shown to reduce the risk of prostate cancer in large clinical trials. Ask your doctor whether you should consider taking one, since you're at increased risk for the disease. There's also intriguing evidence that the cholesterol-lowering drugs known as statins might reduce risk.

Researchers followed 2,447 men for 14 years and found that those who took statins were up to three times less likely to be diagnosed with prostate cancer than those who didn't. They were also less likely to have elevated PSA (prostate specific antigen) levels, which rise when a prostate tumor is present. That doesn't mean you should go out and beg for a statin prescription if you don't need it to lower your cholesterol or reduce your heart disease risk; there's just not enough evidence to warrant it. But if you're already taking a statin, know that it could protect your prostate as well as your heart, probably by reducing inflammation, a known contributor to prostate cancer.

Other drugs that reduce inflammation, such as aspirin and ibuprofen, known as nonsteroidal anti-inflammatory drugs (NSAIDs), appear to lower PSA levels by about 10 percent when taken regularly, according to one recent study, but it's not clear yet whether they lower the risk of prostate cancer. And, of course, taking these drugs long-term comes with risks.

Doctors and researchers used to think that vitamin E and the mineral selenium might help, but a large government study found no benefit to either.

☐ PROSTATE ENLARGEMENT

Does my enlarged prostate mean I'm more likely to develop prostate cancer?

No. There is no evidence that an enlarged prostate increases the risk of prostate cancer.

When is surgery the best bet for an enlarged prostate?

It should be a last resort. For most men, medication is all that's needed to reduce the symptoms of frequent urination, weak stream, and difficulty starting to urinate. Surgery should come into play only if the overgrown prostate is blocking the bladder, preventing you from urinating at all. This can lead to serious complications, including infections and kidney damage. If you find that you're unable to urinate or feel like you have to urinate again soon after you go, you may have some blockage. Other conditions that warrant the knife include blood in the urine and bladder stones, the bladder's version of kidney stones.

WHAT YOU DON'T KNOW

You Don't Have to Treat Your BPH

Unless it's really bothering you and affecting your overall quality of life, you can just live with prostate enlargement, also known as benign prostatic hyperplasia (BPH). In fact, even if you do nothing, it might get better on its own. One review of several studies that followed men with BPH for up to 5 years found that 16 percent had symptoms that never got any worse—and nearly 40 percent improved with no treatment.

What type of surgery is best for an enlarged prostate?

The most commonly performed surgery, and the one with the best track record, is transurethral resection of the prostate, or TURP. The doctor inserts a sharp, looped instrument through the tip of your penis and into the urethra until it reaches the prostate, then uses the loop to strip off the excess prostate tissue and reveal the core of the gland, called the capsule. After surgery, it takes about 6 to 12 weeks for your prostate to grow a new "skin," during which you're vulnerable to bleeding. So no heavy lifting! The procedure takes about 60 to 90 minutes, and you usually stay a day in the hospital to make sure everything is okay. Most men find that the procedure does wonders for restoring normalcy in the bathroom.

An alternative is laser prostatectomy, in which a laser is inserted through the urethra to the prostate and used to destroy the excess tissue. This procedure usually requires an overnight hospital stay. Studies find it's about as effective as TURP with fewer complications, but about 5 percent of men require a second surgery compared with 1 percent of men with TURP.

There are other options, although none have results as good as those with TURP, and some require retreatment as the prostate overgrowth returns.

- *Electro-vascularization.* This is similar to TURP, only instead of cutting away the tissue, the doctor burns it away with a heated roller ball. It's best for men with bleeding disorders or those taking anti-clotting medication.

- *Transurethral microwave therapy (TUMT).* In this outpatient procedure, the doctor inserts a tube with a microwave antenna through the tip of the penis or rectum and uses microwave energy to destroy the prostate overgrowth.

- *Transurethral needle ablation (TUNA).* During this quick outpatient procedure (less than an hour), the doctor uses a tube inserted through the penis and urethra to stick tiny needles into the prostate. Radio waves then heat the needles, destroying the excess tissue. This procedure is a good option for men who don't qualify for surgery or want to make sure nothing happens to their ability to have an erection. However, the results are not as good as with surgery, and you may need a repeat TUNA at some point.

Will surgery for BPH affect my sex life?

It could. Studies find that the risk of erectile dysfunction is about 10 percent with traditional surgeries like TURP, and between 1 and 3 percent with other procedures. But those rates vary considerably, depending on your surgeon's skill. Talk to your doctor about your concerns before surgery. Also ask about the rate of impotence in his patients and if there are specific procedures he can use to reduce the risk.

☐ **PSORIASIS**

Are pills or creams best for psoriasis?

It depends on how serious your disease is. Most people with very mild psoriasis—just a patch here and there—can manage with medications applied to the skin, primarily corticosteroids (though your doctor may choose an injection; a single one can improve a small psoriasis plaque for months), drugs that mimic vitamin D or A, or coal tar.

Generally, however, if you have more extensive disease, topical treatments just don't get the job done (and it's messy to apply that cream everywhere). That's when your doctor will suggest ultraviolet light therapy, also called phototherapy, and systemic medications such as methotrexate (Trexall), acitretin (Soriatane), and hydroxycarbamide (Hydrea), or biologic therapies that target specific components of the immune system, including alefacept (Amevive), etanercept (Enbrel), adalimumab (Humira), ustekinumab (Stelara), and infliximab (Remicade). These come in pills or are given as injections or infusions.

What lifestyle changes can I make to reduce the number of psoriasis flares?

You can slow down and relax, for two reasons. One, stress can trigger a flare. But so can any type of skin injury, such as a cut or scrape you got because you were rushing and fell or bumped into something. Since triggers are different for every person, start by making a list of things you *think* trigger your flares, such as weather conditions, allergens, and specific foods, then avoid them when you can. Also, stay away from beta blockers, lithium, antimalarial drugs, and oral or infused steroids, all of which can make your psoriasis worse.

I have psoriasis and my doctor wants to start me on Remicade. What are the risks and benefits?

Infliximab (Remicade) targets inflammatory substances secreted by certain immune system cells that are linked to psoriasis. The benefits are clear: In several studies, Remicade improved the skin's condition at least 75 percent in as little as 2 weeks compared to just a 3 percent improvement in people taking a placebo. Even better, up to half of participants had nearly

normal skin compared with 1 percent of those receiving a placebo. However, Remicade isn't for everyone. It's used only in people with severe cases because, as an immune-suppressing drug, it may cause life-threatening side effects, including tuberculosis and other lung infections, lymphoma, heart failure, liver damage, and blood disorders. Plus, it requires 2-hour infusions in your doctor's office.

Is it true that having psoriasis raises my risk of heart disease?

Yes, especially if you're a young person with severe psoriasis. The connection: inflammation. In one large study, researchers found that a mild case of psoriasis raised heart attack risk in a 30-year-old by 29 percent; severe psoriasis tripled the risk. For a 60-year-old, a mild case increased risk by 8 percent;

severe psoriasis raised the risk 36 percent. People with psoriasis also have a risk of stroke that's 70 percent higher than that of someone without the condition.

If you have psoriasis, ask your doctor for an hs-CRP (high-sensitivity C-reactive protein) test, which measures a marker of inflammation, and make sure your doctor monitors your cholesterol and blood pressure closely.

☐ **RESTLESS LEGS SYNDROME**

My legs don't move a lot at night but I feel weird, uncomfortable sensations. Could it be from restless legs syndrome?

Most likely it is. The syndrome might be called restless legs, but that restlessness comes from unpleasant sensations in

DRUG-FREE FIX

Weight Loss

If you're significantly overweight and have restless legs syndrome (RLS), the two may be related. One large analysis found that people with a body mass index (BMI) over 30 were nearly one-and-a-half times more likely to have RLS than people with lower BMIs. Another risk factor? Waist size. The bigger your waist, the greater your risk of RLS. The link is the brain chemical dopamine, levels of which are lower in overweight people and those with RLS.

your legs—often described as a burning or creeping or the feeling that insects or small animals are crawling over them. It's these sensations that create the urge to move your legs. Even if you don't move them a lot, that sensation still fits the diagnosis. The other thing to know about restless legs syndrome is that the weird feelings can occur during the day and get worse when you're stressed or lying down, even if you're not trying to sleep.

Don't make light of restless legs syndrome. While it's usually just an annoyance, it could be a sign of iron or folate deficiency, Parkinson's disease, or nerve damage from diabetes. Get your crawly legs checked out.

Are there any drugs to treat restless legs syndrome?

Yes. If your restless legs are caused by low iron levels, expect to take prescription-strength iron supplements. Otherwise, your doctor has a handful of medications to try. Often the drugs doctors turn to if symptoms are moderate to severe are those typically used to treat people with Parkinson's disease, including levodopa (Larodopa, Dopar), pramipexole (Mirapex), and ropinirole (Requip). If symptoms are less severe, your doctor might try an antianxiety drug such as diazepam (Valium), though

these may cause daytime sleepiness. Anticonvulsants, usually used to treat seizure patients, are another option. These include gabapentin (Neurontin) and pregabalin (Lyrica). Side effects may include dizziness and fatigue.

☐ **ROSACEA**

What's the difference between acne and rosacea?

Rosacea usually hits between age 30 and 50. The underlying problem likely involves the blood vessels under the skin. Symptoms include flushing, the appearance of small, broken blood vessels on your face, and, over time, clusters of acnelike bumps on your cheeks and nose, though these are not technically pimples. (The antibiotics that are sometimes prescribed for rosacea are thought to work by fighting inflammation, not bacteria.) If you have acne, you usually have blackheads—the result of clogged pores—which are not present with rosacea. Fluctuating hormone levels likely play a role in acne, which may explain why teenagers and adult women are most at risk. Note that it's possible to have both acne and rosacea at the same time, and that some acne medicines can make rosacea worse.

Are there any natural treatments for rosacea?

Your best bet is to avoid the triggers that cause your flushing and other symptoms. These may include spicy foods, alcohol, stress, harsh soaps, exfoliating products and astringents, washing your face too roughly, hot drinks, and wind and sun exposure.

My eyes feel gritty and are red and watery. Is this related to my rosacea?

Rosacea of the eyes, called ocular rosacea, causes red, swollen, itchy eyes. You may feel as if you always have grit in your eyes. Your eyes may be very sensitive to light, you may develop pustules on or under your eyelids, and your eyelashes may fall out. See a dermatologist or an ophthalmologist if you haven't already.

Self-help measures include humidifying the air at home and work, using artificial tears, and washing your eyelashes with mild baby shampoo (mix a few drops in a cup of warm water). It may also help to place a warm, wet washcloth over your eyes in the morning to unclog tear ducts. In more severe cases, your doctor may plug the tear drainage ducts to keep more fluid in the eye, or destroy the ducts permanently.

I've had rosacea for 10 years now, and the broken blood vessels on my face are making me crazy. What can I do about it?

If medications such as topical or oral antibiotics don't work, a dermatologist or plastic surgeon can attack the broken blood vessels with lasers. Laser therapy can also help with the nose thickening that may occur later in the disease. One small study found that two treatments of pulsed dye laser therapy, the type typically performed, reduced redness 40 to 60 percent and improved flushing, burning, itching, and other symptoms.

Expect to need several treatments, however, and to have some bruising afterward. The bruising is actually a good thing; researchers think it's needed to help reduce the redness and other rosacea symptoms. Laser therapy also stings, although you can probably get by without anesthesia. One caveat: If you've used isotretinoin (Accutane) for your rosacea within the past year, laser surgery is off the table because of an increased risk of scarring.

Another option is intensive pulsed light therapy, which uses a nonlaser light source to minimize broken blood vessels. In one study of 32 patients who underwent one to seven treatments, 83 percent had less redness, 75 percent had less flushing and smoother skin, and 64 percent said they had fewer acnelike breakouts.

☐ **SINUSITIS**

Will antibiotics help my sinusitis?

They could, if your sinusitis was caused by a bacterial infection (viral and fungal infections are other causes), but they're not what your doctor should turn to first. Instead, major medical organizations recommend over-the-counter or prescription decongestants, antihistamines, and saline nasal sprays for acute sinusitis, followed by nasal steroids, if needed, to reduce inflammation and swelling in the sinuses. Antibiotics should be used only in severe cases that don't improve with anything else.

What is the difference between sinusitis and a cold?

While some symptoms are similar—fatigue, feeling run down, congestion—in sinusitis, you also feel pressure, pain, or tenderness behind your ears or cheeks and, in many cases, pain in your teeth and upper jaw. Headache is more common in sinusitis than cold, especially around the eye or temple, as is thick green or yellow mucus. You may also have a fever with sinusitis, which is less likely with a cold.

What are the risks of surgery to relieve my chronic sinusitis?

The primary surgery used to clean out clogged sinuses is functional endoscopic sinus surgery. The surgeon inserts a thin, fiber-optic tube through

AVOID THIS MISTAKE

Turning to Sinus Surgery Too Soon

Sinus surgery probably doesn't work any better for chronic sinusitis than medical treatment coupled with daily saltwater rinses of your sinuses. That's according to one of the only studies to compare the two approaches, in which researchers randomly assigned 90 people with chronic sinusitis to either surgery or medical treatment (3 months of antibiotics, daily nasal rinses with saltwater, and a nasal steroid spray). The message? Make sure you've given everything else time to work before turning to surgery.

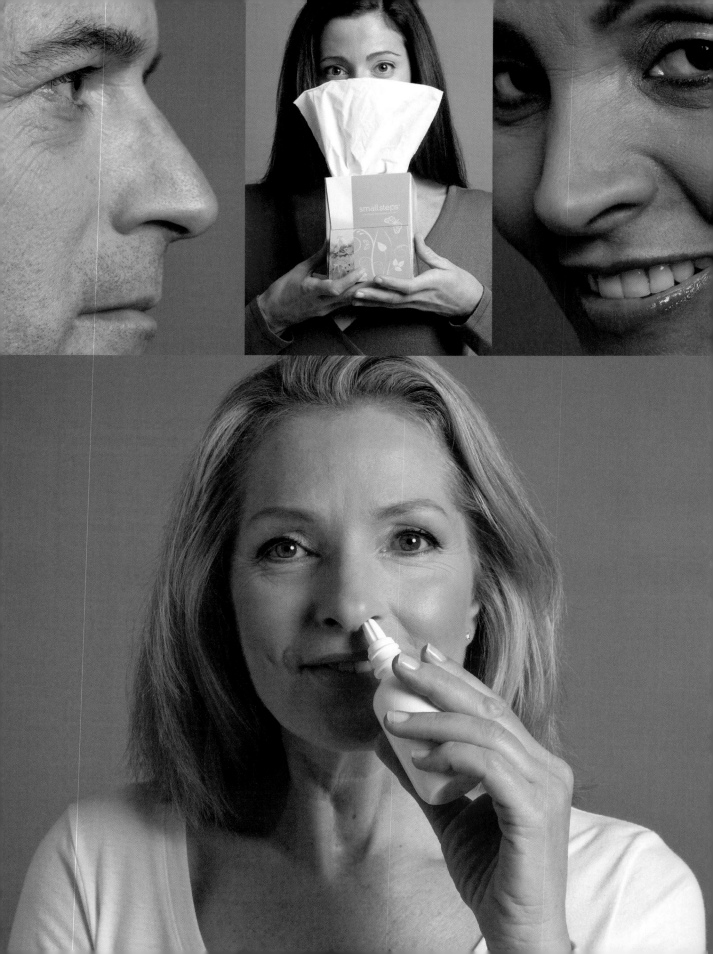

your nose and uses it to feed instruments into the sinus cavities to clear scar tissue and polyps that prevent normal drainage. In severe cases, surgeons use the same infrared technology used to guide the military's so-called smart bombs to make sure they are working in the exact right spot within your sinuses.

Expect some bleeding and discomfort for a few days afterward. Also expect to feel very tired for up to 2 weeks. The greatest risk—albeit a very rare one—is that the surgeon will slip and cut into the brain or optic nerve, both of which are very close to the sinuses.

☐ **SLEEP APNEA**

My husband has sleep apnea and his doctor prescribed a breathing machine, but it keeps both of us up all night. What can we do?

The breathing machine your husband has is called continuous positive airway pressure, or CPAP. It uses air pressure to keep your husband's airways open and prevent the trachea, or breathing tube, from closing or clogging. It is very effective for sleep apnea but, you're right, it can be uncomfortable and even noisy.

Neither of you has to suffer, however. Return to the sleep center where your husband was first fitted and tell the doctor or technician about the problem. A different type of mask or changes in the air pressure can make a huge difference. If your husband has trouble getting used to the mask, have him wear it a few hours during the day when he's in the house. Also have him use the "ramp" setting on the unit so it gradually builds up the air pressure.

Other problems with CPAP and possible solutions include:

- *Nasal congestion.* Spray your nose with a saline solution before bedtime to moisten the tissue. Also add a heated room humidifier or a special CPAP humidifier, available through the sleep center or medical device stores, to moisten the room air. You can also use a nasal decongestant for a few days.

- *Sore throat.* Proper fitting and a humidifier can help.

- *Red eyes or snoring.* The mask isn't fitted properly, leading to air leaks. Return to the sleep center for a refitting or a different type of mask. Also replace the mask and other parts according to the manufacturer recommendations.

- *Rash or other skin problems from mask.* Make sure the mask isn't too tight and is sized properly. Try moleskin or another bandage on the skin under the mask and pads that cover the straps.

My doctor recommended surgery for my sleep apnea. That's scary! Is surgery usually necessary?

Surgery is recommended only for people who can't manage with a CPAP machine or who still have significant symptoms even with CPAP. The most common type of surgery goes by the tongue-twisting name of uvulopalatopharyngoplasty (UPPP). In this procedure, parts of the uvula—the soft tissue that hangs down over your airway—and soft palate are removed, along with your tonsils. It's not terribly effective however, and any improvement usually fades over time. Overall, studies find, surgery just isn't as effective as CPAP.

Are there any options beyond surgery and CPAP?

Yes—through your dentist. People with mild to moderate apnea can use various oral appliances such as a mandibular advancement device, which prevents the jaw from falling down and back during sleep (which causes the tongue to block the throat), and a tongue-retaining device that prevents the tongue from falling back and blocking your airway. Although not as effective as CPAP, they are generally more comfortable and easier to get used to. Ask your sleep specialist for the name of a dental specialist trained in fitting such devices.

Certain lifestyle changes can also help. The most important one is to lose weight if you need to. While it won't cure your sleep apnea, it will improve it significantly. You should also stay away from alcohol, and stop sleeping on your back.

☐ **STROKE**

I think my mother has had a "mini" stroke. What tests does she need?

What used to be called a mini stroke is now referred to by its proper name, transient ischemic stroke, or TIA. The symptoms of TIA resemble those of stroke—numbness or weakness on one side of the body, dizziness or vertigo, and trouble speaking or seeing—but they are temporary and leave no obvious damage behind. That doesn't mean they shouldn't be taken seriously. Your mother has a 10 to 15 percent chance of having a major stroke in the week after a TIA; higher in the weeks and months to follow.

If you think your mother had a TIA, she should see a neurologist who specializes in stroke or be seen at a certified stroke center. Ideally, she should have an MRI or at least a head CT scan within 24 hours of the incident. If it turns out that your mother did have a stroke or TIA, she should receive antiplatelet therapy designed to reduce the risk of blood clots. This can be a daily aspirin (50 to 325 milligrams), a combination of an aspirin and the anticlotting drug dipyridamole (Persantine), or the anticlotting drug clopidogrel (Plavix). Her doctor will determine the best option. She may also receive blood pressure medication, even if her blood pressure is normal. She may need to be hospitalized for a few days so that doctors can monitor her heart and watch for another stroke.

My wife just had a stroke and is in the hospital. When should she start physical therapy?

Ideally, her rehabilitation should begin within a few days of admission. Studies find that starting rehabilitation as soon as people are admitted to the hospital with a stroke significantly improves long-term outcomes. Rehabilitation means more than physical therapy, however. It involves working with you and your wife to set realistic goals, prepare for discharge, and educate you about stroke and stroke prevention. Physical therapy is, of course, critical; one study found that getting 5 extra hours of physical therapy a week in addition to the typical one-hour-a-day, five-days-a-week approach significantly improved stroke patients' ability to walk and use their arms, giving credence to the "more is better" adage when it comes to post-stroke physical therapy.

I had a stroke 2 years ago and I'm terrified of another. What can I do to reduce my risk?

In addition to taking medications to reduce your risk of blood clots and maintain a normal blood pressure, there are numerous lifestyle changes you should have already made to reduce your risk of another stroke.

● *Quit smoking.* Smoking doubles your risk of a stroke, a risk increase that disappears 5 years after you quit.

 AVOID THIS MISTAKE

Using CPAP Only Occasionally

You need to use your continuous positive airway pressure (CPAP) machine every time you sleep, even for naps. And don't forget to pack it (or a smaller version) when you travel.

What Hospital You Choose Matters

Go to a hospital with a dedicated stroke center. Studies find that people treated in such centers are far more likely to receive clot-busting drugs that can prevent death and long-term disability than those seen in emergency departments or by private physicians. If you're over age 60 (when your risk of stroke is greatest), it's worth doing a bit of research to learn which hospitals in your area have certified stroke centers and, if none do, which are connected via telecommunications to a certified stroke center and can provide "telestroke" care—a remote review of your brain scan by a specialist at a stroke center and a videoconference with the doctor at your hospital. You can find a list of certified stroke centers at www.qualitycheck.org/consumer/searchQCR.aspx. Put in your ZIP code, then use the drop-down menu to search for "primary stroke center."

- *Watch your drinking.* If you drink alcohol, you don't have to stop; there's some evidence that a drink or two a day can actually reduce your risk of stroke. Drink any more, however, and you're on your way to another stroke. Studies find that consuming five or more drinks a day increases the risk of stroke by a whopping 60 percent (one drink is 12 ounces of beer, 4 ounces of wine, or 1.5 ounces of liquor).

- *Measure your waist.* If you're Caucasian, more than 40 inches in men and 35 inches in women increases your risk of stroke no matter what your weight or other risk factors. (If you're not Caucasian, check with your doctor about your waist measurement.) The best way to tighten that

measuring tape? Diet and exercise.

- *Increase your heart rate.* Just 30 minutes a day of exercise strenuous enough to get your heart beating faster can reduce your risk of stroke 20 percent. Exercise harder and watch the risk drop another 7 percent. (Check with your doctor about what amount of exercise is right for you.)

Do you have to get to the hospital within 3 hours of a stroke to get that clot-busting drug that can reverse stroke damage?

You're referring to tissue-type plasminogen activator (tPA), the only FDA-approved medication for stroke. The drug has revolutionized the treatment of stroke, slashing the risk of death or severe disability by a third in patients who get it within 3 hours of their first stroke symptoms. Any later, however, and it can increase the risk of dangerous bleeding—or so doctors thought. Now studies find that the drug can be given up to 4.5 hours after stroke symptoms in most patients with no increased risk of bleeding. Still, "time is brain," as stroke doctors like to say. The sooner you get to the hospital, the better.

What if I miss the magic window for clot-busting treatment?

If you're lucky enough to be treated at a stroke center where advanced treatment is available, endovascular surgery may be the best option. In this minimally invasive procedure, doctors thread a tube, called a catheter, through an artery in the groin and all the way up to the site of the clot in the brain. Then they insert a corkscrew-like device to grab the clot and pull it out in order to restore blood flow to the area.

Another procedure, called intra-arterial thrombolysis, involves inserting a tiny tube into the clot and sending clot-busting medicine directly into the clot. The procedure must be performed within 6 hours of stroke symptoms. When done properly on the right patients, it can reduce stroke symptoms by at least 50 percent within the first 24 hours, an improvement so remarkable that doctors call it the Lazarus phenomenon because the patients appear to return from the dead.

Unfortunately, these procedures are all still relatively new and, because of the special training required, are only available at a few regional stroke centers around the country.

☐ THYROID DISORDERS

My doctor says I have an overactive thyroid but I haven't really noticed any of the symptoms. Do you think the diagnosis is wrong?

A blood test to measure levels of thyroid stimulating hormone (TSH) will tell for sure. Low TSH almost always means that you have an overactive thyroid gland, known as hyperthyroidism. Typical symptoms include sudden weight loss, nervousness, excess energy, irregular or rapid heartbeat, sweating, irritability, trembling, feeling hot all the time, problems sleeping, and, sometimes, a swelling at the base of the neck, known as a goiter. Half of all men with hyperthyroidism can't have an erection. But here's the catch: Symptoms in older people may be very subtle and come on

more gradually, so at first, you may not even notice them. Or you might attribute problems such as heat intolerance or a fast heart rate to something else.

What is the difference between Graves' disease and hyperthyroidism?

Graves' disease is a genetic, autoimmune disease in which the immune system produces antibodies that rev up the thyroid gland's production of thyroid hormones. It is the most common cause of hyperthyroidism. People with Graves' disease tend to have an enlarged thyroid gland, or goiter, which appears at the base of their throats, and they may develop eye problems such as double vision, protruding eyes, or irritated eyes. Hyperthyroidism develops for other reasons, typically from

small growths called nodules on the thyroid gland, other autoimmune disorders besides Graves', a virus, taking too much thyroid medication for hypothyroidism, or inflammation of the thyroid, which can occur after pregnancy.

I have thyroid nodules but my doctor says not to worry. Should I worry?

These nodules, which can grow on the thyroid gland, are usually benign (noncancerous) and don't require treatment, unless a large nodule is pressing on your esophagus and interfering with breathing or swallowing or is producing excess thyroid hormone and causing symptoms. In rare instances, however, they are cancerous. To confirm that a nodule is benign, a doctor may order a biopsy (a small needle

WHAT YOU DON'T KNOW

Hypothyroidism May Affect Your Liver

A recent study found a link between liver cancer in women (but not men) who had hypothyroidism for at least 10 years. The researchers compared 420 people with liver cancer to 1,104 healthy people and found that women who had lived with hypothyroidism for at least 10 years were twice as likely to develop the cancer. Thyroid hormones play a major role in the liver, with low thyroid levels increasing the likelihood of "fatty" liver disease, a risk factor for cancer. Plus, people with other risk factors for liver cancer, such as diabetes and hepatitis C, are more likely to have low thyroid levels.

is inserted into the nodule and a sample is taken).

My doctor says I have "subclinical" hyperthyroidism. What does that mean? Do I need medicine?

Subclinical hyperthyroidism is a mild form of hyperthyroidism marked by low levels of thyroid stimulating hormone (TSH) in your blood but normal levels of the two thyroid hormones, T4 and T3. There are usually no symptoms and you wouldn't even know you have it without a blood test. The major risks are bone loss, increased risk of fracture in postmenopausal women, and irregular heartbeat in people over age 60. Thus, preclinical hyperthyroidism is usually treated (with thyroid replacement pills) in older people and in postmenopausal women who are not taking estrogen, while treatment in younger people is dependent on the TSH level and current bone density.

Last year I had hyperthyroidism, and this year I have hypothyroidism. What's going on?

It could be a couple of things. First, get your medication levels checked to make sure that your thyroid production isn't being too suppressed,

which would cause low thyroid levels. If it's not, you could have "silent" or "painless" thyroiditis, in which you first have hyperthyroidism, then hypothyroidism, then you get better, often without treatment. It is thought to be caused by some form of autoimmune disease in which thyroid inflammation stimulates a large release of thyroid hormones. Once that surge of hormone is used up, damaged thyroid cells can't make any more and you plunge into hypothyroidism. Eventually, as the inflammation fades, new thyroid cells grow and the hormone factory whirs to life again. Silent thyroiditis, more common in young women after pregnancy, usually isn't treated unless the symptoms become severe during the hyper phase, which usually lasts for several months. In that case, doctors typically use beta blockers such as propranolol (Inderal) or atenolol (Tenormin) to slow the heart rate, control heart palpitations, and reduce anxiety.

Note that a different type of thyroiditis, called painful thyroiditis, usually occurs after a viral infection and causes pain in the thyroid gland. The front of your throat may be sore to the touch.

☐ **ULCERS**

How do I know for sure if I have an ulcer?

First, the doctor will likely test your blood for the presence of

Helicobacter pylori, the bacterium that causes most ulcers. (The other most common cause of ulcers is taking too much pain medication such as aspirin or ibuprofen.) He may also give you a breath test for *H. pylori.* If you have *H. pylori* and ulcer symptoms—burning or gnawing pain anywhere from your navel to your breastbone that's temporarily relieved by taking an acid-reducing medication—your doctor may just go ahead and treat you for an ulcer.

If necessary, your doctor can get a more definite diagnosis of an ulcer by examining your upper gastrointestinal tract. To do this, he'll put an endoscope, a tube with a camera at the end, down your throat and into your stomach and the upper part of your small intestine. You'll have to fast beforehand. You'll receive an anesthetic and possibly a sedative. Because air is pumped through the tube, you may feel bloated or nauseated afterward, and you may have a sore throat.

I'm taking a daily aspirin to reduce my risk of heart disease but I'm worried about getting an ulcer. How can I protect my stomach?

Ask your doctor if you should consider taking a drug that

reduces the amount of acid your stomach produces. A major study published in the medical journal *The Lancet* found that taking 20 milligrams of famotidine (Pepcid) a day helped prevent ulcers and inflammation of the esophagus in people taking a daily, low-dose aspirin for their hearts. After 12 weeks, the people taking Pepcid were 88 percent less likely to develop an ulcer or inflammation of the esophagus than those taking a placebo. Put another way: Just 5.4 percent of those taking Pepcid developed either condition compared with nearly a third of those receiving a placebo. Don't use this medicine for more than 2 weeks without talking to your doctor, though, since long-term use may cause serious side effects. See page 99 for more information on antacids.

WHAT YOU DON'T KNOW

Acid Blockers May Interfere with Blood Thinners

Researchers recently discovered that proton pump inhibitors (PPIs) commonly used to prevent and treat ulcers, such as omeprazole (Prilosec), esomeprazole (Nexium), pantoprazole (Protonix), and lansoprazole (Prevacid), interfered with the anticlotting effects of clopidogrel (Plavix). The result was a 50 percent increased risk for hospitalization, heart attack, and stroke. Another analysis of the data found that people with diabetes who were taking both drugs had a 44 percent increased risk. The message? If you're taking Plavix and you also need to take a PPI, make sure your doctor knows about the risk and considers other options for your stomach.

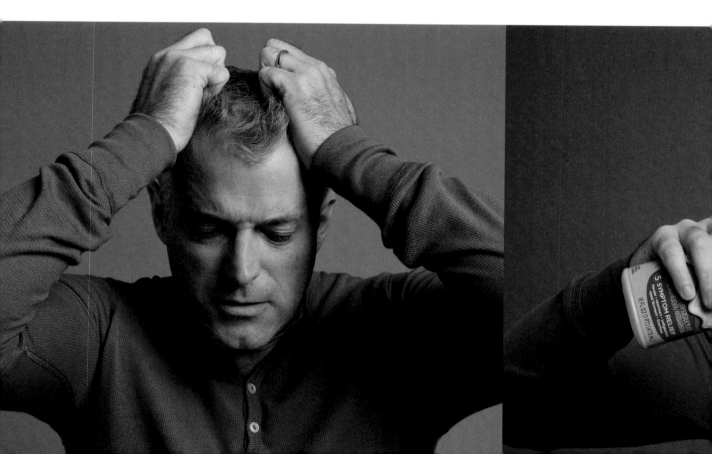

Does eating make an ulcer feel better or worse?

That may depend on where your ulcer is located. Pain from a duodenal ulcer, located in the upper part of the small intestine, often eases right after you eat, only to worsen an hour or two later. Pain from a gastric ulcer, located in the stomach, is often worse after you eat or drink.

Can probiotics prevent or cure ulcers?

They could. There is some evidence that these so-called good bacteria can cling to the stomach lining and prevent *Helicobacter pylori*, the "bad" bacteria responsible for most ulcers, from gaining a toehold. While probiotic supplements don't get rid of the bacteria entirely, they can weaken it. Plus, some studies find that adding probiotics to the traditional three-drug cocktail of antibiotics and proton pump inhibitors typically used to treat ulcers gives the medical treatment an added oomph, increasing the speed at which *H. pylori* bacteria levels drop (a sign of improvement) and reducing side effects.

☐ URINARY TRACT INFECTION

My college-age daughter just told me she is on an antibiotic for her third UTI this year! Why is she getting so many?

It may not be something you want to think about, but the frequent urinary tract infections (UTIs) could be related to sex and alcohol. A study presented at the 2009 American Urological Association meeting compared 181 college women with UTIs to 80 women without infection. Researchers found that recent drinking and

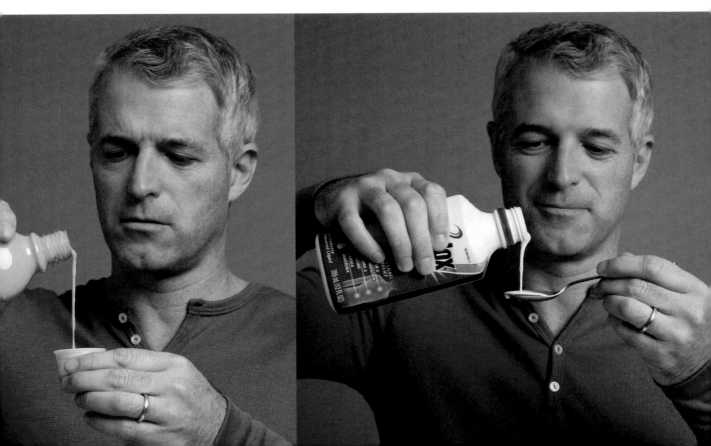

increased sexual activity upped the risk of a UTI, as did using sanitary pads during their periods. Using a diaphragm and spermicide (even condoms treated with spermicide) also increases the risk of UTIs in women with a history of infections.

I have diabetes and get a lot of UTIs. Are the two related?

Yes. Your risk of getting a urinary tract infection (UTI) is more than twice that of someone without diabetes, particularly if you're taking diabetes medicine. The increased risk exists regardless of how well your blood sugar is controlled; it may be related to nerve damage in the bladder that prevents you from fully emptying your bladder, which is an invitation for infection. To help reduce your risk, you should urinate frequently, stay away from spermicides, and, if you get a lot of UTIs, talk to your doctor about taking low doses of antibiotics to prevent them.

How can I reduce my risk of a urinary tract infection?

To prevent infection, urinate after having sex and use a warm, wet washcloth or wipes to clean your vaginal area. Always wipe from front to back after using the bathroom. Wear cotton underwear that breathes rather than nylon underwear that traps moisture. Choose your birth control method carefully; spermicides may increase the risk for infection in some women. You might also try eating yogurt with active cultures several time a week and drinking a large glass of cranberry juice (unsweetened is best) every day.

□ **VARICOSE VEINS**

What can I do about my varicose veins?

Varicose veins don't have to be treated unless they cause pain, blood clots, or skin ulcers (or they're just so ugly that you can't stand it anymore). While surgery to strip out the veins has been the traditional option, today there are several less-invasive approaches, including the ones below.

- *Sclerotherapy.* During this outpatient therapy, the doctor injects liquid or foam into the vein to cause a scar to form, which makes the blood vessel close. It's best for small or medium-size varicose veins (including "spider" veins) and has a rather high recurrence rate, with 65 percent of people requiring treatment again in 5 years. You may need several treatments over several weeks to completely annihilate the vein. It won't work on large varicose veins.

- *Endovenous laser ablation and radiofrequency ablation.* With these procedures, the doctor inserts an instrument into the vein and uses a laser beam or radio waves to destroy it. It can be performed on larger veins and may be done under local anesthesia. You will need 2 to 4 days to recover. Complications include pain, bruising, skin changes, and blood clots.

DRUG-FREE FIX

Weight Loss for UTI Prevention

The heavier you are, the greater your risk of a urinary tract infection (UTI). That's the finding from a study evaluating insurance claims of nearly 100,000 people over 5 years. Obese people were 2½ times more likely to have a UTI and 5 times more likely to have a kidney infection than those who were not obese. The cure? Drop down to a "normal" body mass index below 25.

One analysis of laser procedures, foam sclerotherapy, and vein stripping found that laser procedures were most effective at removing veins, with fewer complications and faster recovery.

Although vein-stripping surgery is rarely performed these days, it still has a place in treatment, particularly for large veins or those that cause skin ulcers. It can be done endoscopically, which involves making one or more small incisions through which tiny instruments can be inserted and used to close off the vein. The surgeon might also tie off the vein and pull it out through the incision. Expect pain, significant bruising, and 1 to 3 weeks of recovery.

My mother had terrible varicose veins. Is there anything I can to make sure I don't get them?

It's a good idea to take precautions, since a family history of varicose veins is a major risk factor for developing them yourself. To reduce your risk:

- *Take breaks.* Standing for long periods of time lets blood pool in your lower legs, putting pressure on blood vessels. Instead, take breaks every 15 minutes or so and sit down with your legs raised.

- *Raise your legs.* When you're sitting or lying down, keep your feet elevated slightly higher than your heart to reduce the risk of blood pooling in your lower legs.

- *Move.* Physical activity that gets your legs moving and strengthens your calf muscles also enhances blood flow.

- *Lose weight.* You'll put less stress on your legs and circulatory system, improving blood flow.

- *Wear flats.* Flat shoes tone calf muscles, which helps move blood through veins and back to the heart.

- *Wear stockings.* Not the sexy black ones, but compression stockings, which apply pressure to the lower part of your legs, forcing blood back toward the heart.

☐ WRINKLES

It's too late for me to stay out of the sun; the damage is done. What else can I do to prevent wrinkles over the next 20 years?

You can still keep out of the sun and slather on sunscreen (and moisturizer) every morning! It's never too late to prevent further skin damage. Also, if you smoke, stop. Smoking is a known cause of

wrinkles and premature skin aging. Heavy smoking and more than 2 hours a day of sun exposure over time makes it about 11 times more likely that you'll develop a faceful of wrinkles compared with someone who doesn't smoke and stayed out of the sun.

You should also sleep differently. So-called sleep lines develop in women who sleep on their stomachs or sides with their faces smushed into the pillow. Instead, try sleeping on your back.

The other option for preventing wrinkles is Botox injections. Botox is a toxin, botulinum, that paralyzes facial muscles, preventing the repeated contractions that can cause wrinkles. But Botox is expensive and the injections must be repeated every few months. Plus, there is little evidence on the long-term effects of repeated injections.

My doctor's office is now advertising the services of a dermatologist who performs cosmetic procedures. Will my face really look better if I spend an hour or so there?

Today there are numerous cosmetic and dermatologic procedures that can be performed in a doctor's office, including Botox injections to smooth

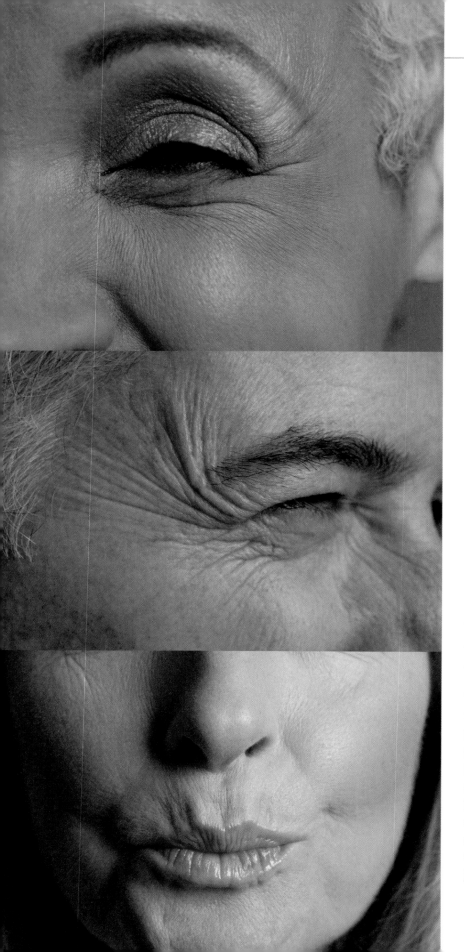

wrinkles, collagen injections to plump up deflated areas, and laser surgery to reduce blood vessels and brown spots. Some procedures, such as microdermabrasion and chemical peels, can even be performed by an aesthetician or other non-MD under a physician's guidance, depending on your state's regulations.

Just because these procedures are done in a doctor's office in less than an hour doesn't mean they are risk-free, however. All have risks, including burning, allergic reactions, bruising, swelling, and redness. And many are temporary; they need to be repeated periodically to maintain the effect. Plus, none are covered by health insurance, so expect to ante up several hundred dollars or more for each procedure.

☐ YEAST INFECTION

I was just diagnosed with a yeast infection during a routine exam. How could I have this and not know it?

Many women have no symptoms of a yeast infection. There is often little or no discharge, and the main symptom is itching. It's much easier for your doctor to spot the signs of swelling and redness in the vulval area (the folds of skin just outside the entrance to your vagina) than for you—not a place that's easy to check out yourself.

Can probiotics help prevent yeast infections?

It looks doubtful. Probiotics are beneficial bacteria, and some women take supplements of them to help prevent a yeast infection after a course of antibiotics, which wipes out good and bad bacteria alike. Without enough good bacteria, fungi that cause yeast infections can gain traction. However, there is no good evidence that probiotics help prevent yeast infections. One study of 235 women prescribed antibiotics found that neither oral nor vaginal probiotics affected their risk of developing a yeast infection during or after their antibiotic treatment. If you're prone to yeast infections while taking antibiotics, ask your doctor to prescribe a dose of the antifungal drug fluconazole (Diflucan) when you start and at the end of the medication course.

AVOID THIS MISTAKE

Diagnosing Your Own Yeast Infection

Yes, the itching and discharge could be a yeast infection—but it might not be. In one study of 95 women who diagnosed themselves, testing showed that just a third actually had a yeast infection; the rest had various other vaginal infections. Pay a visit to your doctor for the correct diagnosis.

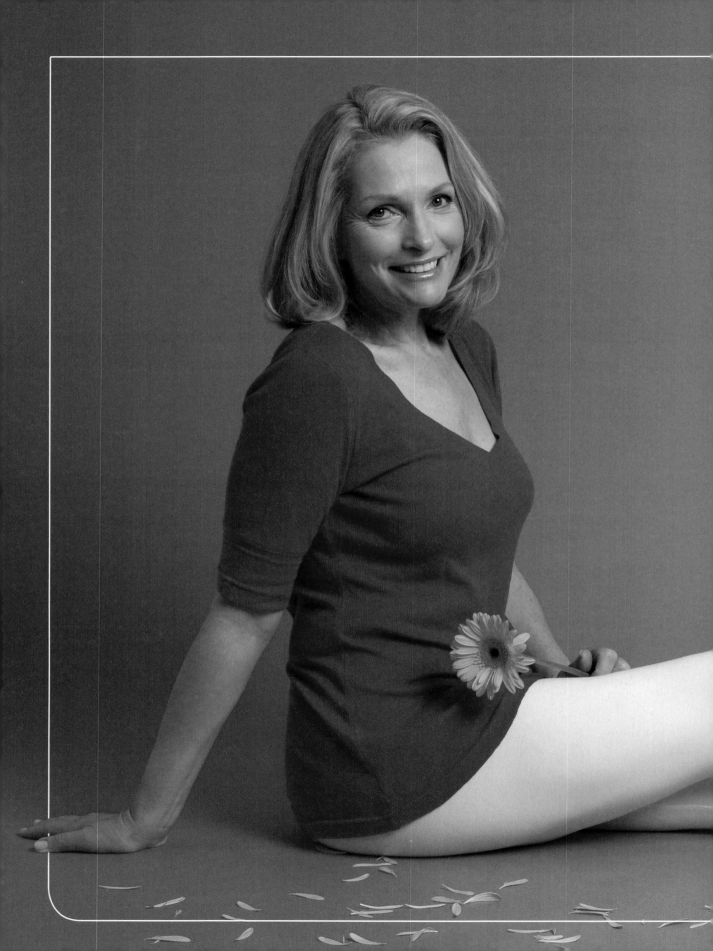

PART FOUR

Medical Tests

From cholesterol tests to colonoscopies, bone scans to mammograms, answers to your questions about being poked and prodded and what it all means.

FAQ Frequently Asked Questions
Medical Tests

My doctor orders a lot of tests. How do I know if they're really necessary?

Although many medical tests provide valuable information, studies show that doctors often order exams that are not likely to detect diseases. There are several reasons why doctors may order a test you don't need.

- *To meet your expectations.* Patients often assume that they need expensive tests; some doctors comply.

- *To avoid getting sued.* Critics charge that too many doctors practice "defensive medicine," that is, they order tests to stay out of court if a patient becomes sicker.

- *They don't know the guidelines.* Busy doctors aren't always able to keep up with changes in guidelines for screening and diagnosing diseases. Or they may simply order a test out of habit.

- *They stand to profit.* If a doctor owns the lab where he sends you for a blood test, he makes money.

If you're concerned about a particular test, ask your doctor why he thinks you need it, exactly what he hopes to learn from it, and how that information might affect the course of your treatment. If you're not satisfied with the responses, seek a second opinion, especially if the test is invasive or involves a lot of radiation (which CT scans do). Ultimately, it's your right as a patient to refuse the test.

If your doctor has ordered a preventive screening test, such as a Pap smear, a colonoscopy, a fasting glucose test, or an exercise stress test, you can find out what scientists have to say about its usefulness for different groups of people on the U.S. Preventive Services Task Force web site (www.ahrq.gov/CLINIC/uspstfix.htm).

Should I ask my doctor for a copy of my test results?

Yes. It's your right to request and receive copies of your test results and other medical records, though sometimes you may need to pay a small fee. And it's a good idea to make such requests: Everyone should keep a personal medical history, and test results are an important part of it. Don't rely on your doctor to maintain a full set of your test results. If a doctor moves, goes out of business, or retires, it may be difficult for you to obtain your records. Keeping your own set ensures that you will be able to provide your new doctor with all of your essential medical information.

Is it okay to use a home medical test instead of going to my doctor's office?

You shouldn't use a home medical test to self-diagnose

any condition. (If you think you're sick, go to the doctor.) But it's okay to use certain tests to monitor an existing condition. Diabetes patients do so routinely when they check their blood glucose levels. And people with high blood pressure who check their blood pressure readings at home in addition to getting it checked at the doctor's tend to have healthier blood pressure levels than people who don't.

You can also purchase home tests for high cholesterol, colon cancer (the fecal occult blood test), infertility, and many other conditions. You can even test your teen for drug use, and find out when you're ovulating. If you decide to use one of these tests, the FDA recommends following these rules:

- *Read all of the instructions carefully* and be certain you know how to perform the test and interpret the results.

- *Store the test properly before you use it;* follow all instructions for collecting and storing the sample.

- *Be aware of what factors might affect the test results.*

- *Check the test's expiration date,* and don't use the test if it's expired.

- *Use only tests regulated by the FDA.*

- *Keep records of your test results.*

- *Don't change your dosage of medication* or otherwise

Sports Drinks Are Better Than Water before a Colonoscopy

The day before a colonoscopy, you must clean out your colon. During this "bowel preparation," you guzzle up to a gallon of formula containing laxatives. Because this process can leave you dehydrated, it's essential to drink plenty of other fluids, too (64 ounces is a good goal). Studies show that patients are less likely to become dehydrated and do a better job of emptying their bowels if they drink Gatorade or other carbohydrate-based sports drink instead of clear fluids such as water. Choose a light-colored variety, such as lemon-lime flavor. Avoid red beverages, which can look like blood during the exam. (People with diabetes should check with their doctors before consuming sports drinks.)

alter your treatment plan based on the result of a home test without talking to your doctor.

Any worrisome test result should be followed up with a visit (or at least a phone call) to your doctor. It's also important to see your doctor for regularly scheduled checkups, no matter what your home test results tell you.

Why do I have to fast before some tests but not others?

Having food in your system can skew the results of certain medical tests, but not others. The most common types of exams that require fasting include:

- *Blood glucose tests.* Elevated blood glucose, or blood sugar, is a sign of diabetes.

Eating a meal that contains carbohydrates causes blood sugar to rise. If you're healthy, your blood sugar drops back to normal within a few hours. But if you have diabetes, your blood sugar remains high. The fasting plasma glucose (FPG) test, one of the tests used to diagnose diabetes, is designed to measure a person's blood sugar on an empty stomach. That's why you can't eat for 8 hours before the having this test.

- *Cholesterol/triglycerides tests.* Lipids are blood fats such as cholesterol and triglycerides that can increase the risk for heart disease. To measure LDL cholesterol, the "bad" kind, labs use a formula that requires measuring your total, HDL ("good") cholesterol, and triglycerides. Your triglycerides rise as much as 20 to 30 percent immediately after a meal, so you need to fast for 12 hours prior to having a cholesterol test that includes triglycerides. Alcohol boosts triglycerides, too, so avoid booze for 24 hours beforehand.

● *Colonoscopies and other GI exams.* Colonoscopies, sigmoidoscopies, abdominal ultrasounds, and upper GI exams use imaging devices to search for cancerous tumors and other evidence of disease in the digestive tract. Having food in your intestines or stomach could block the doctor's view, which is why patients are asked to fast prior to the exam (and, often, to use strong laxatives).

Should I have a genetic test to see if I'm at risk for cancer?

If you have a family history of cancer, such as a parent or sibling who had it, it may make sense. Keep in mind that if you choose to be tested, it's essential to consult with a genetic counselor before *and* after you learn your results. The counselor can explain all aspects of the test, particularly what the results mean. A positive test result is not a death sentence, and a negative result doesn't mean you're home free.

For instance, consider the test for mutations on the BRCA1 and

BRCA2 genes, which indicate an increased risk for breast cancer. If a test reveals that a woman has one of these mutations, she has about a 60 percent chance of developing breast cancer in her lifetime, which is five times higher than a woman who lacks these gene mutations. However, there's no guarantee that she'll develop cancer. Likewise, a negative test result does not mean a woman won't develop cancer, since other gene mutations and lifestyle choices appear to boost the risk for breast cancer, too.

If you don't have a family history of cancer, there's little to be gained from undergoing genetic testing—and potentially some harm. There is no solid evidence that knowing your genetic status will bring any health benefit. Furthermore, because genetic tests don't always offer clear-cut results, you could be exposed to unnecessary treatments that can cause serious side effects. For

instance, the test for BRCA1 and BRCA2 produces ambiguous results 13 percent of the time. Many women who have unclear results do not have an increased risk for breast cancer, yet their doctors may prescribe the drug tamoxifen to help prevent the disease. But taking this drug also makes you more likely to suffer blood clots, develop endometrial cancer, and experience hot flashes.

Should I worry about false-negatives and false-positives?

Don't let your concerns keep you from having needed exams, but keep in mind that almost any clinical test can produce inaccurate results, known as false-negatives and false-positives. A false-negative result occurs when a test fails to detect the presence of a disease. That is, it gives the mistaken impression that a sick person is healthy. A false-positive result occurs when a test detects evidence of a disease where none exists. In other words, it gives the mistaken impression that a healthy person may be sick.

Just about any medical test is capable of producing false-negative and false-positive results, though some tests produce more incorrect or misleading results than others. A false-negative test result can delay detection of a disease, which could prove fatal. False-positive results often lead to unnecessary additional tests, which may be inconvenient, stressful, and painful.

Some commonly used medical tests produce a fairly high portion of incorrect results. For instance, exercise stress testing to detect evidence of cardiovascular disease produces more

false-positives than accurate results in people who have no symptoms of heart trouble. What's more, the lower your risk for a disease, the more likely a positive result is incorrect— a good reason not to ask your physician to order a test "just to make sure." If your doctor wants you to have a medical test, ask about the chances that it will produce a false-negative or false-positive result.

I just had a medical test and my numbers are a little high, but my doctor hasn't done anything. Is that okay?

Sometimes taking no action is the best treatment option,

even when medical tests suggest that a disease may have developed or be worsening. It may simply be that your numbers have not yet risen high enough for you to require an intervention, such as a drug prescription or surgery. However, if the test in question is known to produce a large number of false-positives, your physician may be waiting to see the results from your next round of tests. Also, your high numbers may be a fluke, artificially boosted by something you ate, stress, or some other influence. Many diseases develop slowly, in which case a period of "watchful waiting" is unlikely to do any harm. But don't remain in the dark: If your doctor seems unconcerned about your rising numbers, ask why.

Medical Tests

☐ ALLERGY TESTS

Can a skin prick test diagnose a food allergy?

Skin prick testing, which involves inserting a tiny amount of food extract beneath the patient's skin to see if swelling and redness develop, correctly identifies about 85 percent of people who have a food allergy. The trouble is that it produces a false-positive result—that is, it indicates a food allergy when there isn't one—roughly 60 percent of the time. That's why a positive skin prick test isn't enough to pinpoint which food is causing an allergy. Doctors will consider the history provided by the patient and may perform further tests. These include blood tests such as RAST (radioallergosorbent test), which determine whether a patient's immune system is producing antibodies to a specific food, and a food challenge test, in which the patient swallows capsules containing a suspect food to see if she has a reaction.

Before giving you a skin prick test, your doctor may want you to keep a detailed diary for a few weeks in which you write down everything you eat and any symptoms you develop. The doctor may also ask you to follow an elimination diet that omits certain food groups (such as dairy or wheat) for a few more weeks to see if your allergy symptoms go away.

I had a blood test for my allergies, but my friend was given a skin test for hers. Why?

Blood tests can be less sensitive than skin prick tests, but they're more convenient (though it takes longer to get the results). Also, skin tests, which require training to administer, are usually performed by allergists, whereas a general practitioner is more likely to order a blood test. Finally, some medications can interfere with a skin test result (see "I'm having a skin

All Food Reactions Are Allergies

Fiction. Many food "allergies" are actually a food intolerance. True food allergies occur when the immune system mistakes a specific food or ingredient for a toxin, so it produces antibodies to attack it, causing symptoms such as hives, swelling, and gastrointestinal problems. Food intolerance does not involve the immune system. Lactose intolerance, caused by an enzyme deficiency, is a classic example. In other cases, some people are sensitive to specific foods such as the artificial sweetener sorbitol and preservatives called sulfites (used in dried fruits and wine). In general, food intolerance is far less dangerous than food allergy.

prick test for my hay fever. Do I have to stop taking my allergy medicine?" below). If a doctor doesn't think that you should stop taking the medicine in order to have a skin test, a blood test is a good alternative.

I'm having a skin prick test for my hay fever. Do I have to stop taking my allergy medicine?

A skin prick test can help you determine what you're allergic to so you can try to avoid it. You need to stop taking certain allergy medications, as well as other drugs, before having one. Antihistamines could distort the results by masking an allergic reaction. Stop taking second-generation (non-drowsy) antihistamines such as loratadine (Claritin) 3 to 10 days

before your test. If you use older antihistamines, such as diphenhydramine (Benadryl), stop taking them 2 to 3 days prior to testing.

Just before your test, you may also need to stop taking certain other medications that behave like antihistamines, including drugs used to treat heartburn and ulcers, tranquilizers, older antidepressants, and many others. Check with your doctor.

Stethoscopes Are Germ Magnets

Fact. The stainless steel chest piece of a stethoscope may look clean, but many are swarming with microbial baddies. In one Israeli study, researchers checked 55 stethoscopes belonging to pediatricians and found that 85 percent harbored *Staphylococci* bacteria, including the strain that causes staph infections. Before examining you, your doctor should not only wash her hands but also clean her stethoscope's chest piece with an alcohol wipe.

☐ ANNUAL PHYSICAL

Do I really need a physical every year?

We've all heard stories of people who were diagnosed with a deadly disease just days or weeks after getting a clean bill of health from an annual physical. Clearly, these exams don't reveal everything about what's going on in your body. And if you're generally healthy and feel fine, you may not need them. In theory, annual physicals offer a way for doctors to detect diseases in early stages, when they respond better to treatment. Yet there's surprisingly little evidence that people who see a doctor once a year get sick less often or live longer. The United States Preventive Services Task Force does not recommend routine annual physicals.

Doctors who defend the annual physical say the visit gives them a chance not only to detect potential signs of

Decoding the Annual Physical

There are no standard guidelines for how doctors should conduct routine physical examinations. However, most physicians include the following.

What Your Doctor Will Do	What the Clues Mean
Take your blood pressure	A pressure of lower than 120/80 is your goal.
Take your temperature	Don't worry if it's not 98.6°F; a little higher or lower is still healthy.
Take your pulse	Between 60 and 100 is acceptable. People who are very fit may have a heart rate lower than 60.
Check your respiration rate	If you take more than 20 breaths per minute, you may have a heart or lung condition.
Auscultation	By listening to your body (heart, lungs, intestines) with a stethoscope, your doctor can check for heart murmurs, irregular heartbeat, and other signs of trouble. But auscultation rarely detects evidence of disease.
Palpation and percussion	In theory, tapping your body at specific sites could reveal that your liver is enlarged, for instance, and testing your reflexes with a tap on the knee could detect signs of nerve damage. But these tests almost never find anything wrong.
Give you a good once-over	Doctors can tell a lot about a patient's health just by looking him over head to toe. Your skin can reveal signs of skin cancer; your fingernails can reveal evidence of heart disease and diabetes; and dry skin and brittle hair may indicate an underactive thyroid.
Look in your mouth, eyes, and ears	When a doctor asks you to say "ah," it's to check your gums, throat, tonsils, and other oral structures for signs of trouble. He will likely use an ophthalmoscope to peer into your eyes and an otoscope to check your ears, too.

trouble but also to talk about ways patients can cut their disease risk (though not all doctors actually do). It's an opportunity for the doctor to perform screening tests, such as a digital rectal exam for men and breast exam for women, and to administer or schedule any necessary vaccinations.

The doctor may draw blood and ask the lab to do a complete blood count (CBC) to assess the quantity and quality of cells in your blood, specifically white blood cells, red blood cells, and platelets. But research suggests that the CBC rarely turns up any signs of trouble. A Mayo Clinic study of 1,508 lab tests found that less than 1 percent of the CBCs provided any valuable information. In another study,

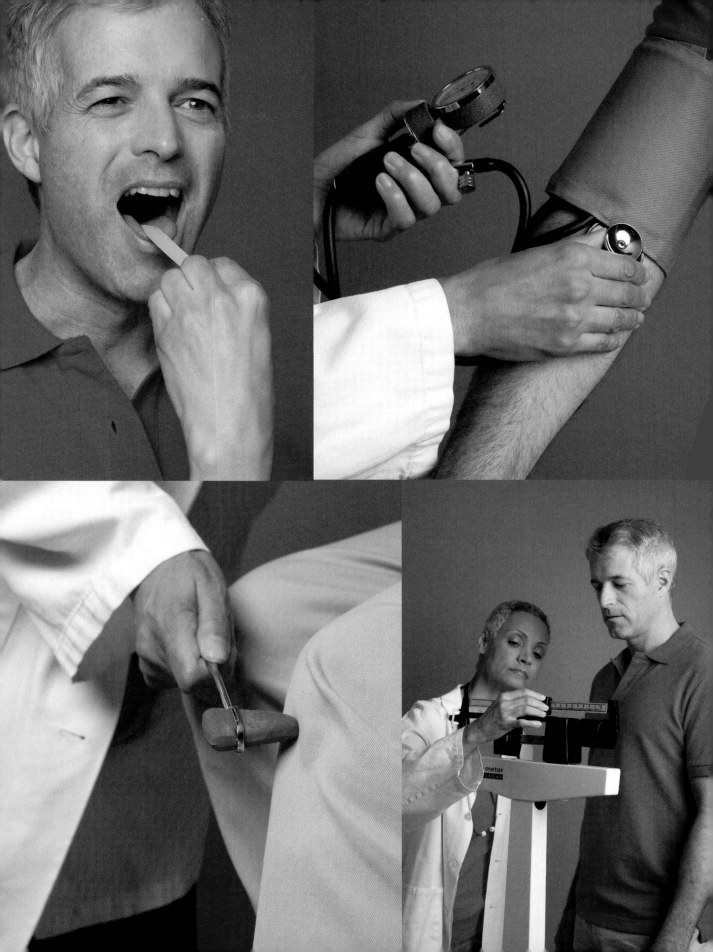

Swiss researchers looked at the records of 1,540 patients who had routine CBCs; just three of the tests found any evidence of a condition that needed treatment. (In each case, the patient had iron deficiency.) Some doctors also use urinalysis, electrocardiogram (EKG), or x-rays as screening tools, but the U.S. government has determined that there is no benefit to performing them on a person who has no symptoms, since they rarely turn up any bad news.

If nothing else, studies show that people who get annual physicals worry less about their health. The best advice? Talk to your doctor and decide how often you should drop in for a routine exam based on your age, sex, and overall health.

☐ ASTHMA TESTS

I've been coughing and wheezing a lot, and I'm always out of breath. Can a test determine whether I have asthma?

Based on your symptoms, there's a good chance that you have asthma, though some doctors will order certain tests to help confirm the diagnosis and rule out other conditions, such as pneumonia or bronchitis. After examining you and taking your medical history, your doctor may give you a spirometry

test. You simply take a deep breath and blow as hard as you can into a machine that records how much air you can inhale and exhale and how fast you can move air through your lungs. If your readings are low for a person of your age, your doctor may ask you to inhale medicine that opens blocked airways. If you perform better on a second spirometry test, and your other signs and symptoms agree with the diagnosis, then you probably have asthma.

☐ BLOOD PRESSURE TESTS

Why did my doctor send me home with this gizmo for measuring my blood pressure?

That gizmo, known as an ambulatory blood pressure monitor (ABPM), provides more accurate information about your blood pressure than a doctor can obtain during an office visit. An ABPM is a blood pressure cuff that's strapped to one arm and attached to a battery-operated monitor worn on the hip. It records your blood pressure repeatedly throughout the day. Patients are usually instructed to wear an ABPM for a day or two.

Doctors often ask patients to wear an ABPM if they suspect "white coat hypertension," or blood pressure that rises artificially due to anxiety during office visits, which occurs in

10 to 20 percent of patients. Many studies show that blood pressure readings from ABPMs are more accurate than those taken in doctor's offices. In fact, some patients initially prescribed blood pressure medication based on measurements taken during office visits are able to stop or lower their dosage after having an ABPM reading. Doctors also use an ABPM to find out if a patient's blood pressure fails to dip at night (as it should) or "surges" in the morning (as it shouldn't); both increase the risk of heart attacks, strokes, and other dangers.

How can I lower my blood pressure reading in the doctor's office?

If possible, sit quietly for several minutes with your feet on the floor (not dangling from the exam table) and take very slow, deep breaths to calm yourself down before your doctor checks your blood pressure.

☐ BLOOD TESTS

Some of the lab results on my last blood test were flagged as abnormal, but my doctor hasn't said anything. Why?

One possibility is that your results were only slightly higher or lower than normal, so your doctor doesn't think there is anything to worry about. A lab report usually lists your test results in one column, next to a column indicating the "reference range," or the range of test values that are considered normal. An abnormal result may mean that you're sick. For instance, an elevated white blood cell count is a sign that you may have an infection, or could even indicate the presence of cancer, while a low count may mean you have a viral infection that affects bone marrow function, a severe infection, cancer of the bone marrow, or certain other conditions. However, a typical complete blood count (CBC) test includes 9 or 10 different measurements of your blood cells' quantity and quality. Even if you're completely healthy, there's about a 50 percent chance that at least one result will be outside the normal range. If some of your numbers are bit off, but you're otherwise in good shape, there's probably no cause for concern—but it can't hurt to ask your doctor for some reassurance.

□ **BONE DENSITY SCANS**

When should I start having bone scans? How often do I need one?

Schedule your first bone scan—which measures the risk for osteoporosis, or fragile bones—right away if you

fall into one of these two categories:
* You are a woman age 65 or older.
* You are a woman over age 60 and you have one or more risk factors for osteoporosis (common risk factors include a family history of bone fractures, smoking, low body weight, and the use of certain drugs). Some doctors advise women with these risk factors to begin screening earlier, after reaching menopause.

Your doctor may recommend a bone mineral density test at a younger age if:
* You have used medications for an extended period that promote bone loss, including steroids (such as prednisone and cortisone), certain antiseizure medications, the contraceptive Depo-Provera, and certain breast cancer therapies—specifically, aromatase inhibitors such as anastrozole (Arimidex).
* You have an overactive thyroid gland (or take high doses of thyroid hormone medication) or overactive parathyroid gland.
* You have a condition that can cause bone loss, such as rheumatoid arthritis or anorexia nervosa.
* You have had other medical tests (such as x-rays) indicating bone loss or fracture of the spine.
* You have experienced early menopause.
* You have lost a significant amount of height.

It's less clear whether routine screening is helpful for men. Some doctors recommend bone scans for men age 70 and older, as well as men over age 50 who have one or more risk factors for osteoporosis.

How often you should return for follow-up bone scans is a matter of debate. If you are at high risk for osteoporosis, your doctor may suggest that you return as often as once a year. Yet other experts point out that it takes at least 2 years for any measurable change to occur in bone density, and that there's no evidence that people who have frequent scans have fewer bone fractures. If your baseline bone scan looks good and you don't have any major risk factors for osteoporosis, your doctor may suggest returning for a follow-up in 3 to 5 years.

Can I have my bone density checked by heel ultrasound or pDXA instead of DXA?

Central DXA is the gold standard for measuring bone density, meaning that it's the best tool doctors have for detecting osteoporosis. In a central DXA (dual-energy x-ray absorptiometry) exam, the patient lies on a table as x-rays measure the density of her spine and hips. The results of a central DXA exam offer doctors the most accurate information about your risk for bone fractures due to loss of bone mineral, the cause of osteoporosis. However, central DXA scanners are large and expensive, so some smaller clinics use alternative methods to measure bone density in the forearm, wrist, finger, or heel. Some of these devices use x-rays (known as peripheral DXA, or pDXA), while others use ultrasound and other imaging technologies. It's okay to have your bone density measured with one of these devices if they are all that's available in your community. However, any abnormal results should be confirmed by central DXA before a doctor diagnoses osteoporosis.

I'm a man with asthma, and I've taken inhaled steroids for decades. Do I need a bone scan now?

Inhaled corticosteroids are one of the most effective treatments for asthma. Unfortunately, these drugs can interfere with cells called osteoblasts, which are needed to form bone mineral. If you have been taking moderate to high doses of inhaled corticosteroids for more than a few years, your bones may be more fragile—and vulnerable to fractures—than would be expected for the average person your age, so you may be at risk for osteoporosis. You may be at even greater risk for bone loss if your asthma has been difficult to control and you have required frequent use of oral steroids to treat severe flare-ups. There are no official guidelines for when users of inhaled corticosteroids should have bone scans, so ask your doctor.

☐ CHOLESTEROL TESTS

If my ratio of total cholesterol to HDL is low, do I still need to worry about a high LDL level?

A low ratio of total cholesterol to HDL ("good") cholesterol is a big plus. It means that your HDL levels are high relative to your total cholesterol. As you may know, HDL scoops up the "bad" LDL cholesterol that clogs arteries and carries it to the liver, where it is processed and eliminated. But even if your HDL levels are high, in many cases, a doctor will still want to see you lower your total and LDL ("bad") cholesterol.

People who have a lot of HDL relative to their total cholesterol are guarded against heart attacks and strokes. For instance, let's say you're a man with a total cholesterol of 200, which is the threshold at which doctors begin to worry. If your

"Bad" Cholesterol: How Low Should You Go?

Whether or not you need drugs and dietary changes to lower your LDL cholesterol—the "bad" kind that increases the risk for heart disease—depends on your overall risk of suffering a heart attack. Your risk is *high* if you have already had a heart attack, you have blood vessel disease (such as peripheral artery disease), or you have diabetes. Your risk is *moderate* if you have two or more risk factors for heart disease, such as obesity, a strong family history of the disease, or smoking). Your risk is *low* if you have one or no risk factors.

If Your Risk for Heart Attack and Stroke Is:	Your LDL Goal (mg/dL) Should Be:
High	100 or lower
Moderate	101–130
Low	131–160

HDL cholesterol is 40—not terribly low, but nothing to brag about—that makes your ratio 5, which means you have an average risk for cardiovascular disease. However, if your HDL cholesterol is a robust 59, your ratio would be 3.4, which cuts the risk for heart disease in half. The flip side: A ratio greater than 5 increases your risk. (Women naturally have higher HDL levels, so a ratio of 4.4 for them confers an average risk; a ratio of 3.3 cuts risk in half.)

If you're under age 40 and a high LDL level is your only risk factor for heart disease—but your HDL is high, too—your doctor may decide that you don't need medications such as statin drugs, since your good cholesterol cancels out the threat. However, if you are over age 40 and have other risk factors, such as diabetes or obesity, your doctor will probably prescribe drugs with the goal of lowering your LDL to below 100 mg/dL (milligrams per deciliter).

I keep reading about VLDL cholesterol. Should I have mine tested?

You probably already have. Very low density lipoprotein (VLDL) is usually measured in the blood test you have as part of a routine physical exam.

Cholesterol travels through the bloodstream in bubbles called lipoproteins. These bubbles also contain triglyceride,

Yesterday's Omelet Will Skew Today's Cholesterol Test

Fiction. Eating eggs may cause your blood levels of cholesterol to rise following a meal, but they return to normal within a few hours. But skip the omelet, and everything else but water, on the day you go to the lab to have blood drawn. The usual recommendation is to fast for at least 8 hours before having your cholesterol checked. It helps to schedule your appointment for first thing in the morning.

another type of blood fat. Different bubbles contain different amounts of these substances. VLDLs contain large amounts of triglycerides, which raise the risk of heart disease just as LDLs do. Knowing your VLDL may help your doctor fine-tune a treatment plan if you are a patient at risk for heart disease.

☐ COLON CANCER TESTS

Is preparation for a colonoscopy as bad as I've heard?

Few people have much good to say about the "bowel prep" required to clean out your colon before a colonoscopy. In general, solid foods are off-limits the day before the exam, though you can sip clear broth and juice. You also need to take powerful laxatives. That often means drinking up to a gallon of fruit-flavored—but still hard-to-swallow—solution containing a substance called polyethylene glycol. (Some

doctors prescribe other laxatives.) Finally, your doctor will probably instruct you to give yourself an enema. Plan on staying close to home once you start your bowel prep, and keep this in mind: Failure to fully clean out your bowel may interfere with the colonoscopy results, meaning you'll have to repeat the procedure.

Most patients find the colonoscopy itself to be relatively painless. In fact, many sleep through it, since patients receive a sedative beforehand to help them relax. To perform a standard colonoscopy, a doctor inserts a slender scope through the rectum and guides it into the large intestine. The scope sends real-time images to a monitor, allowing the doctor to look for colon tumors, polyps (nublike growths that can become cancer), and other signs of trouble. During the exam, you may feel an urge to defecate or a sensation of pressure or fullness. Otherwise, many patients report that colonoscopies are hardly the ordeal they expected.

Is a "virtual" colonoscopy as accurate as a standard colonoscopy?

Not quite, though they are becoming more reliable. Also known as CT (computed tomography) colonography, the virtual colonoscopy is a newer alternative to the standard exam that's less invasive and doesn't require sedation. In a virtual colonoscopy, the patient lies on a table that passes through a CT scanner. The scanner takes multiple pictures that are transformed on the computer into detailed 3-D images of your large intestine, eliminating the need for a scope.

Some early studies found that virtual colonoscopies missed half or more of abnormal growths that would be detected by the traditional exam, possibly because doctors were still learning how to use the technology. However, in the most recent and largest study comparing the two methods, virtual colonoscopies were about 90 percent as accurate as standard colonoscopies for detecting large polyps.

Some people who loathe traditional colonoscopies may be willing to trade a bit of accuracy for less discomfort and inconvenience, such as needing a ride to and from the procedure and taking an entire day off from work (since your doctor will want you to go home and rest while the sedatives wear off)—but you still have to undergo the same bowel-cleansing process required for traditional colonoscopy. Virtual colonoscopies also eliminate the small risk of complications with traditional colonoscopies, which can include bleeding and punctures. The American Cancer Society has given its approval to virtual colonoscopies. But keep these facts in mind:

- Virtual colonoscopies are still significantly less effective for detecting small polyps; in the most recent study, they found 78 percent of those detected by the standard technique.

- If the CT scans show a suspicious growth, you will need a standard colonoscopy to have it removed.

- About 14 percent of suspicious spots on a virtual colonoscopy are false alarms, but require additional tests anyway.

- CT scans use x-rays and expose you to a relatively high level of radiation.

- Virtual colonoscopies must be repeated every 5 years, instead of every 10 years for traditional colonoscopy.

- This new procedure is less invasive, but still requires the insertion of a tube a few inches into the rectum, which fills the colon with air to improve the image.

I still don't like the idea of any type of colonoscopy. Can't I just have a fecal occult blood test instead?

You can, but these tests are not as accurate as colonoscopies, though they are improving. Colon tumors and precancerous polyps can bleed, so the fecal occult blood test FOBT looks for hidden ("occult") blood in a stool sample. For years, the most commonly used FOBT was something called the stool guaiac smear test, which used chemically sensitive paper to detect blood. A doctor can perform this test during an office exam, though there is a home version, too. (Tests use various strategies for obtaining stool samples; one type provides special toilet paper, which you use, then ship to a lab.) A newer type of test does not require you to obtain a stool sample. Instead, you toss a flushable pad into the toilet following a bowel movement and note whether the pad's color changes on a card, which you mail back to a lab. However, some critics say this test is flawed because the color changes can be too subtle to notice.

A bigger concern about the FOBT is that a single test is not very sensitive, probably because colon tumors and polyps bleed intermittently.

AVOID THIS MISTAKE

Scheduling an Afternoon Colonoscopy

Colonoscopies performed in the afternoon not only force you to listen to your stomach grumble all day but also they may be less accurate. A study at the Cleveland Clinic showed that doctors detected polyps in 29 percent of patients screened in the morning, versus 25 percent of patients in the afternoon. Researchers speculated that fatigue may make doctors less likely to spot problems.

In one study, guaiac-based tests found just 24 percent of the advanced colon tumors detected by colonoscopies. FOBTs produce a lot of false alarms, too, since many other conditions (such as hemorrhoids and peptic ulcers) can produce blood in the stool. Any positive FOBT must be followed up with further testing—usually the very colonoscopy you were trying to avoid.

If you still want to use a stool test instead of a colonoscopy, do it every year; it's the best way to increase the test's likelihood of detecting colon cancer. And ask your doctor which type of test to use. Your best bet may be the newest stool test, called the fecal immunochemical test (FIT), which appears to be more accurate than older tests. It's more convenient, too; the older-style FOBT requires you to avoid red meat, citrus fruit, certain other foods, and aspirin 3 days prior to the test. The FIT has no such restrictions. A still-newer stool test doesn't search for blood at all. Instead, it detects DNA shed by tumors and polyps. The fecal DNA test isn't widely used yet because it's very expensive and its accuracy hasn't been fully established.

☐ DIABETES TESTING

When is it okay to have a random blood sugar test instead of a fasting test?

If you turn up in a doctor's office with classic symptoms of diabetes, such as unexplained weight loss, unquenchable thirst, and a frequent need to urinate, your doctor will most likely give you the random blood sugar (RBS) test, also called the casual plasma glucose test. This simple blood test can be performed any time, and no preparation is necessary.

If you have a reading of 200 milligrams per deciliter (mg/dL) or higher, and you are dying of thirst and keep dashing off to the bathroom, then your doctor will diagnose diabetes. However, if you have a reading of 200 mg/dL or higher and only have mild symptoms, your doctor will most likely repeat the test, either a few hours later or on another day, to be certain the diagnosis is accurate. (Some doctors believe that an initial RBS between 140 and 200 mg/dL is cause for concern, and will ask you to return for a follow-up test.) A second reading of greater than 200 mg/dL confirms that you have diabetes. Your doctor may also follow up with the more accurate fasting plasma glucose (FPG) test, which is performed after you have abstained from eating and drinking anything but water for 8 hours. An FPG of 126 mg/dL or higher confirms the diagnosis of diabetes; a reading of 100 to 125 mg/dL means that you have prediabetes, also called impaired fasting glucose, which places you at high risk for developing full-blown diabetes.

What does an oral glucose tolerance test involve, and will I feel sick?

Doctors usually order an oral glucose tolerance test (OGTT) only when truly necessary, given the time and inconvenience involved, and especially because some patients experience nasty

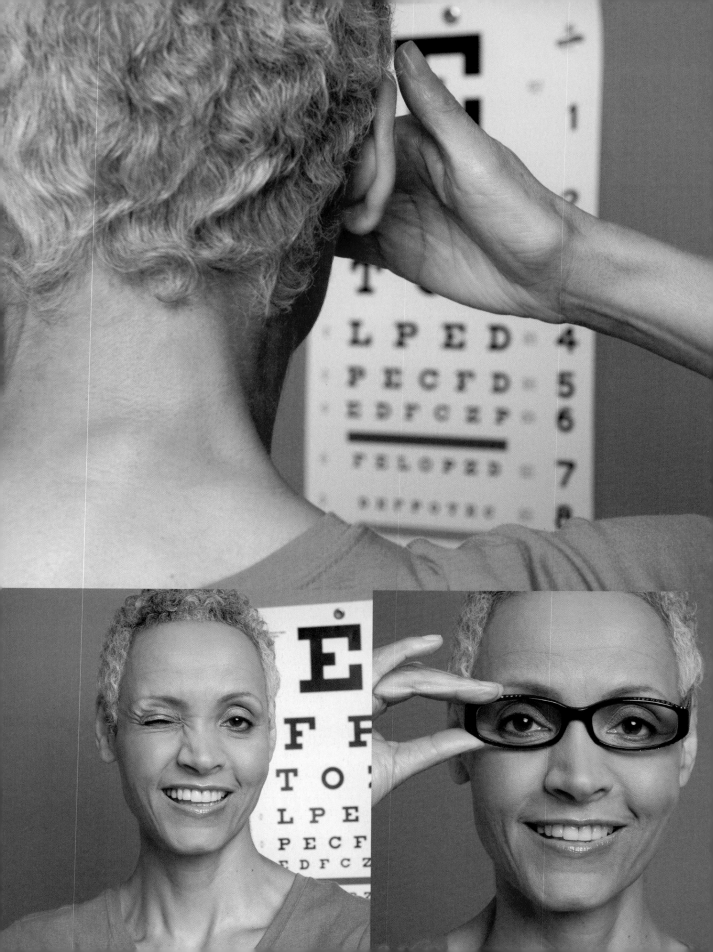

side effects after guzzling the glucose drink, which can include nausea, bloating, vomiting, jitteriness, and headaches.

The OGTT is used to screen for diabetes by measuring your blood glucose after you consume a standard amount of glucose, or sugar. Unlike other diabetes tests, the OGTT directly measures how efficiently your body processes and controls blood sugar. It's primarily used in two circumstances: when a doctor suspects that a pregnant woman has gestational diabetes or when a patient's fasting plasma glucose test result is normal, but other symptoms suggest that he or she has diabetes.

Your doctor will instruct you to fast for at least 8 hours prior to having the test, but otherwise you should eat a normal, balanced diet in the preceding days. The test requires you to quickly drink a very sweet beverage containing a few ounces (75 grams) of sugar, then sit quietly for 2 hours, over which time a nurse or lab technician will periodically take blood samples to test your blood sugar levels. (With pregnant women, the test lasts 3 hours and uses a drink containing 100 grams of sugar.) In a healthy person, blood sugar will rise after consuming the drink, then fall rapidly. However, if your blood sugar measures 200 mg/dL or higher at the 2-hour mark, diabetes is

the diagnosis. A reading between 140 and 199 mg/dL on this test is defined as prediabetes, meaning you are at risk for progressing to diabetes.

☐ **EYE EXAM**

Is an optometrist as good as an ophthalmologist for an eye exam?

Either one of these eye specialists can perform a routine eye exam, but an ophthalmologist may be the better choice in some cases. Optometrists attend a 4-year optometry school and may also spend additional time in a residency program. Ophthalmologists, who are medical doctors, attend medical school for 4 years, then perform a 1-year internship and a 3-year residency. Some spend an extra year or two training in a subspecialty, such as glaucoma or ophthalmic plastic surgery.

If you're in good health, you can feel comfortable choosing either an optometrist or ophthalmologist for an eye exam. However, people who have a family history of eye disease or conditions that can damage vision, such as diabetes or high blood pressure, may prefer to have an ophthalmologist perform their routine vision checkups. You should definitely see an ophthalmologist if you have an eye injury, sudden or severe loss of

vision, or redness or other signs of an eye infection.

I've always had good vision, but lately faces and words on a page seem fuzzy. Is it time for me to get glasses?

Possibly, but be sure to make an appointment soon with an optometrist or ophthalmologist for a checkup that includes a comprehensive dilated eye exam, which can detect signs of vision disorders such as agerelated macular degeneration (AMD). Blurred vision in one or both eyes can be a symptom of a type of AMD called dry AMD.

After having you read an eye chart to check your visual acuity, the doctor will put drops in your eyes to dilate the pupils. Then, using a magnifying lens, he'll examine your retina and optic nerves for evidence of AMD and other diseases, such as glaucoma. To rule out another form of AMD called wet AMD, caused by leaky blood vessels, you may also be asked to stare at a checkered grid to see if the lines look wavy. If your doctor suspects wet AMD, he'll probably order a fluorescein angiogram, which uses dye (injected into the arm) to search for leaky blood vessels. Early detection of AMD is key; there is no cure, but some treatments may slow its progression.

Is it true that an eye exam can reveal brain tumors and diabetes?

Poets say the eyes are the window to the soul, but peering into your peepers can reveal a great deal about your health, too. For example, eye doctors have saved lives by raising brain cancer as a possible explanation when patients complained of blind spots or vision that suddenly turned blurry. A tumor can increase pressure inside the skull, which may cause the optic nerves to swell and impair vision.

Routine annual exams also can detect early signs of systemic health problems. You know those drops your eye doctor uses to dilate your pupils? They allow a clear view of the retinas with the use of a magnifying lens. If your eye doctor detects evidence of hemorrhages, fatty deposits, or other damage to the retina, it could be due to the presence of undiagnosed diabetes.

The American Academy of Ophthalmology recommends getting a baseline eye exam at age 40, though experts disagree on when and how often routine testing is necessary. Ask your doctor how often you should have an eye exam, and schedule an appointment right away if you experience any sudden loss of vision.

WHAT YOU DON'T KNOW

Test Your CRP Twice

If you're going to have your CRP tested, it's a good idea to have it tested twice, at least 2 weeks apart. This way, if something like a cold throws off the first set of results, you won't get a skewed picture of your real inflammation levels. Doctors often take an average of the two results.

□ **HEART DISEASE**

Should I have my CRP tested?

Whether the C-reactive protein (CRP) test provides much valuable information about your risk for heart disease is still up for debate. CRP is produced by the liver in response to inflammation that occurs anywhere in the body. Inflammation can be triggered by anything from a simple infection (such as the flu, herpes, or gum disease) to an inflammatory disease such as rheumatoid arthritis. It can also be triggered by a poor diet, by fat deep in the belly, and by cholesterol particles burrowing into artery walls. Doctors have discovered in recent years that chronic, low-grade inflammation in the arteries appears to trigger heart attacks, leading some to argue that measuring CRP could provide important information about a patient's risk.

Some studies have found that elevated CRP is as bad for the heart as high cholesterol, possibly worse. However, the American Heart Association advises using the CRP test only in borderline cases, when a doctor can't decide whether a patient with a few risk factors for heart disease needs drug therapy or not. Studies show that CRP tests don't offer much valuable information about low-risk patients, who probably don't need treatment no matter what a CRP test shows, or patients who are at high risk, who need drug treatment either way.

My doctor suggested a heart scan to measure the calcium in my arteries. Why do I need one?

Like CRP testing (See "Should I have my CRP tested?" above), heart scans that test for calcium in the arteries are most useful for helping doctors decide how aggressively to treat borderline patients—that is, those who have a modestly elevated risk for suffering heart attacks. If you fall into this category, the results of the scan could theoretically help your doctor decide to prescribe medication such as a statin drug or calcium channel blocker, which may slow the spread of calcification in the arteries.

The scans, known as electron-beam computed tomography, or EBCT, use a specific type of CT scanner to detect calcium in the arteries. Calcium combines with fat and cholesterol to form blockages that can cut off blood flow to the heart and cause angina (chest pain) and heart attacks. Studies show that excess calcium in the arteries increases the risk for heart attack.

Heart scans rarely find much, if any, calcium in the arteries of patients who have no major risk factors for heart disease, so these patients don't need one. And the scans are little use for people who have many risk factors—such as obesity, diabetes, smoking, and close relatives who have had cardiovascular disease—since these people should already be receiving intensive therapy to prevent heart attacks. According to the American Heart Association, heart scans are probably only worth considering for patients who are at intermediate risk for heart disease, defined as people who have a 10 to 20 percent chance of suffering a heart attack over the next decade.

You may fall into that category if you have one or two risk factors for heart disease—if you're a former smoker, for instance, or if you have borderline high

blood pressure. However, these scans aren't without risks. Not only does CT expose you to relatively large amounts of radiation, but the scans often detect suspicious masses in the lungs, which lead doctors to order painful biopsies that usually discover benign nodules. You and your doctor must consider the potential downsides when deciding whether you really need a heart scan.

I have angina and my doctor wants me to have an angiogram. Is this test dangerous?

Angiograms, which x-ray the blood vessels in the heart, are generally quite safe, though they do carry a slightly higher degree of risk than most other heart tests. The gold standard test for people who have

chest pain, or angina, they can detect blockages in the large arteries of the heart, which may cause chest pain and lead to a heart attack. To perform the test, a doctor inserts a slender catheter (a hollow, flexible tube) into a blood vessel, usually the femoral artery in the groin or a vessel in the arm. The doctor then guides the catheter to the heart, where a dye is injected that makes the blood inside the blood vessels show up on the x-ray.

Like any invasive medical procedure, angiograms can cause complications. The most common are minor, such as bruising or bleeding at the site where the catheter is inserted. However, serious complications such as arrhythmia (irregular heartbeat), heart attacks, and strokes can also occur. According to some estimates, major complications

WHAT YOU DON'T KNOW

Angiograms May Miss Heart Disease in Women

Women who have chest pain and undergo angiograms that don't detect an obstructed artery are usually sent home with reassurances that they don't have heart disease. But that might not be true. A 2009 study found that women like these actually had a three-fold increased risk for heart attacks, heart failure, and strokes. According to one theory, women are more likely to develop blockages in the smaller heart arteries, which are less visible on angiograms. The study authors suggest that women who have chest pain should be treated aggressively with statins and other heart medications, regardless of their angiogram results.

happen in 1 in 1,000 procedures, though others put the estimate closer to 1 in 500. Also, some people experience allergic reactions to the dye used. Be sure to tell your doctor if you know that you're allergic to contrast dye, or if you are allergic to iodine or shellfish. Special medications given before the test can help prevent a bad reaction.

If the angiogram detects an obstruction that clogs 50 percent or more of an artery, chances are you'll be referred for further treatment, such as angioplasty, which opens blocked arteries.

☐ **LUNG CANCER**

I was a heavy smoker for years. Should I have a lung scan to check for cancer?

Most doctors think it's too soon to recommend lung scans to screen for lung cancer. Experts already know that chest x-rays are not effective for this purpose; they can detect tumors as small as 1 to 2 centimeters in diameter, but by the time a tumor is that size, it's already too late. Studies show that screening for lung cancer with chest x-rays doesn't lower death rates.

Computed tomography (CT) scans can detect much smaller tumors—but it's not clear whether they save lives. Two large studies in smokers came

to opposite conclusions. One found that CT scans could lower death rates by 80 percent; the other determined that detecting tiny tumors with CT scans made no difference and didn't save lives. Experts aren't sure why these two studies reached such radically different conclusions. It could be due to chance, but there's also the possibility that doctors in the second study detected many small tumors that looked scary, but, in reality, would have remained dormant and never caused full-blown lung cancer. If a scan finds any tumor, small or large, you'll almost certainly have lung surgery, which is not without risks: Twenty percent of patients experience serious complications and 5 percent die.

Before recommending the lung scans, most doctors are awaiting the results from two large trials for detecting lung cancer with CT scans, which will be completed after 2010.

☐ **MAMMOGRAMS**

When should I start having mammograms? And how often do I need one?

That's a controversial topic. For years, most doctors agreed that women should start having annual mammograms at age 40. Many medical organizations, such as the American

Cancer Society and the National Cancer Institute, still make that recommendation, and you should feel free to follow it—you have the right to choose the screening approach that you think is right for you. However, in 2009, the U.S. Preventive Services Task Force, a medical advisory group, looked at new scientific evidence on the value of mammograms and recommended these revised guidelines: Most women should wait until age 50 for their first mammogram, then have the test every other year until age 75. (The task force also determined that breast self-exams do not save lives.)

Why did this group change its recommendation? The task force found that:

● *For women under age 50, the downsides of mammograms outweigh the benefits.*
The risk of breast cancer begins to rise at around age 40, but the disease is still relatively uncommon in women under 50. However, women in this age group who undergo mammograms have an unusually large number of false-positive results—that is, the exam finds many suspicious-looking masses that turn out to be harmless. Most women with false-positive results end up undergoing the anxiety, inconvenience, and pain of follow-up mammograms and biopsies that they don't need.

AVOID THIS MISTAKE

Going Just Anywhere for a Mammogram

If possible, have your breast exam at a radiology center that specializes in mammography. Studies have found that radiologists who read a lot of mammograms detect more breast tumors. They are also less likely to misinterpret normal mammograms, which usually results in a woman having an unnecessary needle biopsy. Some experts recommend having your exam at a facility where the radiologists read at least 15 mammograms per day. It's also a good idea to have all your mammograms at the same facility so that your results can be compared from year to year. (If you don't, ask for your old mammograms and take them with you to the new facility.)

● *For women age 75 and older, there's not enough evidence that mammograms save lives.* The benefits of mammograms have not been well-studied in older women. However, researchers note that women from this age group who find out they have a breast tumor are more likely to die of other causes.

These guidelines don't apply to women who have an increased risk for breast cancer; these women should talk to their doctors about when to begin having mammograms. You may be at increased risk for breast cancer if you've have had a genetic test that indicates that you are; you have undergone extensive chest x-rays; or you have several close relatives (such as your mother or a sister) who have had breast cancer.

Critics of the task force's guidelines note that regular mammograms among women in their forties do save lives— approximately 1 life for every 1,900 women who get screened regularly—and that the potential negatives of early screening—anxiety over a false alarm and even unnecessary biopsies—don't outweigh the potential benefits.

Isn't there a lot of controversy about mammograms and whether they actually save lives?

Keep having those routine mammograms, but it's true—some scientists have raised questions about the exact value of this breast cancer screening tool. Researchers estimate that mammograms have doubled the number of women diagnosed with early-stage breast cancer. That sounds like a huge breakthrough, but here's the catch: There has been a mere 10 percent drop in the number of women diagnosed with cancer that has spread beyond the breast, the point at which breast cancer becomes life-threatening.

If early detection is so important, why hasn't it dramatically lowered the number of women diagnosed with advanced breast cancer? Some doctors say that many of the breast tumors detected by mammograms are essentially harmless —if they had gone undetected, they would have never spread to other organs and turned deadly. Meanwhile, they speculate that mammograms haven't prevented more cases of advanced breast cancer because they *miss* many potentially lethal tumors that spread too fast to be detected by routine screening.

Keep in mind that mammograms do save lives—they cut the risk of dying of breast cancer by about 20 percent among women ages 50 to 70. No one has recommended forgoing them.

I have dense breasts. Is a regular mammogram good enough or should I have a digital mammogram, or even an MRI?

Standard mammograms are x-rays of the breasts, which are reproduced on large sheets of film. Digital mammograms use x-rays, too, but the images are stored and viewed on computers, which allows a doctor to enlarge and sharpen them. As a result, they produce fewer inconclusive results and are less likely to make retesting necessary. Large studies show that both techniques are effective, but suggest that digital mammography is more accurate if you:

- Are under age 50
- Have dense breasts
- Are approaching menopause or you had your final menstrual period within the last 12 months

If dense breasts are your only issue, you probably don't need an MRI. Women who should talk to their doctors about breast MRIs are those who've tested positive for a gene mutation that greatly increases the breast cancer risk, and those who have already been diagnosed with cancer in one breast. About 10 percent of women diagnosed with cancer in one breast have a tumor in the other breast that is not detected by mammography.

MRIs use radio waves and magnets to produce detailed images of body tissue, and studies show that they can detect about 90 percent of these hidden tumors.

I'm on hormone replacement therapy. Will that affect my mammogram?

Some doctors advise women who take hormone replacement therapy (HRT) for menopause symptoms to stop a month or two before having a mammogram. The reason: HRT increases breast density, which can make it harder to interpret mammograms. Tumors may be missed, and suspicious masses may lead to more unnecessary biopsies. However, a 2009 study found that women who continued HRT were no more likely to have abnormal mammograms that required further testing than women who went off it. Some experts point out that women who have reached menopause tend not to have dense breasts to begin with, so the modest increase from HRT may not matter.

☐ METABOLIC SYNDROME

Is there a test for metabolic syndrome?

There is no one test for this condition, which is actually a cluster of several different conditions, including excess belly fat, unhealthy cholesterol and triglyceride levels, high blood pressure, and high blood sugar. If you have metabolic syndrome, you have an increased risk for developing heart disease and type 2 diabetes. Doctors diagnose it when you have three of the following five risk factors:

- *Waist circumference:*
41 inches or more for men;
36 inches or more for women

- *Triglycerides:*
150 mg/dL or higher

- *HDL ("good") cholesterol:*
39 mg/dL or lower for men;
49 mg/dL or lower for women

- *Blood pressure:*
135/85 mm Hg or higher

- *Blood glucose:*
100 mg/dL or higher

☐ OVARIAN CANCER

Is the blood test for ovarian cancer accurate?

Ovarian cancer cells contain high levels of a protein called CA-125. A simple blood test can measure CA-125. But many conditions other than ovarian cancer cause CA-125 to rise, including endometriosis, uterine fibroids, pancreatitis, pelvic inflammatory disease, and liver disease, as well as several other forms of cancer. CA-125 rises during normal menstruation and if you become pregnant, too. For these reasons, the CA-125 test is not effective for early detection; just 50 percent of women who test positive have stage 1. (It's more effective at finding later-stage cancers, but these cancers may have already spread to other organs.) To make matters more confusing, CA-125 does *not* rise in up to one in five women with ovarian cancer.

Some doctors may advise women who have a close relative who had ovarian cancer or who have tested positive for the BRCA1 and BRCA2 gene mutations to have the CA-125 test, since these so-called breast cancer genes also increase the risk for ovarian cancer by about 10- to 30-fold. However, there's no evidence that the test saves lives in these women. The blood test does have a clear role in diagnosing ovarian cancer in women who have symptoms of the disease. If imaging tests reveal that a woman has a mass in the pelvic area, a CA-125 reading of 65 or greater means there's a 90 percent chance she has ovarian cancer. Also, doctors use the CA-125 test to track how a patient's disease is progressing and how well treatments are working.

☐ **PAP SMEARS**

Is it true that older women can stop getting Pap tests?

Yes, though some older women may need to continue having this test that screens for cervical cancer. Young women have long been advised to start having annual Pap tests within 3 years of their first sexual activity, though the American College of Obstetricians and Gynecologists (ACOG) says it's okay to wait until age 21 because cervical cancer is extremely rare among teens. (Starting at age 30, women who have had three normal

Pap tests in a row can get screened every 3 years.) Women can stop getting Pap tests between the ages and 65 and 70 if they have had three or more normal test results in a row and no worrisome tests in the last decade, since cervical cancer is rare past middle age.

There are exceptions, however. Plan on continuing to have routine Pap smears if:

- You have had cervical cancer
- Your mother took the synthetic form of estrogen called DES (diethylstilbestrol) while carrying you
- You have HIV
- Your immune system is weakened for any reason

Most women who have had a total hysterectomy can stop having Pap tests, too, though some doctors recommend continuing to have them if you have had invasive cervical cancer or have been exposed to DES.

Is the HPV test better than a Pap test? Should my doctor use both?

The human papilloma virus (HPV) test appears to be superior to the Pap test, but many doctors continue to use the latter, or order both tests, for several reasons.

HPV is a common virus that comes in many different forms and can be transmitted through

sex. It's usually harmless and disappears on its own, but some types of HPV can cause cell changes that lead to cervical cancer. The HPV test searches for DNA evidence of infection by the most dangerous forms of this virus.

Side-by-side comparisons show that the HPV test does a better job of detecting cervical cancer than the Pap test. In one study of more than 10,000 women, the HPV test detected abnormal cells that could become cervical cancer with 96 percent accuracy, compared to just 55 percent for the Pap test.

Despite the HPV's edge, many doctors are reluctant to stop using the Pap test, which led to a 70 percent drop in cervical cancer deaths since it came into wide use in the early 1950s. HPV tests are still relatively new, so there are no long-term studies proving that they reduce the risk of dying from cervical cancer. If you're over age 30, your doctor may want to give you the Pap test and HPV test. (The HPV test produces too many false alarms in women under 30 to be used for routine testing.) Both tests can be performed at once and, when combined, detect evidence of cervical cancer 100 percent of the time.

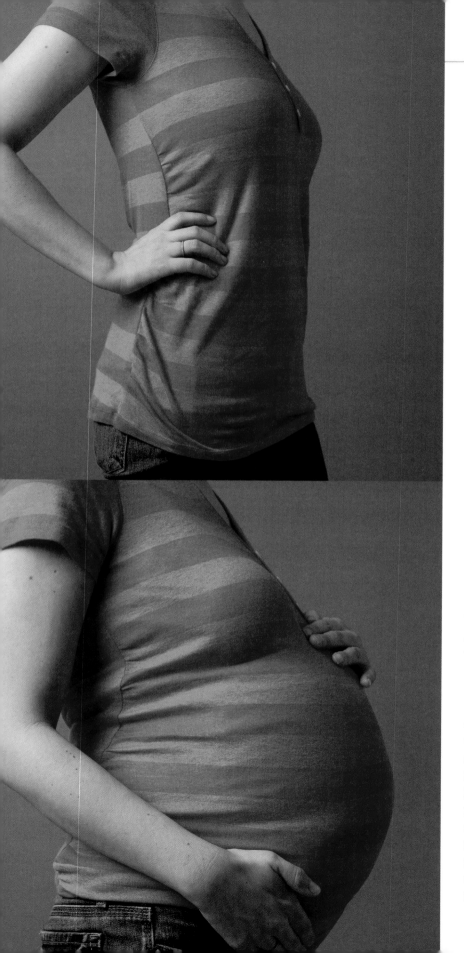

My home pregnancy test was negative. Does that mean I'm not pregnant?

Not necessarily, so plan on repeating the test. Most home pregnancy tests work by detecting the presence of a hormone called human chorionic gonadotropin (hCG) in a woman's urine. Typically, the user holds a test strip in her urine stream or collects the urine in a cup to test. A positive result is often indicated by a stripe, plus sign, or other symbol that appears in a window on the test strip.

The makers of many home pregnancy tests claim that their products are highly accurate and can detect hCG on the first day of a missed period. But at that stage, hCG levels are usually very low, so a positive test result may be faint, causing it to be mistaken for a negative. Also, hCG isn't produced until a fertilized egg implants in the uterus, which doesn't occur until after the first day of a missed period in about 1 out of 10 women. Finally, keep in mind that some tests are more sensitive than others, and that human error is always a possibility. For these reasons, any negative test should be repeated a week later (when hCG, if present, will have risen). If you can't wait, call your doctor, who can administer a blood test.

Is amniocentesis safe for my baby and me?

Amniocentesis is relatively safe, but it does carry a small degree of risk. Amniotic fluid is a watery liquid that surrounds a fetus in the uterus during pregnancy. In amniocentesis, a doctor inserts a fine needle into the uterus to withdraw a sample of this fluid, which can be analyzed to diagnose chromosome abnormalities (such as Down syndrome), genetic disorders (cystic fibrosis, for example), or neural-tube defects (such as spina bifida). Amniocentesis may be used for other reasons, too, such as determining whether a fetus's lungs have matured.

Doctors use ultrasound to guide insertion of the needle, so it rarely jabs the fetus. A more justified concern is miscarriage, a somewhat more common complication. At some clinics, roughly 1 woman in 200 who has amniocentesis suffers a miscarriage, though that happens far less often (closer to 1 woman in 400) at facilities that routinely perform the procedure. This risk

needs to be weighed carefully when choosing to have amniocentesis.

If you're concerned about the risk of miscarriage, you may want to ask your doctor about alternatives to amniocentesis, which include:

- *Multiple maternal marker screening.* This blood test, also called a triple or quadruple screen, measures levels of three or four substances (depending on which version your doctor uses) that may indicate that a fetus has certain birth defects, such as Down syndrome or spina bifida.

- *Ultrasound.* Doctors use ultrasound at various stages of pregnancy; one application is to examine whether a fetus has thick neck skin, which can be a sign of Down syndrome.

☐ **PROSTATE EXAMS**

I've heard that PSA tests aren't very accurate for detecting prostate cancer. Should I still have one?

Your doctor may turn the question back on you: What do *you*

want to do? That's because this test can detect prostate cancer, but many doctors think it rings too many false alarms to be useful as a screening tool, which is why they're encouraging patients to help make the decision.

The prostate specific antigen (PSA) test measures blood levels of a protein that rises when you have a prostate tumor. However, conditions such as prostatitis (inflammation of the prostate) or an enlarged prostate can raise PSA, too. Some 65 to 75 percent of men who find out they have high PSA and undergo needle biopsies—which can be scary and painful—do not have prostate cancer.

What's more, some doctors believe that the PSA test is overly sensitive, detecting tumors that would otherwise have never caused any trouble. This form of cancer can grow slowly, and autopsies show that many old men die of other causes, unaware that they had malignant prostate tumors. Doctors don't yet have a reliable way to distinguish a slow-growing prostate tumor from one that's aggressive and potentially lethal. As a result, men who learn they have prostate cancer often end up undergoing unnecessary surgery, radiation, and other treatments that can cause erectile dysfunction, urinary incontinence, and other troublesome side effects.

A 2009 study involving 76,693 men found no evidence that having a PSA test reduces the

WHAT YOU DON'T KNOW

Morning Is the Best Time for a Pregnancy Test

To increase the accuracy of a home pregnancy test, use it on your first visit to the bathroom in the morning. Urine has a higher concentration of hCG, the hormone that indicates pregnancy, when you wake up.

Having Sex before a PSA Exam

Ejaculation can cause PSA levels to rise, so men should abstain from sex for at least 48 hours before having blood drawn for a PSA test. (Some doctors suggest 72 hours to be on the safe side.) In a University of Michigan study, researchers found that PSA levels rose after ejaculation in 88 percent of the subjects and didn't return to baseline for 48 hours on average.

risk of dying from prostate cancer. The test may make more sense for men who are at high risk for prostate cancer, including African-American men and men who had a close relative (a father, brother, or son) diagnosed with prostate cancer before age 65. If several close relatives developed prostate cancer at a young age, start talking to your doctor about PSA tests when you turn 40.

My doctor found something during a rectal exam. But my PSA levels are normal. Do I need a biopsy?

Probably not. Some doctors will order biopsies whenever they find a suspicious mass with a digital rectal exam (DRE), regardless of your PSA results. But these exams (in which a doctor inserts a gloved finger into the rectum and examines the prostate) correctly detect prostate cancer in only about 1 case in 10 when PSA levels are normal. Due to the low odds of finding cancer,

doctors usually don't order a biopsy in a case like yours. (Some doctors will order one if your PSA levels are on the high side of "normal.") Even if your doctor doesn't order a biopsy,

expect him to pester you about scheduling routine prostate cancer screenings and to watch your PSA levels closely.

☐ SKIN BIOPSIES

I need to have a skin biopsy. Will it leave a scar?

Yes, though in some cases it will be barely noticeable. Doctors take a skin biopsy, or tissue sample, when they suspect cancer or some other skin disease. There are three basic types of skin biopsies.

The PSA Test: Reading the Numbers

A PSA of 4 ng/mL (nanograms per milliliter) or higher indicates a heightened risk for prostate cancer, according to the American Cancer Society. However, the PSA exam isn't perfect: Many men who have elevated levels are cancer-free, while a small number who actually have the disease test negative. Some doctors use PSA velocity—that is, how fast PSA rises over time—and other variations on the exam to determine whether a man needs a biopsy.

PSA Value (ng/mL)	What It Means
3.9 or lower	**Low risk.** About one in seven men with prostate cancer have a PSA of 3.9 or lower.
4.0 to 10.0	**Borderline risk.** About one in four men with prostate cancer have a PSA in this range.
10.1 or higher	**High risk.** More than half of men with prostate cancer have a PSA of 10.1 or higher.

- *Shave.* A doctor uses a scalpel or razor to remove a suspicious growth by paring it away, along with the uppermost layers of skin underneath it. A shave biopsy usually leaves a small saucer-shaped scar.

- *Excision.* A doctor uses a scalpel to remove a portion of skin a few millimeters wide surrounding a growth. Excision biopsies usually require stitches and leave straight-line scars.

- *Punch.* A doctor uses an instrument shaped like a slender cookie cutter to extract a small cylinder of skin. Stitches are often unnecessary; if so, just one or two do the job. Punch biopsies tend to leave very modest scars.

Any doctor with proper training can perform a skin biopsy. However, if you need a tissue sample taken from your face or another highly visible part of your body, consider having the procedure performed by a plastic surgeon or dermatologist.

☐ **THYROID TESTS**

My TSH test came back normal, but I still think I might have thyroid disease. I've heard about the free T4 test. Should I have it?

The thyroid stimulating hormone (TSH) test is highly accurate, so having the free T4 test in addition is unlikely to add much to your diagnosis. TSH prompts the thyroid gland to make two types of thyroid hormones, known as T3 and T4. A low TSH level almost always means that you have an overactive thyroid gland, or hyperthyroidism. Symptoms may include nervousness, trembling, excessive perspiration, weight loss, and, in women, irregular menstrual periods. High TSH usually indicates that you have an underactive thyroid, or hypothyroidism. Symptoms include sluggishness, weight gain, a puffy face, brittle hair, constipation, and sensitivity to cold.

The TSH test is so reliable that it's often the only one a doctor orders. Normal results are usually interpreted to mean that a patient's symptoms must be due to some cause other than a thyroid problem. However—and this is very rare—TSH levels may be normal in people who have hypothyroidism caused by a tumor or other problem in the pituitary gland or hypothalamus (the brain region that controls the pituitary gland). For that reason, some doctors may order a test of free T4 (thyroxine) in patients who have normal TSH levels and symptoms of hypothyroidism A reading lower than 4.5 mcg/dL (micrograms per deciliter) may mean you have hypothyroidism.

In patients with a known thyroid disorder, a doctor might order a free T4 test in addition to a TSH test to help monitor thyroid function.

Why does my doctor want me to have a thyroid scan?

Doctors order thyroid scans for several reasons, but one of the most common is to detect nodules, or knobby growths, on the thyroid. Most thyroid nodules are cysts and other benign (noncancerous) masses; in only about 1 percent of cases are they cancerous. A doctor may discover signs that you have thyroid nodules during a routine physical exam, or the nodules may turn up on imaging tests (such as carotid ultrasound) for other conditions. Before ordering a thyroid scan, a doctor will usually perform a fine-needle biopsy to extract cells and fluid from nodules. If the results of the biopsy are not clear, a thyroid scan is usually the next step.

Before the exam, the patient swallows a capsule containing radioactive iodine, or is injected with this substance. The thyroid naturally soaks up iodine, and "tagging" the iodine with radioactive isotopes makes it possible for the scanner to create an image of the gland. Nodules that take up a great deal of iodine are considered "hot," an indication that they're overactive (producing too much thyroid hormone). Hot nodules are unlikely to be cancerous. "Cold" nodules take up little iodine; a small percentage of these are cancerous. A growing number of doctors are using high-resolution thyroid ultrasound (which produces better images) in addition to standard scans to help diagnose nodules.

Cancerous nodules are always surgically removed. Noncancerous nodules may be removed if they are causing hyperthyroidism, pain, or other symptoms. Women tend to have more thyroid nodules, but these growths are more likely to be cancerous in men.

☐ VASCULAR DISEASE

An old friend of mine suffered a ruptured abdominal aortic aneurysm. Should I get screened?

Only men ages 65 to 75 who smoke or used to smoke should be screened for abdominal aortic aneurysm (AAA). The aorta is the largest artery in the body, about the thickness of a garden hose. It starts in the heart and descends all the way through the abdomen. Arteries and smaller blood vessels that branch from the aorta deliver blood throughout the body. Aneurysms, or bulges, can form in the aorta, especially in the portion that passes through the abdomen. If an abdominal aortic aneurysm ruptures, the prospects are grim: Seventy to 80 percent of victims die before reaching a hospital.

Doctors often discover AAAs in patients by accident, while evaluating some other abdominal condition. If they're large enough to pose a clear threat, they can be surgically repaired. The most common method is to cut away the aneurysm and replace it with a tube-shaped graft. In a newer procedure, doctors insert a graft with metal coil called a stent into the aneurysm; over time, the aneurysm shrinks around the stent graft.

Ultrasound does an excellent job of spotting them, and studies show that screening can reduce the risk of dying from a ruptured AAA by as much as 43 percent in some groups. If you do get screened and receive a clean bill of health, there's no need to be screened a second time.

My legs and feet feel fine, so why does my doctor want to test for peripheral artery disease?

Testing for peripheral artery disease (PAD) shows whether your lower limbs are nourished by adequate blood flow and may help diagnose the condition before symptoms emerge. PAD is a general term for narrowing and hardening of blood vessels outside the heart. It can occur anywhere in the body but frequently afflicts arteries and veins in the legs and feet. The main symptoms are pain and tightness,

especially when you walk or exercise. However, you may not feel like anything is wrong until PAD has reached an advanced stage.

A simple exam called an ankle-brachial index (ABI) test compares blood pressure in your ankle and arm, producing a result in the form of a ratio. An ABI of 0.95 or lower means you have PAD. A 2008 study in the *Journal of the American Medical Association* found that people with an ABI of 0.90 or lower doubled their risk for having a fatal heart attack or dying of other causes over a 10-year period. Some doctors feel that the ABI test may help identify patients at risk for heart disease who would otherwise be missed by traditional cardiovascular tests. However, it's still far from clear whether tests for PAD should be used in routine screening for heart disease.

☐ VITAMIN AND MINERAL TESTS

Should I get my blood tested to see if I'm deficient in any vitamins or minerals, just in case?

Some doctors who practice alternative or integrative medicine routinely screen patients' blood for vitamin and mineral deficiencies. There are also companies advertising on the internet that offer to analyze

✋ AVOID THIS MISTAKE

Getting Your Iron Tested in the Afternoon

Your iron level naturally fluctuates throughout the day. If you need to have your iron levels checked, get tested in the morning. Your blood concentration of iron is highest then, so you'll get a more accurate reading. Don't eat beforehand and skip taking iron pills or any supplements containing iron for 24 hours before the test.

your blood to determine which dietary supplements you may need. (Not surprisingly, those companies often offer to sell you the very same supplements you're allegedly lacking, too.) As a rule, there's little to be gained by having a routine blood screen for nutrient deficiency. However, there may be some specific exceptions. For instance, a growing number of doctors are testing patients for vitamin D deficiency as part of their routine health screening, thanks to mounting research suggesting that low levels of this nutrient increase the risk for fragile bones, heart disease, and other conditions.

My doctor suspected vitamin B_{12} deficiency, but my test came back at the low end of the normal range. Does that mean I have some other condition?

Despite the "normal" test result, it's still possible that you have vitamin B_{12} deficiency. Low levels of vitamin B_{12} can lead to anemia, nerve damage, mental health issues (such as depression, irritability, and memory problems), and other symptoms. The obvious way to measure this deficiency is to measure vitamin B_{12} levels in the blood. However, studies show that up to 50 percent of patients with low levels of vitamin B_{12} in their body tissue have a normal concentration of the nutrient in their blood. In borderline cases like yours, some doctors would do a follow-up test to measure a metabolite (a substance produced during metabolism) of vitamin B_{12} called methylmalonic acid. It rises in the early stages of vitamin B_{12} deficiency. If not caught and treated, vitamin B_{12} deficiency can cause irreversible nerve damage.

☐ X-RAYS

How often do I need dental x-rays?

That's up to your dentist, but the American Dental Association recommends these guidelines.

- All new patients should have a complete set of x-rays.

- If you don't have cavities and you're a model patient—that is, you brush and floss regularly—your dentist should take a set of posterior bitewing x-rays (that is, of the back teeth) every 2 to 3 years. Some dentists may suggest annual x-rays.

- If you have cavities or other dental problems, you may need x-rays every 6 to 18 months. The ADA recommends more frequent x-rays for children and teens.

I had to have a series of x-rays for an injury. Should I be worried about getting cancer from all the radiation?

X-rays do expose the body to radiation, but most use a low dose, and the increased risk for cancer is small. Keep in mind that you are exposed to low levels of radiation in the atmosphere every day—from the sun and electronic devices, for example—though medical x-rays are by far the greatest source over a lifetime. Avoiding unnecessary x-rays makes sense, but the benefits of a diagnostic x-ray almost always outweigh the risk. For example, mammograms (which use

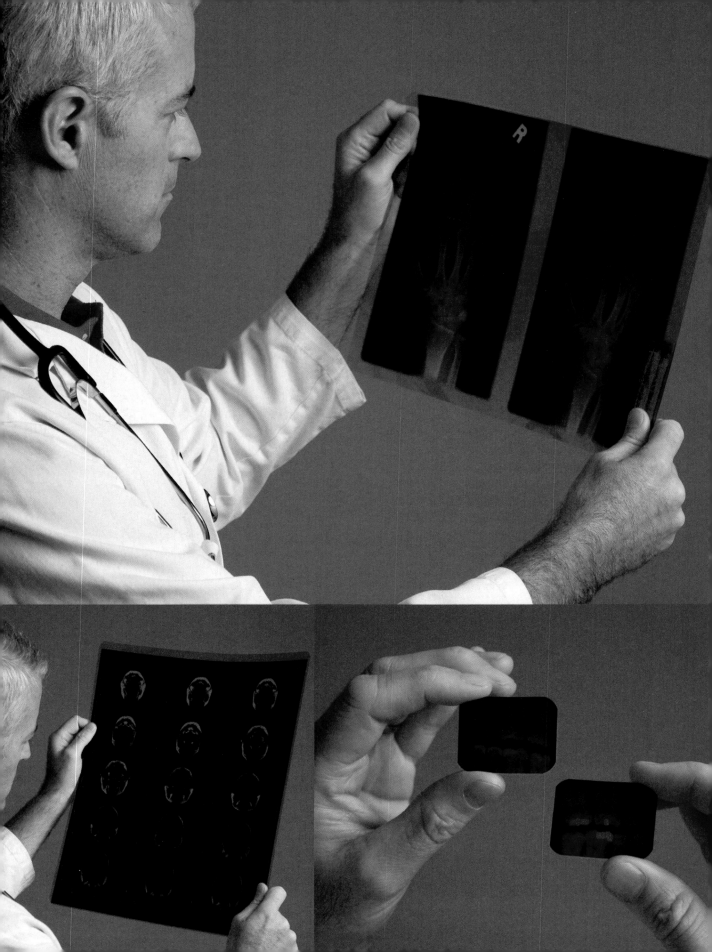

x-rays) save lives by detecting breast cancer at a treatable stage, but a single exam only increases a woman's lifetime cancer risk by about 0.002 percent. Experts estimate that medical x-rays account for about 0.5 to 3 percent of cancer cases worldwide.

That said, CT scans use higher doses of radiation than traditional x-rays and are more likely to increase cancer risk. (See "What about CT scans? Aren't they more dangerous than x-rays?" below.)

What about CT scans? Aren't they more dangerous than x-rays?

Computed tomography (CT) scans use x-rays, too, but they involve higher doses of radiation (one CT scan of the chest, for instance, is like having 100 chest x-rays), so they are more likely than a single x-ray exam to increase your risk for cancer. For instance, experts estimate that 1 additional cancer case occurs for every 800 middle-aged people who undergo a cardiac CT scan. How much a CT scan increases your risk of cancer depends on your age, the body part being scanned, and other factors. CT scans can provide doctors with important diagnostic information, so it's critical to balance their modest risks against their benefits. Find out how much a specific x-ray or CT scan increases your cancer risk at www.xrayrisk.com.

WHAT YOU DON'T KNOW

Recordkeeping Can Help You Avoid Unnecessary X-Rays

Every time you have an x-ray (including at the dentist), write down the type of exam, the date, the referring doctor, and where the x-ray is stored. This information may allow a physician examining you to refer to a previous x-ray instead of ordering a new one. Also, your doctor can compare a fresh x-ray to an earlier image to note how a medical condition has changed. You can find an x-ray wallet card at www.fda.gov (search within the site for "x-ray record card").

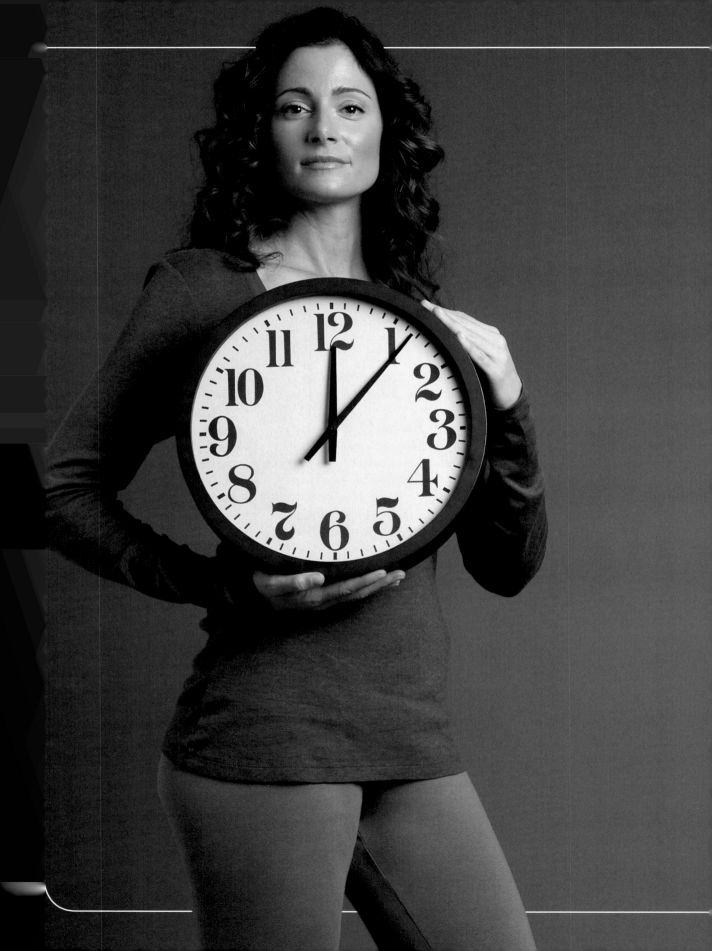

PART FIVE

Quick-Action Guide

From dog bites to bee stings, heatstroke to heart attacks, what to do when the unexpected occurs. Read this chapter ahead of time and you'll always be prepared for what may come.

FAQ Frequently Asked Questions

Quick-Action Guide

How do I know if I'm dealing with a true emergency?

If you have to ask, then it's probably the real thing. Don't doubt yourself, says Bret Nicks, MD, an emergency physician and assistant medical director at Wake Forest University Baptist Medical Center. "Although some people are reluctant to believe they are facing serious circumstances," Dr. Nicks says, "year after year, only 10 to 12 percent of visits to the emergency room are in error." In other words, trust your instincts. But if you're looking for further confirmation, a good sign that you need professional help is when a situation feels out of your control. It might entail bleeding you can't stop, a victim who is unconscious, signs of stroke (such as slurred speech), a seizure or a sudden and severe headache in someone who doesn't have a history of either, or extreme pain in the chest, left arm, or jaw. With burns, any wound that covers an area larger than your hands placed side by side demands a trip to the emergency room.

I have a big gash— how do I know if I need to be stitched up? Do I need to go to the ER?

Small cuts are easy: Soap and water, a little antibiotic ointment, and a bandage. But there's considerable gray area for bigger ones. Here are the four situations in which a cut should probably be sewn up.

1. The cut is on your face or some other visible part of your body (a professionally treated wound is less likely to scar).

2. The cut is deep—look for yellowish tissue when you wash it out. You're seeing the fatty subcutaneous tissue, and if dirt or bacteria reach that area, the result could be a serious infection.

3. You can't easily pinch the cut skin together, or it won't stay closed when you do.

4. The cut is in an area of your body that regularly flexes and moves (stitches or other closure options can prevent it from reopening).

If you can't control the bleeding with direct pressure, call an ambulance. It is best to have wounds cared for as soon after the injury as possible. With most wounds, you have 6 to 8 hours to get to an emergency clinic and have the wound cleaned and sewn up before it starts to close on its own. After that (and in the cases of a particularly dirty slash), doctors are reluctant to stitch because they could trap bacteria and cause a serious infection. While most lacerations are well-managed by emergency physicians, some cuts on your face or near your eyes may require a plastic surgeon's care; an emergency physician can help make that determination.

I'm not sure if I should drive myself, or my loved one, to the ER or call an ambulance?

The first thing to ask yourself is whether the circumstances have you too upset to drive safely. No? Then the American College of Emergency Physicians has some guidelines to help you decide whether to get behind the wheel or call for help.

- Do you think the victim's condition could become life threatening?
- Are you worried that moving the victim could cause further injury?
- Would distance or traffic conditions cause a delay in getting the victim to the hospital?
- Would the victim's condition prevent you from concentrating on the road?

If all the answers are no, then you can—and should—drive to the ER, rather than call an ambulance.

What can I expect when I call 911?

You'll be flustered—thankfully, no one has to make this call so often that they get good at it. Some of the questions you'll be asked will seem superfluous. For example, you'll be asked for your name, phone number, and the location of

FACT OR FICTION

You Can Call 911 on a Cell phone That Isn't Activated

Fact. Cell phone companies are required by law to put 911 calls through from any phone that has power and can receive a signal. For this reason, an old cell phone is an excellent addition to the first-aid kits you keep in your car and boat (remember to recharge the battery from time to time). Just be aware that because there is no number assigned to the phone, there's no way for 911 to reach you should you be disconnected; you'll have to redial.

the victim. Although dispatchers have technology that can pinpoint your whereabouts, they're required to confirm that information with you. People calling from home should be ready to describe access to the room and floor where the victim is located. Likewise, if you're calling about a car accident on a freeway, you'll need to know where the closest exit is and whether you're on, say, the southbound or northbound side. There will be pauses as the dispatcher takes down the information, but let him lead the conversation and don't hang up until he tells you to. Although the length of the call may make you feel impatient, rest reassured that the dispatcher has already notified emergency services and that help is on the way.

Parents should practice imaginary calls with their children so that the kids will know what to do should they need to dial 911.

The ambulance is on the way. What should I do while we're waiting?

First, make sure the victim is comfortable by offering support for his head or helping him to a seated position (provided he's conscious). Cover him with a blanket or jacket if he's exposed to weather. At home, your door may need to be propped open while paramedics come and go, so put your pets somewhere safe before the emergency medical technicians (EMTs) arrive. Turn on the porch light at night. Check your driveway—do you need to move your cars so the ambulance can pull closer to the door? Then trace the path through the house to the victim: Is it clear? Move tables or chairs so that the EMTs will be able to wheel the gurney through. Just remember to keep checking on the patient as you prepare.

I've heard there's a new type of CPR that's easier. How do you do it?

In a move designed to take the "ick factor" out of cardiopulmonary resuscitation (CPR), the American Red Cross removed the mouth-to-mouth breathing that was once a part of CPR. "Breathing into another person's mouth was a significant barrier for many people," says Dr. Gordon Ewy, MD, professor and chief of cardiology at the University of Arizona College of Medicine. "Studies have demonstrated that chest compression alone is enough to keep someone alive until medical help arrives," he says. The new method is easy to memorize and perform. Here are the steps to follow if an adult collapses, stops breathing, and is unresponsive.

1. Call 911, or have a bystander do it.

2. Place the victim on the floor, face-up.

3. Put one hand over the other on top of the victim's chest between the nipples.

4. Press down on the chest, compressing it about 2 inches, and then release so that the chest can rebound upward.

5. Repeat this 100 times a minute. (Remarkably, the beat of the Bee Gees song, "Stayin' Alive," is about the right speed.) This will be vigorous and tiring work, so take turns with another bystander, if possible.

6. Continue until the paramedics arrive.

For drowning victims and children, the mouth-to-mouth breathing of traditional CPR is still required. See the question "How do I treat a drowning victim?" on page 352 for more information.

I've seen those defibrillator machines in malls and restaurants but I'd be terrified to use one. Could I hurt someone?

Though training through the American Red Cross or another certified first-aid training group is strongly recommended, automated external defibrillators (AEDs) are designed to be easy to use and safe. Many of the machines have a recorded voice that will guide you through the steps. AEDs can take the victim's pulse and analyze whether a jolt is actually necessary, so you don't have to worry about shocking someone who doesn't need it. They typically have diagrams instructing you where and how to check for a pulse, attach the wires, and place the pads.

If someone is available to do CPR, have her perform it while you set up the AED. Make sure the victim's chest is dry and relatively free from hair (often the AED case will contain a razor for shaving the areas where the electrodes will be placed). Place the pads on the victim's chest as instructed, then turn on the AED. Wait to see if it indicates that a shock is needed. If it is, have everyone stand clear and then press the

WHAT YOU DON'T KNOW

It Pays to Put Your Cell Phone on ICE

Imagine you're driving alone and you're in an accident that leaves you unconscious. How will EMTs or emergency room doctors reach your emergency contact? Most Americans don't carry that information in their wallets. So, first, fill out a card with the name, phone number, and your relationship to the contact and put it in your wallet. But also create an "ICE" (In Case of Emergency) entry in your cell phone address book. More and more, paramedics and emergency room staff will check your phone for ICE. If you can attach notes to your address book entries, put in any medications you're taking, any drug allergies, and whether you have a chronic condition that may require special treatment.

Top Mistakes Never to Make in an Emergency

Don't...	Because...	Do This Instead
Move someone who has been in a serious fall or accident	Her neck or back might be broken, a broken rib could puncture a lung, or you could make a break much worse.	Leave her where she is. If the person is in danger (a car fire, for example), recruit three or four bystanders to help you lift the victim without altering the relative position of her body, especially the neck.
Begin first aid without calling 911 first	Even though your instinct is to help the victim first, he needs professional help to arrive as quickly as possible.	Make the call or instruct a specific bystander to do it.
Refuse medical treatment after you've been in an accident	Your body releases adrenaline and other pain-killing hormones in an emergency, and they can mask the pain from serious injuries.	Listen to the medical staff on the scene. Take their advice, especially if they want to take you to the ER for further observation.
Pull a knife, piece of metal, or stick out of a deep wound	You could damage organs or trigger uncontrollable bleeding.	Carefully place a cloth or bandage around the object to stanch the bleeding, and keep the person as calm and still as possible until help arrives.

shock button. Immediately resume CPR for 2 minutes, after which the AED will check the pulse and heart rhythm to see if another jolt is necessary. Continue until the machine gives a "no-shock" message or until the paramedics arrive.

What can I do ahead of time so I'm prepared for a medical emergency?

Have well-stocked and up-to-date first-aid kits in your home, car, RV, boat, and any other residence. You can find complete kits in most drugstores; just make sure it includes:

- Over-the-counter painkillers such as ibuprofen, acetaminophen, and aspirin
- Medical adhesive tape
- Antiseptic cleanser
- Gauze in rolls and squares ranging from 2 to 4 inches
- Elastic bandage
- Bandages of various sizes
- Safety pins
- Instant cold packs
- Latex gloves
- Tweezers
- Blunt-tipped bandage scissors
- Thermometer
- Aloe vera gel and calamine lotion for burns and insect stings
- Antihistamine such as diphenhydramine (Benadryl)

You'll also want to write down all your local emergency numbers—ambulance, hospital, poison control, primary physician and pediatricians, fire, police—and keep them in the kit. Include directions to the local hospital in case an out-of-town guest or babysitter needs to drive you or your children there. While you're at it, put in medical consent forms for everyone in the family along with each member's medical history and a list of current medications and allergies.

Quick-Action Guide

☐ **ALLERGIC REACTIONS**

The last time my son was stung by a bee, he got a rash and the area swelled a bit. If he gets stung again, what are the signs that he's in danger?

First, discuss the initial reaction with his pediatrician. He may prescribe medications or refer your son to an allergist for further testing. Although his first reaction wasn't too severe, the next time could be very different, and the right medication will help keep him stable in an emergency.

A serious reaction often starts with wheezing or a high-pitched whistling as airways constrict. Other common signs are pale, cool, and clammy skin; anxiety; confusion; difficulty swallowing; swelling in the face, lips, and tongue; and nausea that may be accompanied by vomiting or diarrhea. This is what's known as anaphylaxis, an overreaction by the body to an allergen. At this point, he could slip into anaphylactic shock, which is characterized by a big drop in blood pressure, heart palpitations, difficulty breathing and a loss of consciousness.

If your son is sensitive to bee venom, he should also be wary of cross-reactivity to other insects, such as yellow jackets and centipedes.

My friend just ate something she's deathly allergic to. What should I do?

First give her a Benadryl or other antihistamine if you have one handy. Ask whether she has an EpiPen (epinephrine auto-injector) with her. It's something everyone who is highly allergic should always have handy. She may be able to inject herself or at least be able to tell you how to use it. But wait until she's actually showing signs of a reaction before using it. If it's been years since her last exposure, there's a chance she might have outgrown her allergy, and epinephrine is hard on the body, so it shouldn't be used when it's not necessary. The minute she begins to struggle to breathe or her tongue, lips, or face begins to swell, give the injection and dial 911. If she collapses, roll her onto her back and elevate her feet higher than her head while you wait for professional help.

If you spend a lot of time with someone who carries an adrenaline injector, consider taking a first-aid course in the use of the device.

☐ **BITES AND STINGS**

What's the best way to treat a bee or wasp sting or a spider bite?

For a bee or wasp sting, remove the stinger by scraping it with a credit card. You can use tweezers, but you'll need to grasp the stinger as close to the skin as possible to avoid squeezing more venom into your body. After washing the area with soap and water, you can ice the wound to relieve pain. If the sting starts to redden or spread, or fails to get better over the next several days, make an appointment with your doctor. It may be infected.

Most spider bites are merely an annoyance that will cause some minor irritation or itching. Wash the site and keep an eye on it for infection. But if you're bitten by a black widow, brown recluse, or some other type of poisonous spider, seek

emergency care at a hospital or medical clinic. Catch the spider if you can (without getting bitten again, of course) so the care provider can identify it. You can kill it, just don't squish it beyond recognition. Wash the bite, apply gauze, and then keep a cold pack or ice wrapped in a dish towel or cloth on the area for 10 to 15 minutes every half-hour until you can get help. The bites are rarely deadly, but you may feel sick.

I just found a tick on me. How do I remove it? Should I save it?

About 20,000 new cases of Lyme disease are diagnosed each year in the United States. The disease isn't something to take lightly since it can lead to arthritis and other chronic conditions. And Lyme is only one of several tick-borne ill-

nesses; the most severe is Rocky Mountain spotted fever, found in many states outside the Rocky Mountains, which, after an incubation period of 5 to 10 days, can trigger high fever, headaches, muscle pain, and rashes on the hands or feet. Untreated, it can be fatal.

To remove a tick, use tweezers and grasp the tick as close to your skin as possible. Gently pull it straight out (don't twist because you could leave parts of the tick in your skin). Try to avoid using your fingers because you could squeeze infected fluids into your body. Save the tick in a plastic ziplock bag in case you develop symptoms or the classic bull's-eye rash or other symptoms (see "Ticks and Bug Bites on page 32). Always check yourself when you come back from walks in the woods because the sooner you remove a tick, the lower your risk for contracting an illness.

 FACT OR FICTION

Rabies Requires a Series of Painful Shots to the Stomach

Fiction. Though you will get a series of injections, the treatment is far less distasteful these days. Remarkably, there's still no cure for rabies, and once an infection sets in, it's almost always fatal. The shots you'll get are antiviral: They're designed to keep the virus from taking hold. For that reason, they must be started as soon as possible after a bite. The first shot is given near the bite; over the next 28 days, you'll get 5 or 6 more shots in the arm. That sounds much better than 12 or 24 or 36 shots in the belly, as playground lore would have it.

I've heard cat bites can easily become infected—how should I treat one? What about a dog bite?

Fluffy's bite is more likely to cause an infection than Rover's, but you should treat them both with care. If the bite isn't too bad, handle it like you would any minor cut: Wash it out with soap and warm water, apply some antibiotic ointment, and cover it with a bandage. Also, check that you've had a tetanus shot in the last 10 years. Not sure? Get a booster within 72 hours of being bitten.

Wild animal bites—or a bite from a domestic animal you don't know—are a different matter because rabies is a concern. Call Animal Control to capture the animal for evaluation; this may require having someone follow the animal until they arrive. Clean the wound with soap and water (the Centers for Disease Control and Prevention reports that thorough wound cleansing alone can greatly reduce your risk of infection) and seek emergency help. If the bite is bleeding profusely, call 911 and apply pressure to the wound; let emergency crews clean a deep, hemorrhaging bite.

☐ **BLEEDING**

How do I tell if someone's losing too much blood? How do I control the bleeding?

A victim's life may be at risk if the blood loss doesn't stop or diminish after the first couple of minutes. To control bleeding, place a clean cloth or a large bandage directly over the wound and press firmly on the area. (The exception is a head injury—just cover the area that is bleeding and hold the cloth or bandage firmly in place; pressing too hard could cause brain damage if the skull is fractured.) If the wound is to an arm or a leg, raise the limb above the level of the heart, unless you suspect that the limb is broken. Keep applying firm pressure. Should the bandage or cloth become saturated, don't remove it; simply place another bandage on top of it and continue to press down.

If the blood is still coming fast and help isn't in sight, you can slow the bleeding on an arm by compressing the brachial

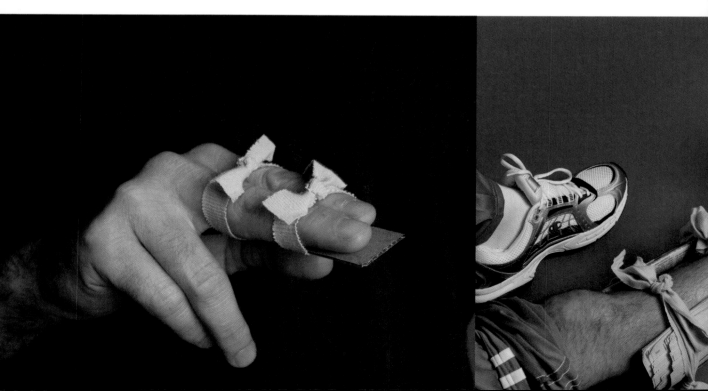

artery. It's located on the inside of the upper arm, between the bicep muscle (on top) and the triceps (underneath the bicep). Press down with four fingers on the artery and watch the bleeding to see if it slows or stops. Keep pressing until the ambulance arrives. For a wound on the leg, lay the victim on his back and apply pressure with the heel of your hand to the femoral artery, near the groin on the inside of the leg.

☐ **BROKEN BONE**

What if I have to move someone with a broken bone?

Only move a fracture victim as a last resort. But if you're miles from help or the person is in danger where she is (on a road or near a fire, for example), there are ways to move her with minimal to no harm. Find any stiff material at hand—a stick, a rolled-up newspaper—and, using a piece of cloth from a torn-up shirt, sheet, or towel, bind the stiff material to the fractured limb in the position you found it, or one that causes the least discomfort to the victim. Don't try to reset or straighten the limb. (One exception: If help will be a long time coming and blood doesn't seem to be getting to the injury—the skin is cold and gray below the fracture—you can try *slowly* straightening the arm or leg to restore circulation.) Don't bind it too tight. Ask the victim if her skin feels numb. If it does, or if the limb goes cold and loses color, ease the binding on the splint.

Keep these tips in mind when splinting: You can bind a broken finger to its neighbor, or stabilize a broken leg by splinting it to the other leg. A fractured ankle or foot should be wrapped in a pillow or soft clothing, but be sure to leave the shoe on as it can help control swelling (and pulling it off could do more damage).

Once the injury is splinted, recruit bystanders to help you move the victim. The key is to keep the victim in the same relative position in which you found her. If there's no one to assist you, try gently maneuvering the victim onto a large towel or blanket, and then carefully pull the blanket to slide her to safety.

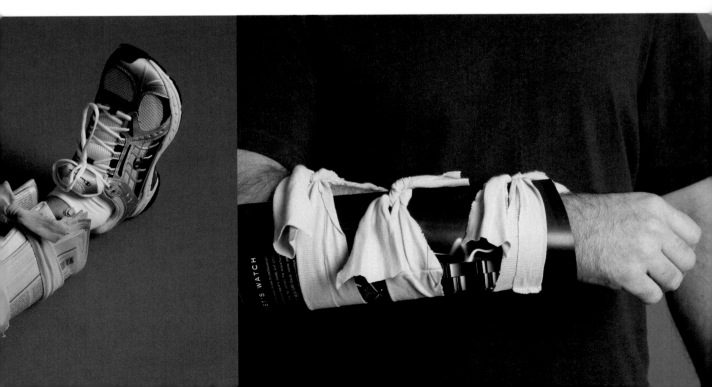

My kids scream bloody murder anytime they fall. Is there an easy way to tell if they have a broken bone?

Kids have a way of commanding attention for the slightest boo-boo, but you—and they—will know when they're really hurt. Their fussing will be difficult to dismiss—in fact, they may seem to be in shock from the pain. Assuming the limb or joint isn't obviously out of alignment, check the injured area for swelling or other signs of deformity. Your child will be in a lot of pain and extremely reluctant to use the broken limb. Don't encourage him to move around because it could make the break worse. Instead, keep him calm, splint (see "What if I have to move someone with a broken bone?" on page 347) and support the injury, and apply ice wrapped in a towel to the injury for 10 to 15 minutes every half-hour until you can get to a doctor. Avoid direct ice-to-skin contact, which could cause further damage.

Is it true that there's nothing a doctor can do for a broken toe? Should I even bother making an appointment?

A badly broken big toe demands a doctor's attention. If it doesn't heal properly, the toe could interfere with your gait and upset your balance. But for the rest of your little piggies—especially the one that went "wee-wee-wee" all the way home—you probably don't need to seek immediate medical attention. Your doctor won't do much more than offer comfort and pain relief. It may help to loosely tape the toe to its neighbor. Be sure to rest the injured foot and ice it with a cold pack or ice wrapped in a dish towel or cloth for 10 to 15 minutes every half-hour. Keep it elevated as much as possible for the first few days following the injury. For comfort, wear a hard-sole shoe when walking during the healing period. If, after a few days, the pain doesn't lessen or continues to worsen, you feel numbness or tingling, or the skin turns blue or gray around the injury, seek medical care: The blood supply to the toe may be affected, and you could be in danger of losing it.

WHAT YOU DON'T KNOW

NSAIDs Can Slow Bone Healing

When you're on the mend from a broken bone, avoid pain relievers known as nonsteroidal anti-inflammatory drugs (NSAIDs): aspirin, ibuprofen (Advil), and naproxen (Aleve) are over-the-counter versions. These drugs ease pain by blocking substances known as prostaglandins. Unfortunately, your bones need prostaglandins to knit properly, and several large studies suggest that NSAIDs may interfere with healing. In one study, patients using NSAIDs took up to 2 months longer to recover from a fracture than patients who avoided this class of drugs. Your best choice for pain relief from a broken bone is acetaminophen (Tylenol), which acts on pain centers in the brain. Save NSAIDs for headaches, sprains, and other aches and pains.

☐ **BURNS**

What's the right way to treat a burn from grease or a fire?

Wash off the grease if any remains, and run cool—not cold—water over the burn. Don't use ice; research has found that it's no better than cool water, and it has the downside of damaging the surrounding skin and delaying healing. Forget butter or other types of grease, because they do nothing for a burn and can actually trap heat. Remove any burned clothing unless it's embedded in the burn itself. Apply some antibiotic cream and take a dose of an over-the-counter painkiller. If the injury is larger than two hands side by side and involves blistering or charring, or it's affecting the eyes, mouth, hands, or genitals, it's time for a trip to the ER.

What about a chemical burn?

If the person has been burned by a dry chemical, such as the powdery acid on a battery, don gloves to protect your hands, brush off any visible powder, then remove the victim's clothes and jewelry and have him shower off in lukewarm water for 15 to 20 minutes. Keep your head turned through the process to protect your eyes (or wear protective eyewear), and have the victim shut his eyes. If the person has been burned by wet chemicals, such as bleach, put him in the shower for the same amount of time (15 to 20 minutes). Again, if the burns cover an area larger than two hands side by side or are in sensitive areas like the eyes, hands, mouth, or genitals, seek medical care. Be sure to tell the doctor what type of chemical caused the burn.

I got a really bad sunburn and now I feel sick. Is it related?

Almost certainly. The nausea is probably linked to dehydration,

and if you are unable to drink liquids or keep them down, your doctor may want to put you on a saline drip to bring your fluids up. That will handle the nausea, but you're in for a world of hurt over the next few days. Try over-the-counter drugs such as ibuprofen and naproxen to manage the pain and inflammation. Alcohol-free aloe vera gel (check the ingredient label) can also ease pain and swelling. Cold compresses and cool baths or showers will provide some temporary relief. To avoid infection, don't pop any blisters. And use more caution in the sun—there isn't a lot of difference between severe sunburn and burns from heat or chemicals in terms of damage to your skin.

□ **CHEST PAIN**

I have chest pain. How do I know if it's heartburn or a heart attack? Should I wait and see?

Don't hesitate to call 911. A heart attack can start slowly with a clot blocking blood flow to the heart, but as the minutes tick by, the heart muscle is suffering permanent damage.

The telltale signs of a heart attack include feelings of fullness, pressure, or squeezing in the chest, and the sensation may come and go. Pain may spread to the shoulders, neck,

jaw, arms, or back, and you could feel light-headed and suffer nausea and heavy perspiration. The sudden onset of unexplained anxiety, weakness, or fatigue is also a sign. Women are more likely than men to experience vague symptoms such as shortness of breath, nausea or vomiting, and jaw or back pain. Youth—relatively speaking—is no reason to disregard these symptoms, especially if you're female. Heart attacks are up 32 percent in the last decade among women under the age of 50, which is troubling in light of a 2007 study that found more than half of women under the age of 55 who suffer a heart attack ignore their symptoms for more than an hour.

Should I give someone aspirin if I think they might be having a heart attack?

Yes, but only after calling 911. The usual dose is one full-strength aspirin (325 to 500 milligrams) or four baby aspirin; the 911 operator will guide you. The victim should chew the pill so that it will enter the blood-stream more quickly.

Given after a heart attack, aspirin can reduce the risk of dying by 20 to 30 percent. The protection comes from aspirin's anticlotting effect: It helps restore and maintain blood flow until surgeons can reopen arteries.

When I cough or breathe deeply, the side of my chest burns. Is that a heart attack?

Figuring out the difference between heart attack symptoms and other chest pain issues is tricky, and most emergency physicians would rather you be safe than sorry. Always seek medical help first and question your symptoms later. That said, what you're describing sounds more like a broken rib. If you've fallen recently or bumped into something, probe your chest for tender spots. If you can identify a particularly sensitive area, you probably have a dislocated or broken rib. You should still see a doctor, but you don't need an ambulance.

☐ **CHOKING**

Can I assume that if someone's coughing and can't stop, they're choking?

Actually, loud coughing is a pretty good sign that the person will be okay. Real choking is almost silent, and the victim may be clutching at his throat with both hands in what's known as the universal distress signal for choking. Keep your eye on the cougher, though, because food or some other obstruction may be making its way to his windpipe. Offer water, ask him if he's choking (a person who isn't will be able to tell you so), and be ready to offer assistance if the person does start to choke.

How do you perform the Heimlich maneuver?

For adults, the technique is relatively simple. But before you start, check that the person really needs the procedure. She won't be able to breathe or talk, and when you ask if she's choking, she'll nod yes. Before you start, have someone call 911. Get behind the victim, make a fist with your hand and place it thumb-end against the stomach, just above the navel and below the rib cage. (For a pregnant women or an obese person, place the fist over the chest.) Reach around with the other hand, place it over the fist, and pull back and up sharply six to ten times, quickly. If necessary, repeat until the lodged food comes free or until paramedics arrive. Children older than a year get the same procedure, but you'll want to use less force.

Heimlich for infants is very different. Sit down and place the infant face-down on your forearm, supporting the head and neck with your hand. Rest your forearm on your thigh, and check that the baby's head is lower than the body. Now deliver up to five sharp blows with the heel of your hand to the infant's back, between the shoulder blades. Turn the baby face up and check

for obstructions in the mouth. Repeat, if necessary.

I'm afraid of breaking someone's ribs during the Heimlich maneuver—what are the chances?

It happens, say emergency experts, and no one is sure how often. But if you don't perform the Heimlich maneuver, the chance that a choker will die is pretty close to 100 percent. Victims will happily trade a broken rib for almost certain death.

☐ **DROWNING**

I often lifeguard when my children and their friends play in our pool. I should watch for a lot of splashing or listen for yelling to see if a kid is in trouble, right?

Though it's counterintuitive, you need to watch for the kid who is motionless and quiet. Yes, people scream when they think they're in danger, but at least you know they need help. Assist the noisy one, if necessary, but the one who needs lifesaving treatment is the kid not making any noise, and floating face-down.

Keeping kids safe in and near water is a big job and begins with continuous monitoring.

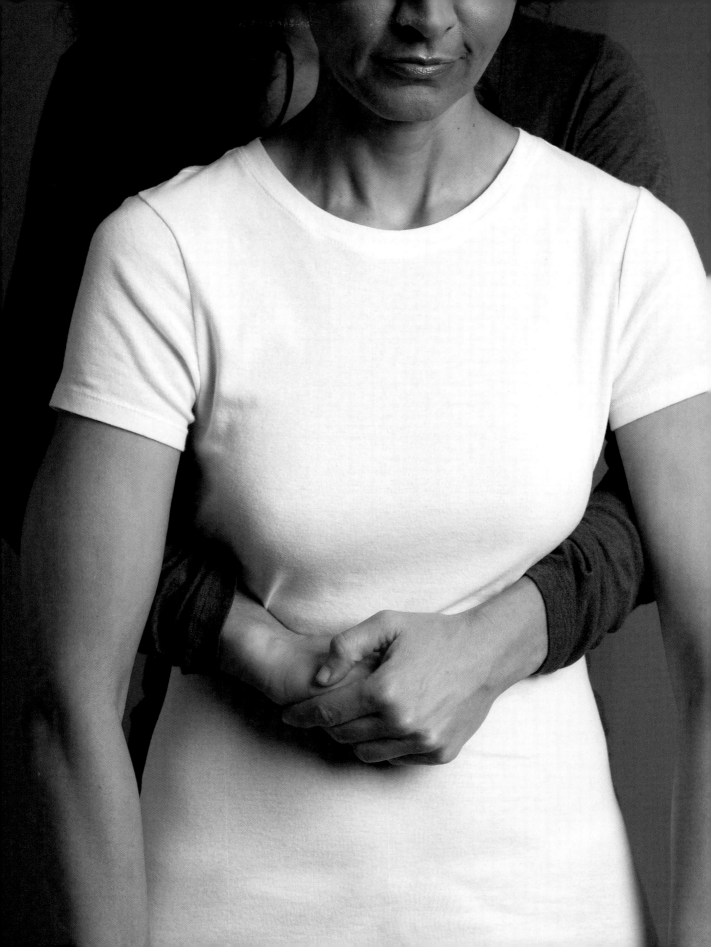

Drowning is the second leading cause of death for kids between the ages of 1 and 14 (car accidents is the category leader), and toddlers under the age of 4 account for 80 percent of home drownings. Make sure you're up-to-date on CPR training, and consider taking lifeguard training from your local chapter of the American Red Cross. Of course, if you have a pool at home, it should be properly fenced in.

How do I treat a drowning victim?

Have someone dial 911 right away while you begin CPR. For someone who has drowned, you will need to give rescue breaths in addition to chest compressions. Gently tilt the victim's head back while lifting the chin up to help clear the airway. (If there is concern for a possible neck or spinal injury, just lift the jaw.) Breathe in normally but not deeply, pinch the victim's nose, then place your mouth over his and give a rescue breath. The victim's chest should rise; if it doesn't, reposition the head to help clear the airway. Give

2 rescue breaths followed by 30 chest compressions, 2 more breaths, 30 more compressions. (See the question "I've heard there's a new type of CPR that's easier. How do you do it?" on page 342 for directions on administering chest compressions.) Keep it up until help arrives or the victim regains consciousness.

☐ **ELECTRIC SHOCK**

My husband likes to do his own electrical work. If he gets shocked, what should I do?

Before he starts his next project, have him show you where the circuit breakers are in the house. If he should get a jolt, the only way to safely interrupt the charge is by throwing the breaker. Under no circumstances should you touch him if he's still in contact with electricity, or you'll end up in the same condition. Once the power is off, check for a pulse and breathing, and call 911 and start CPR, if necessary. If he's

responsive, search him for broken bones and bad burns that might require emergency treatment.

To avoid this situation altogether, take action *before* your husband gets hurt: Remind him that electrocution is the fifth leading cause of on-the-job deaths in the United States, and try to convince him to leave rewiring to the professionals.

What can you do for someone who has been struck by lightning?

The victim will likely be unconscious, may be burned, and will need emergency care right away. Call 911, then begin CPR if the person isn't breathing (watch the chest to see if it's rising and falling). Treat the burns as you would a burn from a hot surface such as a stove or fireplace: Remove clothing around the burn unless it's actually embedded in the wound and run cool—not cold—water over the area.

Should the person survive, chronic troubles may emerge due to damage to the brain. Lightning-strike victims can lose short-term memory and struggle to handle multiple tasks, and they may find themselves unable to handle the demands of their jobs. As a result, they can withdraw, become irritable and angry, and slip into depression. Anyone who survives a lightning strike should get regular checkups

 WHAT YOU DON'T KNOW

How Long the Brain Can Survive without Oxygen

If a victim stops breathing, whether it's due to drowning, a heart attack, or choking, you have about 6 minutes after breathing stops before brain damage begins. You may have more time if the event occurred in very cold water.

with a physician and consider seeing a therapist. A support group such as Lightning Strike and Electric Shock Survivors International (www.lightning-strike.org) could also be helpful for the victim and his family.

☐ EYE INJURY

I was cleaning the bathroom and some cleanser splashed in my face. How long should I rinse my eyes?

If it was just a drop or two, rinse your eyes for at least 15 minutes under the faucet. Turn your head to the side with the injured eye facing up and hold it open under the flow. Flushing it with running water is more likely to clean out the chemical than submersing the eye using an eyecup or in a stopped sink. (You can start the flushing with saline solution if you have some handy. It's a little easier on the eye.) If, after 15 minutes, your eye still hurts, your vision seems affected, or it was a large exposure, head to an emergency room.

Acids in cleaning products, garden chemicals, and solvents can leave a haze on the cornea (the transparent covering over your iris and pupil) even after flushing, but the eye will usually recover. However, alkaline substances like drain cleaners, lime, and lye will not only per-

AVOID THIS MISTAKE

Stepping into a Flooded Basement

It doesn't take much water to conduct electricity, so if there is water in your basement, play it safe and call your electric company. They can send someone out to assess the situation and shut down the power, if necessary. If your basement floods regularly, consider buying a generator to power your sump pumps and wet vacs. That way you can begin your cleanup without having to use house power.

Natural gas is another concern should your basement flood. If the water puts out the pilot light on your furnace or hot water heater, gas could accumulate and all it would take is a spark to trigger an explosion. Call your gas company to turn off the lines to your house, and wait until the air clears before you start cleaning up.

manently damage the cornea but they can continue to damage the eye after treatment. In the future, be sure to wear eye protection when cleaning with chemicals or gardening with pesticides.

My wife was gardening and a bunch of dirt and bark blew into her eyes. She thinks she has something stuck in one. Should she rinse her eye?

Definitely not. If her eye has been cut, the risk that you could introduce bacteria and trigger an infection is very high. She needs to be careful not to rub the eye even though the

impulse will be strong. Place gauze over both eyes (by keeping the good eye still, you can help prevent further damage to the injured one), and drive her to the emergency room, where a doctor can safely remove the debris and administer antibacterial eye drops. If she needs an eye specialist, the emergency room staff will have one on call.

I hit my head and now I'm seeing flashes of light. Will those pass?

Those flashes of lights may be a symptom of retinal detachment and, without treatment, this condition almost always leads to blindness. The visual flashes are caused by an improper stimulation of the eye's retina or optic nerve, which the brain interprets as light. Those flashes indicate that you need immediate medical assessment and diagnosis to prevent or minimize any vision loss.

Detached retinas can sometimes occur after a blow to the head, but they're also associated with risk factors including being nearsighted, undergoing cataract surgery, having glaucoma, or simply growing older. An ophthalmologist can surgically reattach the retina, but success in restoring vision depends on catching the detachment early.

☐ FAINTING

What causes fainting? Should I call a doctor if I faint?

Typically, fainting isn't a medical emergency, but you still may want to talk to your doctor about the episode. This brief interruption of blood flow to the brain can result from many conditions, including low blood pressure, an irregular heartbeat, low blood sugar, or stress. If you're with someone who has fainted, lay him on his back and elevate his legs above the level of his heart. Check to see if he's breathing by watching to see if his chest rises and falls. Loosen any belts, ties, or other restrictive clothing. When the person comes around, have him rest and remain quiet for a few minutes before allowing him to stand. If you're the one that feels faint, quickly sit

down and put your head between your legs until the blood flow returns to normal. (Lie down if there's nowhere to sit, and elevate your feet above your head, if possible.) Wait until you feel better before trying to stand again.

If fainting is accompanied by chest pain, an irregular heartbeat, or trouble speaking, you should seek an immediate medical assessment. The spells could be a sign of heart rhythm problems, a mild stroke, or blockage in your arteries.

☐ HEADACHES

I get bad migraines from time to time. Are there symptoms that indicate I might need to go to the ER?

Headaches usually aren't a sign of something serious, but there are exceptions. Even if you regularly have migraines, pain that is considerably worse than any you have previously experienced calls for an emergency room visit. Get emergency help for a sudden and violent headache or any head pain that wakes you from sleep, gets worse over a 24-hour period, is accompanied by slurred speech or a change in vision or coordination, is the worst sudden headache you've ever had, is associated with a fever, or interferes with your daily activities. The source of the pain could be anything from bleeding in the

brain to a tumor in your spine. Whatever it is, you need to get it diagnosed quickly.

I recently turned 50 and have begun to get throbbing headaches in my temples. Is that just a normal part of aging?

There are several possible reasons for the pain, but the most troublesome is temporal arteritis, inflammation in the lining of your arteries in your temples. While this isn't necessarily an emergency situation, you should seek help quickly because the condition could blind you. Other signs of temporal arteritis include headaches that worsen when you chew and gradually worsening vision.

While the cause isn't clear, temporal arteritis may be due to a faulty immune response, severe infections, or large doses of antibiotics. Whatever the cause, the inflammation can limit blood flow to vision cells, starving them of nutrients and oxygen. (Women, by the way, are two to three times more likely than men to get temporal arteritis.) Your doctor may order scans for a closer look at your arteries, but the only way to diagnose this condition is with a biopsy of the artery tissue to check the lining. Corticosteroids are the treatment of choice; the drugs reduce inflammation, and you'll feel better within days.

☐ HEAD INJURY

My daughter banged her head in a fall and has a big, raised bump. Now she's running around and playing. Should I still take her to the doctor?

If she seems fine, you probably don't need to. The trouble signs to look for after a knock on the head—especially in children—are persistent crying, a headache that won't go away or gets worse, loss of balance, mood changes, persistent vomiting, and unconsciousness. In adults as well as kids, watch for sleepiness, unequal pupil sizes, convulsions, slurred speech, and confusion or agitation. Any of these symptoms could indicate an intracranial bleed (which puts pressure on the brain) or concussion (the brain was shaken within the skull). Depending on the history and symptoms, an

emergency physician may do a scan of the brain to identify internal injuries. While there's nothing a doctor can do for a concussion—and most people recover without medical intervention—if there is evidence of bleeding or further injury, you'll need to see a neurosurgeon for further treatment.

☐ HEAT EXHAUSTION/ HEATSTROKE

I can't tolerate hot weather like I used to, and my doctor warns me about heatstroke. What is it?

It's true that as you get older, you lose your tolerance for hot weather. The body relies on perspiration and blood circulation to cool itself. With age, circulation becomes less vigorous, and the body's ability to regulate internal temperature breaks down. (Babies are also at higher risk for heatstroke

because their cooling system isn't operating at peak efficiency yet.) So watch for the symptoms of heat exhaustion: Pale, clammy, dry skin (people with heatstroke stop sweating), weakness, dizziness, headaches, nausea/vomiting, and a racing, weak pulse. As the victim's temperature rises, her organs and brain could suffer permanent damage leading to changes in mental status and neurologic dysfunction (signs of stroke). If you suspect heatstroke, call 911 and get her out of the sun quickly. To bring down her temperature, consider using a fan, sponging her with cool water, or even applying ice packs to her trunk. Don't give her medications used to treat fever, such as aspirin or ibuprofen, because her organs won't be able to process them and the drugs could cause further damage. Salt pills and any drinks containing alcohol or caffeine will also worsen her condition.

Sometimes in the summer, when I've been working in the garden all day, I feel weak and dizzy, and occasionally the muscles in my legs cramp up. Should I be worried?

This sounds like garden-variety (sorry) heat exhaustion. It means that you're dehydrated

FACT OR FICTION

If Someone with a Head Injury Falls Asleep, They Could Go into a Coma

Fiction. The only reason to keep a person with a head injury awake is to observe her symptoms, say the experts at the American College of Emergency Physicians. And if you're too worried about the victim's symptoms to let her go to sleep, then you should take her to the ER. Otherwise, wish her good night and sweet dreams.

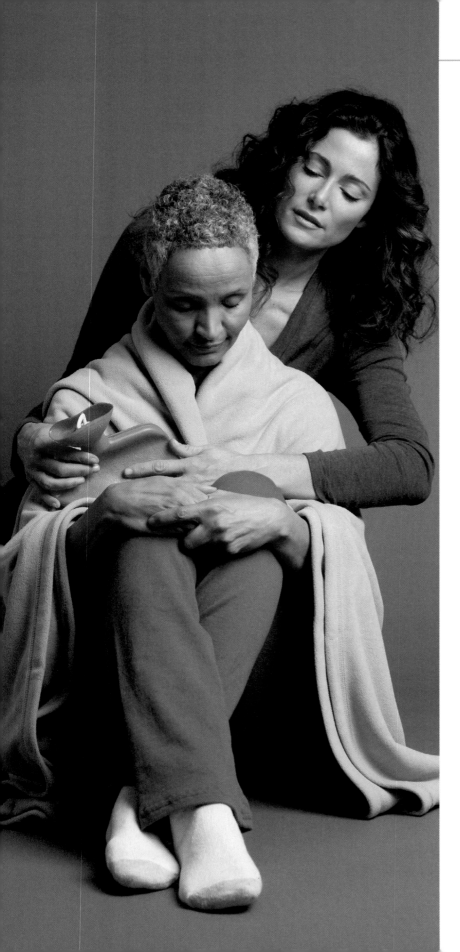

and your internal temperature may be starting to rise. To protect yourself, limit your time in the sun to 45 minutes out of every hour, and then take 15 minutes inside to cool off and replenish your fluids. (You might even want to start with 30 minutes of work in the sun followed by 15 minutes of cooling off.) When you're in the sun, wear a wide-brimmed hat and lightweight loose clothing and sip ice water or a sports drink frequently. If you find that you are feeling dizzy or suffering from cramps anyway, move to a shady spot or head inside to climate-controlled air. Drink plenty of fluids and, if you still feel woozy, consider a cool shower or sponge bath.

☐ **HYPOTHERMIA**

I like to hike, even when it's rainy and cold. Do I have to worry about hypothermia?

Believe it or not, your risk of hypothermia can be higher in a cold rain than in snow because your clothing can get soaked through, leaving you much wetter than if you were hiking in, say, much colder conditions and dry snow. Also, people heading outdoors in the snow tend to be prepared, wearing quality waterproof coats, gloves, hats, and shoes. A light rain may not seem very threatening,

WHAT YOU DON'T KNOW

Watch Out for the "Umbles"

"Umbles" is a mnemonic device for remembering the signs of hypothermia: Stumbles, fumbles, mumbles, and grumbles, all of which indicate a breakdown in coordination and consciousness. Hypothermia often sneaks up on people. By remembering the umbles, you may be able to spot the symptoms in yourself early enough that you can take action before the condition worsens.

and you could be tempted to brave it in a nylon shell or sweater. But if you get wet, all it takes is cool temperatures or a brisk wind for hypothermia to set in.

How do I recognize when someone is going into hypothermia?

Hypothermia begins with shivering, which is a response to the core temperature cooling—the body is trying to generate heat. Next is a loss of coordination in the fingers, an unsteady gait, and uncontrollable shivering. As hypothermia progresses, the victim may start slurring his speech and seem confused. Irrational behavior, such as wanting to disrobe, begins to set in as the brain becomes affected. As the body can no longer compensate for the temperature losses, shivering may cease; the body is moving into a state of hibernation, stopping blood flow to the limbs in an attempt to keep the core warm. If the victim is still

exposed to the elements, there's no way his body will be able to sustain core temperature, and death will soon follow.

Hopefully for the victim, long before this occurs, emergency services will be on the way. For someone in the mild stages of hypothermia, adding more layers of clothing or changing them into dry clothes, sheltering them, and giving them food and drink can be enough. But if a person is

confused and shivering uncontrollably, you'll need to take more drastic measures until help arrives. Remove wet clothing and dry the victim off, then wrap him tightly in dry blankets or a sleeping bag. If you have instant heat packs, place them near major arteries on each side of the neck, under the arms, and on the groin. If he's capable of drinking, give him a sports drink or sugar water to help kick-start his metabolism.

☐ POISONING

What is the Poison Control Hotline? How can it help me?

Write this number down next to your phone, and make sure everyone in the family knows it's there: 1-800-222-1222. That's the National Poison

AVOID THIS MISTAKE

Giving Ipecac Syrup to Induce Vomiting

Syrup of Ipecac is made from an herb that contains alkaloid substances that trigger vomiting when they come into contact with mucous membranes in the throat. Unfortunately, several studies over the last two decades have found that vomiting doesn't actually remove poison from the stomach. To complicate matters, some of the side effects of Ipecac, such as lethargy, are similar to the symptoms of poisoning, making diagnosis of the patient difficult for doctors. Even worse: There have been several cases of accidental Ipecac overdose. If you have Ipecac in your medicine cabinet, throw it out.

Control Hotline, and operators are there 24 hours a day, 7 days a week. No matter what someone swallows, inhales, or sprays in his face, the experts at the hotline can help. If you call, be ready to describe the poison, the type of exposure, and how long ago it happened, along with the victim's age and weight. An operator will walk you through the next steps based on the exposure described. They will instruct you whether additional care is needed in an emergency department or whether care at home will be appropriate.

☐ SEIZURE

My friend has epilepsy. If she has a seizure, should I let it pass or call 911?

For people with a history of seizures, the only reasons to call 911 are: The episode lasts longer than 5 minutes, the victim has injured herself during the seizure, she's struggling to breathe, she has a fever, or confusion persists after the seizure ends. Emergency staff should also handle seizures in people with diabetes or chronic conditions such as multiple sclerosis. But someone with a history of epilepsy who is suffering a seizure similar to ones he's had in the past doesn't need emergency medical attention.

What should I do while the seizure is happening?

Your first job is to make sure that the person is safe. Don't try to restrain her. Instead, move furniture and other hard objects out of reach, loosen any clothing around the neck (ties, scarves, a high-necked blouse), and roll her on her side in case she vomits; place a pillow or a rolled up piece of clothing under her head. Observe the victim closely: Time the episode on your watch, note what her limbs, head, and eyes are doing, and

how long it takes her to return to normal consciousness. This information will be useful both for the victim and her doctor to track the progression of her condition and the effectiveness of her antiseizure medications.

☐ SPRAINS AND STRAINS

I stepped off a curb and landed awkwardly, but I'm pretty sure it's just a sprain. Do I have to see a doctor?

Did you hear or feel a pop? Are you unable to move your ankle without a lot of pain? If the answer is yes to either of those questions, you've probably sprained your ankle. Make an appointment to see your doctor. You're not looking at an emergency, but you may need your doctor to prescribe a brace or even put you in a cast. The pain is from a pulled or torn ligament, the fibrous tissue that attaches one bone to the next (they help hold your skeleton together). A joint with a stretched or torn ligament may need to be immobilized with a cast or splint until the tissue can heal. If you are unable to place weight on the injured ankle or have deformity about the ankle, head for the ER.

A strain, on the other hand, usually refers to an overstretched muscle or tendon (these attach muscle to bone).

?? FACT OR FICTION

Seizure Victims Can Swallow Their Tongues

Fiction. Despite what Hollywood has taught us, it's physically impossible to swallow one's own tongue, and forcing your fingers or a spoon or spatula into someone's mouth is only going to injure you and the victim. At times, a seizure sufferer may sound like he's gagging on his tongue, but by rolling him onto his side, you'll help keep his airways clear.

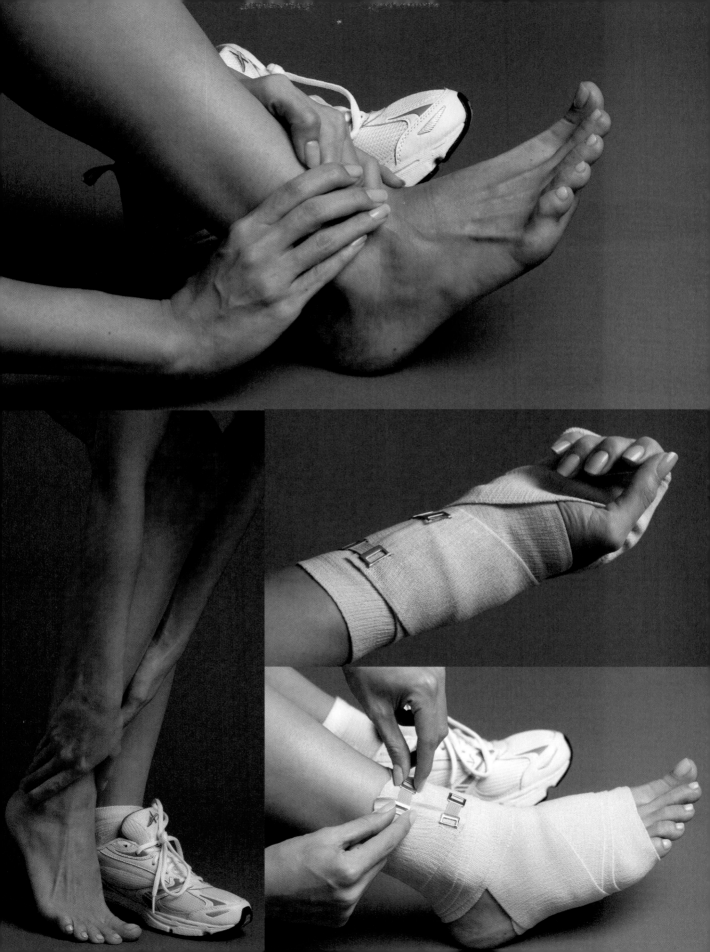

While less serious, a strain should still be treated with care; immobilize the injured area and go easy on it for at least 72 hours. With either a strain or a sprain, make an appointment to see a doctor if you don't start to feel better within 2 to 3 days.

Do I put ice or heat on a sprain?

Applying heat may feel good at first, but it will increase swelling in the injured area, decrease your mobility, and prolong the pain. The proper treatment is RICE: rest, ice, compression, elevation. This acronym will guide you when treating a sprain or a strain. The rest should extend 24 to 48 hours; use a cold pack or ice wrapped in a dish towel or cloth on the area for 10 to 15 minutes every half-hour until you can get help. Avoid direct ice-to-skin contact. Continue icing four times a day for the first 48 hours after the injury; gently wrap the joint in an elastic bandage such as ACE when you're not icing it; and finally, keep the injured joint elevated above your heart for the first 24 hours. RICE will help keep swelling down.

Is it true that a sprain hurts more than a broken bone?

Not usually, unless the broken bone is only a hairline fracture. Generally, a broken bone will make its presence known through your inability to move the limb or area without intense, shooting pain. A sprain may cause substantial swelling and pain in the injured joint. And sprains frequently require as much, if not more time than fractures to heal completely and return to normal function.

☐ **STROKE**

My elderly father suddenly had trouble speaking for several minutes, but then the problem passed. Should I take him to the doctor?

Yes. Your dad probably had a mild stroke, known as transient ischemic attack (TIA). The symptoms, which can include weakness on one side of the body, numbness or tingling all over, sudden vision trouble, vertigo, or as your father experienced, trouble speaking, usually last no more than 20 minutes. But any stroke is considered a very serious event. TIAs are often an indication that a much more debilitating stroke could happen in the very near future. And getting timely treatment for a stroke can mean the difference between debilitating damage or even death and a potentially full recovery. People who get appropriate treatment within 3 hours of suffering a full-blown stroke are far more likely to recover most or all of their mobility, speech, and muscle control, compared to victims who delay treatment.

If I suspect that someone has had a stroke, should I give her aspirin?

No—that works with a heart attack, but it could make matters worse with some types of stroke. Aspirin thins the blood, which is helpful for strokes caused by a blocked artery. But because bleeding in the brain is another possible cause, the last thing you want to do is increase that blood flow. Dial 911 and be sure to tell the dispatcher you suspect a stroke. That will allow the responders to make sure the proper equipment and drugs are ready on arrival. Write down the time that symptoms first began, as this will directly impact the type of care that can be considered in the ER. When treating a stroke, every second matters.

Index

eggs:
   cholesterol tests results and, 319
   eating raw, 83
   health benefits of, 73
electric shock, quick action for, 352–53
electric toothbrush, 14–15
electrolyte imbalance:
   from diarrhea, 245
   pain from, 55
electron beam computed tomography (EBCT), 325
emergencies:
   advance preparation for, 343
   mistakes to avoid in, 343
   quick action for, 344–60
   what constitutes an, 340
   who to call in, 53
emergency room, getting to, 341
emphysema, similar signs for lung cancer and, 269
endometrial ablation, for heavy menstrual cycles, 277
endovascular surgery, 297
endovenous laser ablation, 302
enemas, 237
energy level:
   boosted by dietary supplements, 159
   diet linked to, 78–79
enlarged prostate, 68
   decongestants as risk with, 106–7
   incontinence caused by, 43
   medications for, 289
   surgery for, 289–90
   treatment not always needed for, 289
epigallocatechin-3 gallate (EGCG), 90–91
epilepsy, helping during episode of, 358
erectile dysfunction:
   causes of, 39, 138
   vitamins and supplements for, 167

erectile dysfunction medications, 39, 138–39
   comparing oral, 136, 138
   lifestyle change vs., 138
erythromycin, Cialis interaction with, 138
esophagus, heartburn damage to, 252–53
Estring, 276
estrogen patch, 288
evening primrose oil:
   for breast tenderness, 216
   for eczema relief, 166
   for PMS, 178
   potential drug interactions with, 190
exercise, 19–22
   as beneficial for osteoporosis, 21, 283
   blood sugar levels and, 242
   cancer risk lowered by, 220
   for CFS patients, 227
   colds from intensive, 230
   with congestive heart failure, 234
   in COPD therapy, 229
   in diabetes management, 242
   doctor's approval for, 19, 21
   eating before, 19
   HDL cholesterol raised by, 74
   immunity boosted by, 27
   mental, 205
   optimal amount of, 19
   overeating after, 19
   as pain relief, 151
   as part of arthritis management, 210
   strategies for depression, 240
   stroke risk lowered by, 297
   to decrease incontinence, 43
   when quitting smoking, 29
exercise stress tests, 256
expiration dates:
   on drugs, 96, 137
   on medical tests, 309
external otitis, 57
eye drops, 58, 109–11
   effectiveness of OTC, 109–11
eye exams, 323–24
   when to get, 323

eyes, eye problems, 22
   "floaters," 55, 69
   gritty feeling in, 58
   injuries to, 353–54
   ocular rosacea, 292
   possible reasons for, 58
   quick action for injured, 353–54
   red or itchy, 58
   see also vision, vision problems

F

face masks, as flu prevention, 23
fainting, faintness:
   after eating carbs, 72
   possible reasons for, 58
   quick action for, 354
fasting, 79
   before medical tests, 309–10
fasting tests, for diabetes, 321
fatigue:
   dietary boosts for, 78
   from statins, 134
   possible reasons for, 58–59
   vitamins and supplements for, 167
fecal impaction, 51
fecal occult blood test, 320–31
feet:
   antiperspirants used on, 40
   diabetes-related problems with, 244–45
   peeling skin on, 65
fever:
   avoiding antidiarrheals during, 109
   as flu symptom, 53
   mild vs. serious, 59
   in pneumonia vs. bronchitis, 286
   possible reasons for, 59
   as strep symptom, 66
feverfew, for headache relief, 168
fiber:
   in coffee, 75